GNVQ Advanced
Health and Social Care

Liam Clarke • Bruce Sachs • Peter Waltham

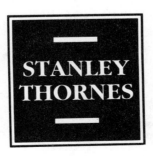

STANLEY THORNES

First published in 1994 by:
Stanley Thornes (Publishers) Ltd
Ellenborough House
Wellington Street
CHELTENHAM
GL50 1YD

Reprinted 1994

A catalogue record for this book is available from the British Library.
ISBN 0 7487 1693 9

Typeset by GCS, Leighton Buzzard
Printed and bound in Great Britain by The Bath Press, Avon

Contents

Acknowledgements

We would like to thank all the students and clients who have taught us the real essence of care. We have listened!

Liam Clarke
Bruce Sachs
Peter Waltham

The authors and publishers are grateful to the following for permission to reproduce material:

Alzheimer's Disease Society, page 171 (right); BNA, pages 44, 235; British Diabetic Association, page 131; British Heart Foundation, page 124; Butter Council, page 205; D.C. Thompson & Co., page 117; Daily Mail, page 214; Down's Syndrome Association, page 114; Educare for photographs from the *Caring for Mary* video workbook, pages 9, 11, 31, 37, 47, 53; Gloucestershire Royal Hospital Special Care Baby Unit, page 251; Gloucestershire Social Services Department, page 171 (left); Health Education Authority, pages 6, 104, 108, 184, 187, 213; Hulton–Deutsch Collection, page 148; John Birdsall, 234/ Age Concern, 238, 291, 286/Age Concern, 294; Kanga's Pouch Day Nursery, page 304; Mansell Collection, page 227; Milk Marketing Board, pages 124, 205; Multiple Sclerosis Society, page 211; National Asthma Campaign, page 95; National Osteoporosis Society, page 73; Nick Oakes/Age Concern, page 275; Pharmacia Ltd, page 205; Sainsbury's plc, pages 103, 187; Stroud District Council, page 205; Terrence Higgins Trust, pages 205, 209; Guardian News Service Ltd, page 260; Ulrike Preuss/Age Concern, page 267; WRVS, pages 254–6.

Every effort has been made to contact coypright holders and obtain permission to reproduce material prior to publication. We apologise if anyone has been overlooked.

GNVQ Advanced Health and Social Care: Summary of units

Unit 1 Access, equal opportunities and client rights

Unit 1 Access, equqal opportunities and client rights

1.1 Investigate attitudes and other social influences on behaviour

1.2 Investigate discrimination and its effects on individuals

1.3 Describe how equal opportunities are maintained

Unit 2 Interpersonal interaction

2.1 Communicate with individuals

2.2 Promote communication within groups

2.3 Analyse clients' rights in interpersonal situations

Unit 3 Physical aspects of health

3.1 Examine how body systems inter-relate

3.2 Investigate human disease

3.3 Investigate the components of healthy diet

Unit 4 Psychological and social aspects of health and social care

4.1 Investigate the development of individual identity

4.2 Investigate threats to maintaining individual identity

4.3 Investigate the relationship of social and economic factors to health

Unit 5 Health promotion

5.1 Prepare a plan of health promotion advice

5.2 Present health promotion advice to others

5.3 Identify different types of risk to health

Unit 6 Structure and practices in health and social care

6.1 Investigate the structure of health and social care provision

6.2 Investigate the impact of legislation and funding on provision and priorities

6.3 Investigate ways in which services within health and social care operate

Unit 7 Care plans

7.1 Describe the development of care plans

7.2 Describe methods of assessing client need

7.3 Identify the purpose of monitoring and evaluation approaches within care plans

Unit 8 Research in health and social care

8.1 Investigate types of research used in health and social care

8.2 Construct a structured research instrument to survey opinion

8.3 Investigate methods of interpreting information

GNVQ Core skills: Summary of levels

	Communication	Application of numbers	Information technology
Level 1	**1.1** Take part in discussions with known individuals on routine matters. **1.2** Prepare written materials in pre-set formats. **1.3** Use images to illustrate points made in writing and in discussions with known individuals on routine matters. **1.4** Read and respond to written material and images in pre-set formats.	**1.1** Gather and process data at core skill level 1. **1.2** Represent and tackle problems at core skill level 1. **1.3** Interpret and present mathematical data at core skill level 1.	**1.1** Input information into specified locations. **1.2** Edit and organise information within individual applications. **1.3** Present information in pre-set formats. **1.4** Evaluate features and facilities of given applications. **1.5** Deal with errors and faults at level 1.
Level 2	**2.1** Take part in discussions with a range of people on routine matters. **2.2** Prepare written material on routine matters. **2.3** Use images to illustrate points made in writing and in discussions with a range of people on routine matters. **2.4** Read and respond to written material and images on routine matters.	**2.1** Gather and process data at core skill level 2. **2.2** Represent and tackle problems at core skill level 2. **2.3** Interpret and present mathematical data at core skill level 2.	**2.1** Set up storage systems and input information. **2.2** Edit, organise and integrate information from different sources. **2.3** Select and use formats for presenting information. **2.4** Evaluate features and facilities of given applications. **2.5** Deal with errors and faults at level 2.
Level 3	**3.1** Take part in discussions with a range of people on a range of matters. **3.2** Prepare written material on a range of matters. **3.3** Use images to illustrate points made in writing and in discussions with a range of people on a range of matters **3.4** Read and respond to written material and images on a range of matters.	**3.1** Gather and process data at core skill level 3. **3.2** Represent and tackle problems at core skill level 3. **3.3** Interpret and present mathematical data at core skill level 3.	**3.1** Set system options, set up storage systems and input information. **3.2** Edit, organise and integrate complex information from different sources. **3.3** Select and use formats for presenting complex information. **3.4** Evaluate features and facilities of applications already available in the setting. **3.5** Deal with errors and faults at level 3.
Level 4	**4.1** Take part in, and evaluate the effectiveness of, discussions with a range of people on a range of matters. **4.2** Prepare, and evaluate the effectiveness of, own written material on a range of matters. **4.3** Use and evaluate the effectiveness of own use of images to illustrate points made in writing and in discussions with a range of people on a range of matters. **4.4** Read and respond to written material and images, recognising the factors which influence own interpretation.	**4.1** Gather and process data at core skill level 4. **4.2** Represent and tackle problems at core skill level 4. **4.3** Interpret and present mathematical data at core skill level 4.	**4.1** Set system options, set up storage systems, and prepare and input information. **4.2** Set up and use automated routines to edit, organise and integrate complex information from different sources. **4.3** Set up and use automated routines to format and present complex information. **4.4** Evaluate the features and facilities of applications already available in the setting and the features and facilities of new applications. **4.5** Deal with errors and faults at level 4.
Level 5	**5.1** Lead, and evaluate the effectiveness of, discussions with a range of people on a range of matters. **5.2** Prepare, and evaluate the effectiveness of, own and others' written material on a range of matters. **5.3** Use and evaluate the effectiveness of own and others' use of images to illustrate points made in writing and in discussions with a range of people on a range of matters. **5.4** Read and respond to written material and images, recognising the factors which influence own and others' interpretations.	**5.1** Gather and process data at core skill level 5. **5.2** Represent and tackle problems at core skill level 5. **5.3** Interpret and present mathematical data at core skill level 5.	**5.1** Set up storage systems for use by self and others, and set up processes to be used by self and others for preparing and inputting information. **5.2** Set up and use automated routines for self and others to edit, organise and integrate complex information from different sources. **5.3** Set up and use automated routines for self and others to format and present complex information. **5.4** Evaluate for use by self and others the features and facilities of applications already available in the setting and the features and facilities of new applications. **5.5** Deal with errors and faults at level 5.

Introduction

In September 1992 the first groups of students embarked on pilot programmes for the new General National Vocational Qualifications. Not only was it a new qualification but it also introduced a greater emphasis on student-directed study. For the pilot groups in Health and Social Care, there was no single text to support them in this task.

This book is primarily aimed at students in schools and colleges who are following an Advanced level GNVQ in Health and Social Care. It covers all of the mandatory units and as such will support students registered with any of the awarding bodies: City and Guilds, BTEC or RSA. It will also provide background reading and vital underpinning knowledge for candidates for NVQs in care.

While this book comprehensively supports the structure and content of the mandatory units, we have developed the material beyond minimum requirements in order to allow what may otherwise appear to be disjointed elements, to be put into a proper vocational context.

We have placed an emphasis on active learning with activities and case studies used to illustrate and expand upon the contents of each unit. How the book is used will to some extent be determined by the way in which the GNVQ is tackled. There is no true hierarchy of the mandatory units although we would recommend that the chapters related to Unit 8 Research into Health and Social Care are read before attempting to carry out any surveys for other units. We would also suggest that Chapters 1 to 4 should be read before undertaking any work experience in care environments. Students should also be acquainted with the methods of assessment used for GNVQs, so that work may be planned with assessment in mind. A brief section on assessment is provided.

Each chapter concludes with revision questions and an assignment. The revision questions are based on the knowledge and understanding for the units. Seven mandatory units in Health and Social Care will be subject to external testing. At the time of writing, the unit Interpersonal Interaction has been identified as one that will not.

The assignment at the end of each chapter has been designed to address some of the elements specified for each unit, and will provide evidence not only of achievement, but also in support of grading.

The Advanced GNVQ in Health and Social Care is a challenging and worthwhile achievement. It will provide the student with a thorough knowledge of Health and Social Care, and an opportunity to experience working in care settings. As a qualification, it may provide the means directly into employment for some. For most, it will provide access to higher education, including courses toward social work and nursing qualifications. The vocations and professions included within Health and Social Care are some of the most personally rewarding jobs there are. They require special people, willing to devote themselves to the well-being of others. The authors of this book have considerable direct professional experience in the Health and Social

Care industry. We know how important this work is, and the devotion that one should possess in order to succeed. We dedicate this book to all those who use it, for the purpose of making a better, more caring world for all people. Good luck, and work hard!

Liam Clarke
Bruce Sachs
Peter Waltham
January 1994

Assessment for GNVQ

What is a General National Vocational Qualification (GNVQ)?

GNVQs are new alternatives to A levels or GCSEs, and can be taken at three levels:
- **Foundation GNVQs** Equivalent to four GCSEs at grades D–G, these normally take one year of full-time study.
- **Intermediate GNVQs** Equivalent to four or five GCSEs at grades A–C, these normally take one year of full-time study.
- **Advanced GNVQs** Equivalent to two A levels, and sometimes referred to as 'Vocational A levels', these are normally taken over a two-year period of full-time study.

Eventually, there will be four levels of GNVQs – Foundation, Intermediate, Advanced and Higher (equivalent to level 4 NVQ, HND and Degree).

GNVQs may be gained unit by unit, developing the knowledge and skills required for further study or the workplace, including general skills in numeracy, communication and computing. These broadly based qualifications are the same throughout the country.

How is a GNVQ structured?

A GNVQ is made up of:
- **mandatory vocational units**
- **optional vocational units**
- **mandatory core skills units**.

Additional vocational and core skills units may be added. All GNVQ units are of equal size and value, and each unit is composed of elements. Credit is awarded for each unit separately. Unit credits are accumulated for the full award. Strictly speaking, GNVQs do not require the student to learn in any particular way, or within a specified time period. However, your college or school will have devised organised programmes by which you can obtain the knowledge required within particular time scales.

Each GNVQ unit consists of performance criteria and range statements:
- **The performance criteria** describes the specific competencies which you will be required to demonstrate in being assessed.
- **The range statement** describes the different circumstances in which the performance criteria must be applied.

How are GNVQs assessed?

Assessment for GNVQs focuses on what you have actually achieved. This is referred to as outcome-based assessment. Your work will be assessed by assessors after you have provided them with evidence of your achievement. An **assessor** is a teacher or lecturer who has demonstrated competence in judging work presented by the student against the standards set nationally for GNVQs. The assessors will judge the evidence you have presented for each element of each unit, and ensure that your work meets the required national standards.

Verification is the process by which assessment is inspected to ensure that it is consistent within the college or school, and consistent with national standards. Your college or school will have a system, utilising **internal verifiers**, to ensure this, and this system is externally double checked by **external verifiers** appointed by such bodies as BTEC, City and Guilds or RSA.

A GNVQ is assessed on the **evidence** provided by the student. Evidence consists of all work presented by the student which is believed to satisfy performance criteria and range statements.

Evidence which will be assessed consists of:

- **Internal Assessment**   This is the assessment that takes place within your college or school. Projects, assignments, tests, testimonials, and more, are organised into a **Portfolio of Evidence**, which is subject to internal and external verification. Your school or college will support you in preparing your portfolio. Internal assessments must also provide evidence of achievement of core skills in Communication, Application of Number, and Information Technology.

- **External Assessment**   This may consist of short answer or multiple-choice question tests, or case studies and assignments, that will be set externally for each mandatory vocational unit. These tests will assess your knowledge and understanding of concepts, principles and relationships which underpin the vocational area. Each written test will last one hour, and will consist of approximately 40 questions or items. The pass mark for tests will normally be 70 per cent.

External testing will take place on a number of occasions each year and there is no restriction on the number of times you may resit a test. Your college or school will provide you with test specifications and model tests, which will help you to understand what should be learned and what will be assessed. The model tests will also help you to become accustomed to the style and format to be used in the external tests.

All awarding bodies must ensure that assessment can be undertaken by all students, including those with learning difficulties or disabilities. If you have a particular problem in being assessed, you must tell your school or college as soon as possible.

What grades are there?

Each GNVQ unit, when assessed as complete, will be given a **pass**. To gain the GNVQ you must pass all the required units and pass the external tests also.

Upon completion of all the units required for the GNVQ award, a mark of **pass**, **merit**, or **distinction** will be awarded. (Individual units are not graded as merit or distinction.) To obtain a merit or distinction your portfolio must show that you have consistently exhibited skills in:

- **planning**
- **information-gathering and information-handling** and (at level 3)
- **evaluation.**

Your assessors will give you every opportunity to develop these skills. Your final grade will depend on the quality of evidence that you have demonstrated in your portfolio of evidence.

Is it possible to appeal against the assessment decisions of the assessors?

Each school or college *must* have an appeals procedure which will deal effectively with any complaints that a student may have. Students may appeal on the grounds that *an assessment procedure was not properly carried out* or that *an outcome (pass) was not carried out* in a proper manner. The diagram shows an example of an appeals system.

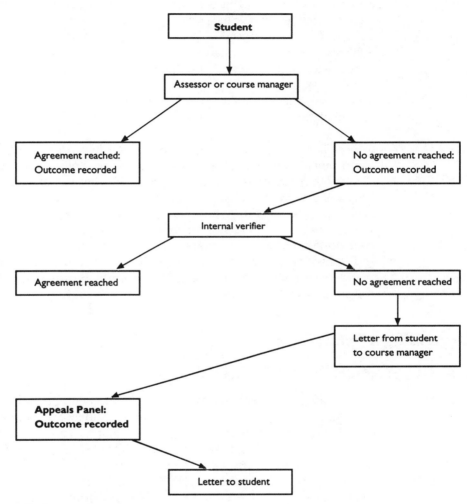

An example of an appeals system

Preparing for assessment

Your portfolio of evidence and the external test for each unit will need to be complete and passed in order for the unit to be credited toward the full GNVQ award. Evidence may be obtained in a variety of ways including:

● **Practical tests**   Be familiar with what you will be tested on, and have ready all equipment and materials you will need. Do not rush, and work to health and safety guidelines.

- **Assignments and projects** Plan your time carefully, and discuss your work with your teacher or lecturer. Be sure that you fully understand the aims of the activity, and ensure that your work is well presented.
- **Observations** (either on work-placement or in college) Ensure that you know precisely what it is you have to do. Try not to feel uncomfortable about being watched. Discuss beforehand with your assessor.
- **Oral questioning** This is a common way to assess the range. Make sure that you know what it is that will be asked, and ask for questions to be repeated or rephrased if you do not understand.
- **Written tests** Understand the process of revision, and start early. Good and complete course notes are essential. Always read instructions carefully, and plan your time.
- **Self-assessment** Make careful notes about all that you do. These notes may count as evidence. Even activities and achievements outside school and college may contribute.
- **Evidence of recent, previous experience** Records of achievement, testimonials and much more may be accepted as evidence. Your college or school will provide you with guidance and support in organising this type of evidence.

Be familiar with the units, elements, performance criteria, and range statements that make up the GNVQ for which you are studying. You may find that a single item of work may provide evidence for more than one unit. Such planned work can make your portfolio of evidence simple and efficient. Always check for gaps in your skills and knowledge, and work on them. The more you practise and revise, the more confident you will be. Your college or school and the teaching staff are all there to help and support you. Use them!

Organising a Portfolio of Evidence

What is a portfolio?

A portfolio is a convenient way to keep a record and to present the evidence that you have collected. It is a permanent record of the evidence of your achievements over the period you have taken to complete your course. This evidence will allow you to demonstrate to your assessors that you have achieved the skills, knowledge and understanding to gain the GNVQ qualification.

Your portfolio should be organised into a number of sections, each section perhaps containing evidence for each GNVQ unit. It will also contain forms which will be completed by you and your assessor. These forms will contain basic information about the status of the evidence with respect to individual GNVQ units.

Your portfolio must have an index which will allow your assessor and the internal and external verifier to find evidence for any element of competence, and may also have sections on personal information and any other evidence which you feel may help in your assessment.

Providing evidence for your portfolio

There are two types of evidence:
- **Performance evidence** Sometimes called direct evidence, this may consist of a

report, an assignment, a product or an assessor's observation of the candidate.

- **Supplementary or indirect evidence** This may consist of photographs, videos, audio tapes, written or oral questioning, tests or references from workplace supervisors.

Evidence should arise as a result of the work you have agreed to complete during discussions with your assessor. As explained, evidence that you have demonstrated the required knowledge over the appropriate range could be found in an assignment, essay or record of the answer you gave to oral questions on the subject. How much and what evidence you require will be discussed with you and should form the basis for an **Individual Action Plan** (IAP). This IAP, which should form the basis of your activity, could be the completion of an assignment, or a plan to visit a company or establishment to obtain information.

Whatever the nature of your evidence, these records should be kept in the appropriate section of your portfolio, cross referenced against the performance criteria for each element of the unit.

REMEMBER!

- A piece of work can provide evidence for more than one element or unit.
- Present your portfolio in a professional manner.
- All the evidence you are providing should be sufficient (enough), authentic (your own work) and relevant (tests what the performance criteria asks to be tested).
- The assessor or internal verifier should find the portfolio easy to read, understand and access. The index should identify what the evidence refers to.
- The documentation should be fully legible.
- Before you present evidence, remember that you will be asked questions about it by your assessor and the internal and external verifier.
- You should be very familiar with your portfolio as you may be asked to discuss the contents with an internal or external verifier.

I   Socialisation, attitudes and values

What is covered in this chapter

- The influence of socialisation on attitudes and values
- Sources of socialisation
- The development of attitudes and values
- The client's rights and entitlements in health and social care

These are the resources you will need for your Access, Equal Opportunities and Client Rights portfolio:
- examples of policy statements regarding clients' rights and care workers' attitudes
- example of a client's complaints procedure
- your written answers to each of the activities in Chapter I
- your written answers to the review questions in Chapter I
- your completed survey for Assignment I.

The influence of socialisation on attitudes and values

The ways in which people assimilate values

Social attitudes are learned through a process of association. We are all driven by basic needs that need to be satisfied. When we behave in ways that satisfy needs, the behaviour, or response, is rewarded or reinforced. We are then likely to use the same behaviour again and again to satisfy the need. In a social context, if we behave in ways that meet with the approval and praise of those around us, those behaviours will be reinforced.

Many of our attitudes are shaped by the responses of those around us. Thus, the attitudes of the social class we belong to are likely to be adopted by us because we are socially rewarded by the approval of others. Similarly, our gender, race and religion will all play a role in shaping our attitudes, as all of these constitute social groups that will reward certain attitudes, and disapprove of others. For example, social class may determine our views about education and work. Our gender may influence beliefs about roles within the family, or safety in the streets. Our race may influence the realistic expectations we may have about being treated fairly in employment, or our tastes in music and food. Religion is a major shaper of attitudes, as it often constitutes an organised system of beliefs about right and wrong. Most of these attitudes will be learned within the context of the family.

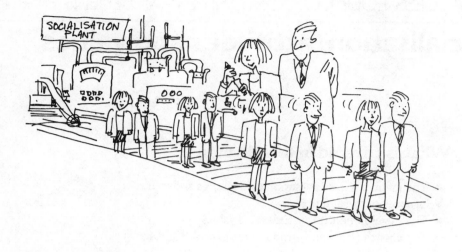

Most societies tend to reproduce their social kind from generation to generation

Activity

a In small groups of three or four, define your own religious attitudes.

b How do you believe that these attitudes may help or hinder your activities in supporting a client?

Examples of issues which you may wish to consider are euthanasia or contraception.

The learning process described above is called **socialisation.** Our personalities are shaped and developed through social contacts with other people. The process starts when we are infants and progresses throughout our lives. We come to behave, to feel, to evaluate and to think similarly to those around us. Most societies tend to reproduce their social kind from generation to generation. However, the process is complex and not fully understood. We all know of examples of lack of socialisation – for example, the child who rebels and adopts a lifestyle completely different from her parents! Socialisation is explained in more detail in Chapter 7.

Sources of socialisation

Socialisation is influenced by two groups in society:

- **membership groups**, such as a person's culture and social class where socialiation occurs through one-to-one contact with family (the strongest socialising influence, and the most studied), friends and neighbours
- **reference groups**, which are perhaps the most personally significant influencer of attitudes.

Membership groups

- **Family** The family is the best-known and strongest socialising influence. Parent's essentially wish to guide the child's acquisition of values, behaviour and personality characteristics into what the culture considers appropriate. Parents direct the child's learning toward what the culture defines as desirable characteristics and behaviour. At the same time, undesirable behaviours and values are inhibited.

The inhibition of undesirable behaviours in the child is referred to as **repressive socialisation**. Repressive socialisation usually begins during the child's second year. The child is asked to stop making so much noise at dinner, to stop jumping up and down on the bed, and to curb tantrums. Repressive socialisation emphasises obedience and respect for authority.

On the other hand, some parents soon begin to move away from this socialising technique towards **participatory socialisation**. This gives children freedom to try things out for themselves, and explore the world on their own terms.

Participatory socialisation is child-centred, rather than parent-centred. Children are more likely to be motivated by their desire to be like someone they respect, love and admire. This is called the **process of identification**.

Early socialisation is probably most readily accomplished through a combination of both techniques. Rewards and punishments are both effectively used. However, as the child gets older, the acquisition of values and behaviours is more likely to be product of identification with a model.

> Children watch what you do.
> So watch what you do!

Both types of socialisation are not quite randomly distributed in society, but are correlated with socio–economic level and education. The evidence indicates that repressive socialisation is more characteristic of the working class, while participatory socialisation is found more commonly in the middle class.

The socialisation that occurs within the family develops notions of what is right and wrong. It also determines the level of importance put on traditional roles. Importantly, the family have a powerful influence on the value of education. Religious beliefs are also largely socialised through the family.

- **Culture** Culture is the set of beliefs and values that people regard as natural and normal in a particular society, for example the expectations of people in the UK are very different from those of Chinese people. The values of our society are taught to us in the family and in school, and are communicated to us through television and newspapers.
- **Sub-culture** There are variations within a national culture that are determined perhaps more locally, or related to special interests or lifestyle. The attitudes of people from Yorkshire, for example, may differ from those of Londoners. Examples of lifestyle sub-cultures are punks, hippies and travellers. Race and religion may also be sub-cultural influences. For example, African and Caribbean culture will influence the attitudes of that sub-culture in Britain, and Chinese culture will influence the attitude of the UK's Chinese community. Religions such as Judaism and Islam rely on sub-cultural influence on an international level in order to remain intact.
- **Social class** Divisions in labour and education create other sub-cultures known as 'social class' (see Chapter 2, page 24). Social class is characterised by values and attitudes acquired through contact with others in a particular class. Some young people, for example, go to special, privileged schools with the intention of socialising them into particular class attitudes and behaviours.
- **Peer groups** Peer groups have a strong influence on attitudes, as they may be simultaneously membership *and* reference groups (see below). Peer groups are formed by individuals with a common interest or identification. A good example is the friends

3

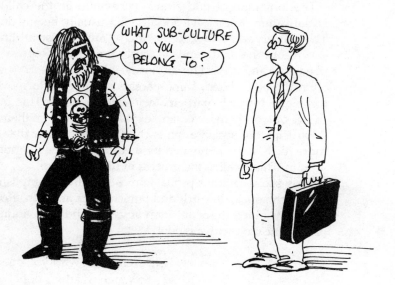

you choose when you are young. They are likely to influence your attitudes toward school work, the music you like, the way you dress, and even the way you express yourself both verbally and non-verbally. Later in life peer groups may be identified more in relation to vocation or profession. Teachers, for example, may relate as a peer group, members often dressing alike, and possessing similar views.

Activity

a In small groups, make a list of other peer groups that influence dress and appearance. Examples may be based on age, profession, or social groups.

b Do you think that the groups you identified are stereotyped by their dress and appearance?

Imposed membership groups These include elderly people, disabled people, unemployed people and mentally ill people. Health and social care services have been largely ignorant of the importance of reference groups (see below) to people's own sense of identity. Hence, access to care services is often determined by establishing the client as a member of a group with a negative label (i.e. imposing a membership group upon them) that stresses their 'abnormality'. These are not likely to be the membership or reference groups that the individuals would choose for themselves.

> Putting individuals into groups creates a language for us to describe them. Language determines attitudes. This has been well-documented by sociologists such as Goffman (1961), psychiatrists such as Laing (1960), and neurologists such as Sacks (1985). Sacks describes how we use a language describing deficit, shortcomings and problems for users of health and social care services, and how our language does not describe the capabilities, potential or hopes of clients.

Reference groups

- **Aspirational reference groups** These are groups with whom the individual may have little or no contact, but whose standards and attitudes are aspired to. The individual will have internalised the values of the group to which he wishes to belong (i.e. to which he 'refers'), and wants to be perceived as a member of. Such aspirations are often associated with upward mobility through the class structure. For example, young medical students often will quickly internalise the conservative values of the medical profession, to which they hope to belong. Some people may value flashy cars, and expensive clothes, because they want to be rich one day.
- **Imaginary reference groups** This is where people adopt what they believe to be either the values of the future or the past. They might fancy themselves as 'ahead of their time' or 'longing for the good-old days'. The slow uptake of services and benefits by elderly people may reflect former cultural attitudes about self-reliance.
- **Dissociative reference groups** This is where the individual, in rejecting a group's values, makes choices that put him at odds with the group. This phenomenon is seen in some people who offend, where the challenging of cultural values is rewarding, as it reinforces the image with which they wish to be perceived.

Reference groups are important to understand, as more than any other influence, they direct our decisions and choices. Individuals are fiercely loyal to their reference group, and strongly influenced by particular people who represent its values. Such a particular person might be a teacher, an employer or a minister. It might be a politician, an actor, a sporting personality or a member of the royal family. We are socialised not just into who we are, but who we would like to be.

Activity

a Work in groups of three or four. Individually determine which social class you 'believe' you belong to, and how this has influenced your attitudes. Ways of determing your 'actual' social class will be discussed in Chapter 2.

b Do the same for other membership groups, and then reference groups. Make sure that you understand the differences between these groups and how they affect you.

c Compare your answers with others in the group, and draw conclusions. Make a note of the conclusions to contribute to a summary session involving all of the class.

The development of attitudes and values

Attitudes

> An attitude is an organised and consistent manner of feeling, thinking and reacting towards people, social issues, groups, or any event in one's environment.

Attitudes consist of thoughts, beliefs, and feelings. We develop our attitudes through the process of socialisation. The process of coping and adjusting to our social environment creates attitudes which regulate our reactions or behaviour.

Attitudes can become inflexible and **stereotyped** (see also pages 147–8). If a person's attitudes become firmly set, he is then too ready to categorise people and events.

Individuality is not recognised or examined. Fixed or stereotyped attitudes reduce the potential richness of a person's environment.

The large social system that surrounds us, with its many races, religions and classes, has shaped who we are. We live in a multi-cultural society that is constantly changing, and health and social care services must reflect this fact. All groups make contributions to the overall values of society, and every individual is affected by these values and attitudes.

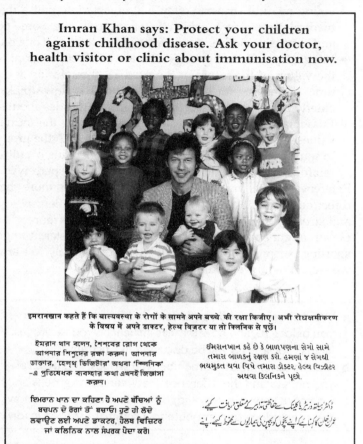

We live in a multi-cultural society. Health and social care services must reflect this fact

Activity

In small groups, identify the contributions of various cultures to your school or college environment. Discuss how these contributions have helped widen your experiences.

In health and social care, understanding the attitudes of potential service users is important, because it helps those who provide services to provide them in a more acceptable manner. Some Asian families, for example, will not find residential care acceptable for elderly people, as they believe care of the elderly is a family responsibility. Many families will not accept help from social workers, as they do not accept the view of themselves as a 'problem' family. Such a label may be incompatible with their reference group. In order for all people in society to have equal access to care services, the attitudes and perceptions of service users should be given the highest regard.

Our own attitudes as carers must also be constantly re-evaluated. It takes conscious effort not to allow attitudes to develop into **prejudices** (see page 147). We are not fully conscious of most of our attitudes, and how they affect other people.

Our attitudes may change as we become exposed to more social situations. We incorporate attitudes that seem appropriate for belonging to groups that we consider important (reference groups). Attitudes are particularly resistant to change if:

- they have been learned early in life
- they help to satisfy needs
- they are integral to one's personality and style of behaving.

Behaviour

Much of our behaviour is influenced by the attitudes we hold. They affect our judgements and perceptions, our reactions to others, and our basic philosophy of life. Attitudes organise themselves into patterns of activity which define our personalities. This activity is called **behaviour**. Behaviour is the observable responses that an individual makes according to his attitudes. The term 'observable' is important because although the attitudes and values themselves cannot be observed, our responses to them can. (For more about observable behaviour, see page 306).

Values

> Values are principles, standards or qualities considered worthwhile or desirable.

As with attitudes, an individual's values can be observed in their behaviour.

Although it is difficult to change attitudes, and hence values, some vocations, such as health and social care, require much attention to be paid to them. The caring professions support a single value base, and in fact there is a Value Base Unit (Unit 0) for the National Vocational Qualifications (NVQ) in Care. It is hoped that by stimulating thought and discussion, and exposing carers to a wide variety of situations, attitudes may be developed that are consistent with the value base.

The Value Base unit
The Value Base unit for the NVQs in Care addresses five elements:

- anti-discriminatory practice
- confidentiality
- individual rights
- personal beliefs and identity
- effective communication.

Activity

Divide the class into five groups, each group taking one of the five elements that make up the Value Base unit. Discuss the contents of the element assigned with reference to professional practice in care settings. Make notes of your discussion and report back to the whole class.

Such discrimination results in exploitation and abuse. It disenfranchises groups of people from mainstream society. The dominant value system in a society often perceives the only worthwhile culture and attributes to be those positively valued by the majority of citizens. In the UK, this tends to be white, middle-class, Anglo–Saxon, Protestant, intelligent, young and healthy.

Discrimination is not restricted to particular groups in society. It is aimed at anyone who, for whatever reason, possesses attributes which are not culturally valued. On the basis of having such 'negative' attributes, assumptions are made about the individual. Such ignorance and intolerance is wide-spread throughout society. **All of us are likely to be both victims and perpetrators of discrimination.**

Activity

In small groups, discuss ways in which each of you have been discriminated against. Consider not just your race, but your age, sex, disability, etc.

Most of us will be acquainted with some forms of discriminatory practice, such as racism and sexism. There has been much media attention focused in these areas. However, the problem of discrimination is far more extensive. What links all forms of discrimination is the concept of intolerance. It is not unusual to be suspicious of those not like us in appearance, beliefs, background, and much more. The real challenge in developing anti-discriminatory practice in the caring services is in developing a more tolerant attitude to differences between people. If the underlying cause of intolerance is fear, then the objective of anti-discriminatory practice must be to remove the fear.

Activity

a In groups of three or four, discuss the sorts of ways in which individuals may be different from each other.
b When your group has agreed, write these differences down in a list. Decide what positive points and what negative points are associated with each difference.

Types of discrimination

In the last activity, you may have listed some of the more common bases of discrimination:

- **Age** The culturally valued age to be in UK society appears to be between 18 and 35. The views of children tend to be disregarded. Much of the interaction between parents and children is corrective in nature. People over 35 will begin to experience the effects of discrimination in the job market. Elderly people are largely written off as being of little use, and prone to disease and deterioration.
- **Class** There is considerable evidence that discrimination on the basis of social class is widespread. Significant differences exist in educational opportunities, work and health care. A key indicator of class is the UK is accent. (See page 24 for a classification of social class.)
- **Culture** There are many sub-cultures in the UK based on race, religion, place of origin, lifestyle, and more. In fact, much discrimination is cultural discrimination. There is much intolerance of lifestyles which are not considered to be the 'norm'.

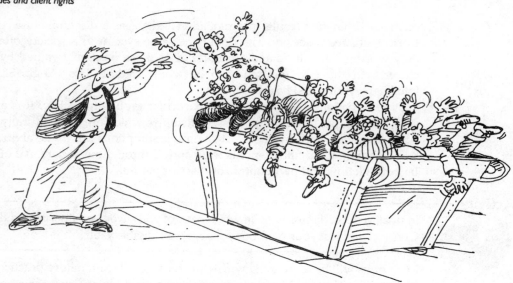

Elderly people are largely written off as being of little use, and prone to disease and deterioration

- **Gender** We are all aware of discrimination on the basis of gender. Women are still generally paid less than men, and are excluded from certain occupations. Both men and women are victims of sexual stereotyping, are expected to behave in certain ways, and fulfil particular roles.
- **Health status** Those in our society suffering from chronic, recurring or terminal health problems are often excluded from social and employment opportunities. They may also be perceived as 'problems' by health and social service agencies, and considered to be a burden on social security budgets.
- **HIV status** In recent years, we have seen much fear and ignorance about HIV and AIDS. Those who are HIV positive have been assumed to be homosexuals or drug addicts, and there is much irrational fear about having contact with them.
- **Marital status** Assumptions are still made about individuals on the basis of whether they are married or not. Married men are seen to be more conventional and trustworthy. Married women, on the other hand, may be perceived as an employment risk, because they are likely to want or have children.
- **Cognitive ability** Those of low cognitive ability are often perceived as being unable to participate in society. If employable at all, they are often exploited on ridiculously low wages. Children of limited cognitive ability are frequently abandoned by the educational system, and are often removed from main-stream education into 'special' units.
- **Mental health** Those people experiencing mental health problems are frequently treated with suspicion. They are often perceived wrongly as being violent or dangerous. Attempts to house some individuals with mental health problems in the community sometimes results in protests and anger. Similarly, they are often denied decent employment opportunities.
- **Offending background** It is not uncommon to find that someone who has made a mistake, and has been in prison, is denied employment, and sometimes housing.
- **Physical ability** Those of limited physical ability are frequently denied access to public places, and suitable housing. Physically disabled children are sometimes denied main-stream education.

- **Place of origin** Those of a place of origin other than the UK, often have different customs, beliefs and diet. Their experiences are often invalidated, and they are put under considerable pressure to appear to be British. Sometimes, they must disguise their accents and abandon their native dress in order to 'integrate'.
- **Political beliefs** Although the UK may be more tolerant of diverse political beliefs than some other nations, political allegiances are still frequently the basis on which many assumptions about individuals are made. Extremism, of any kind, is frowned upon.
- **Race** The colour of one's skin is still an overwhelming source of discrimination. The human species is racially diverse, but this is not always reflected in communities, education or employment. Racism remains one of the major sources of discrimination in the world.
- **Religion** Many different religious beliefs and practices can be witnessed throughout the UK. Rather than being a source of interest and education, religious differences are regarded with suspicion and hatred. Religious differences have been the cause of many wars throughout the world.
- **Responsibility for dependants** Discrimination exists, primarily in the employment, market against those who have children to care for, as they are perceived to be less reliable. There is also some discrimination against men by the legal system in custody disputes.
- **Sensory ability** We live in a world that assumes everyone can see and hear. The needs of those who cannot are sometimes not considered in the provision of services.
- **Sexuality** We live in a society that is largely intolerant of anything other than heterosexual relationships. Homosexuals are treated with suspicion and sometimes violence. They were legally considered to be mentally ill until the 1960s. In addition, certain behaviours are perceived as promiscuous, or out of the ordinary, and are not tolerated by society in general. Those perceived to be sexually different from the 'norm' are denied both employment and social opportunities.

The list above is not exclusive, but it is easy to see that there is a risk of discrimination wherever individuals or groups are perceived to be different from the norm, or what is commonly encountered and valued in mainstream society.

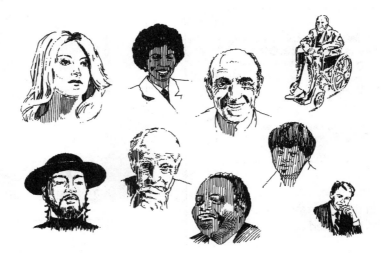

What are your assumptions?

Activity

a In small groups, identify which groups of people are associated with HIV.
b Why does this association exist? Is it justified?

Overt and covert discrimination

Discrimination may be **overt**, in that it is clearly articulated, public and obvious. For example, advertising for a job and stipulating that applicants should be under 40 years of age (ageism). Much overt discrimination is a societal problem and is legislated against. More often, however, discrimination is **covert**, in that it is hidden and subtle.

Activity

WAREHOUSE PERSON

Due to recent company expoansion a further person is required to assist in our fabric warehouse.
Working within a team , the person we require should be flexible, ages 23-35, and be able to work on their won initiative. A knowledge of goods in/despatch procedures would be advantageious as well as the ability to work well under pressure.
In return we offer an excellent salary, bonus and pleasant working condition in the heart of the Cotswolds.

Production Manager c£ 27,000
Shift Manager c£20,000

A major brand leader in East Anglia requires two ambitious career minded managers for a high volume 3 shift food packing operation.

You will have a degree or appropriate qualification and will be:

Production Manager

With 3 shifts reporting to you, you will be in your late 20's to early 30's and able to demonstrate a track record of change management in a modern production enviornment.

Shift Manager

Aged early to late twenties, you are probably looking for you first major career move.

Both positions command an attractive salary and a relocation package.

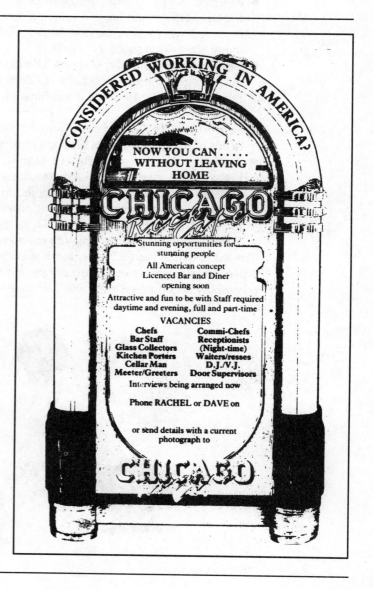

Here are three examples of discrimination in the job market. Identify who is being discriminated against.

Case study

In September 1993 the press reported a case in which Mr Green, a black insurance salesman, and his pregnant white girlfriend, Miss Jones, were awarded £24,233 by an industrial tribunal after they had been simultaneously dismissed from the sales department of the company for which they both worked.

The tribunal was told that when Miss Jones informed her employer that she was pregnant, he swore at her and refused to allow her to attend ante-natal classes (her right in law) saying, 'I ain't running a charity, I'm running a business.' He gave her additional work to do at home, saying that if she had done so 'instead of playing with that black', she would not have become pregnant. He referred to her as a 'slag' and a 'stupid cow', among other abusive terms. His business partner was equally abusive towards her.

When Miss Jones was five months pregnant, she was sacked along with Mr Green. She said that 'they did everything ... to make me walk out of my own accord.' The company claimed that the couple were made redundant after a fall in orders, but later admitted to the tribunal that staff numbers had actually increased from 20 to 40 after the redundancies!

The award of £24,233 covered injury to feelings and loss of earnings. The case was the first since the European Court of Justice had removed the limit of £11,000 on awards for injury to feelings. The tribunal chairman described the treatment received by Mr Green and Miss Jones from their former employers as 'grotesquely offensive' and said it had made them both feel disadvantaged.

Activity

In small groups, discuss and summarise the issues raised by the case study above.

Covert discrimination is difficult to legislate against because it largely results from negative pre-judgements expressed through individual attitudes and language. Much of this is discussed in Chapters 3 and 4, as body language, tone of voice, and choice of words are all important. An important rule of thumb is never to describe an individual or a group by turning an adjective into a noun. For example, instead of 'the elderly', use 'elderly people'. Instead of being a 'schizophrenic', a person is 'having schizophrenic experiences'. The words we use to describe social disability in individuals and groups is explanatory, but does not diminish their essence as humans. All health and social care deals with people with problems – not just problems. Because covert discrimination is such a problem, discriminated-against groups may still find attitudes and access to services less than even-handed in spite of legislation.

Activity

In small groups, determine five examples of both covert and overt discrimination. Make sure you understand the difference.

The effects of discrimination on society and on individuals

The effects of discrimination on society are profound. Instead of the enjoyment of a multi-

Activity

In small groups, decide what attitudes care workers should have in order to provide quality service. Make a list of these, and discuss why each is important. Consider both social care and health care settings.

The values and attitudes of care workers can only be expressed through interpersonal interaction. The values and the behaviours appropriate to care have been established in the Value Base unit for the NVQs in Care (see below).

The Value Base and interpersonal skills

Health and social care is a service that not only requires a great deal of technical skill in physical care, but also considerable skill in emotional and psychological care. The style of help is of equal importance to any physical support offered. Indeed, some care services, such as mental health, are wholly dependent on proficiency in emotional care. All users of care services have emotional needs, so the ways in which care workers respond to them are crucial.

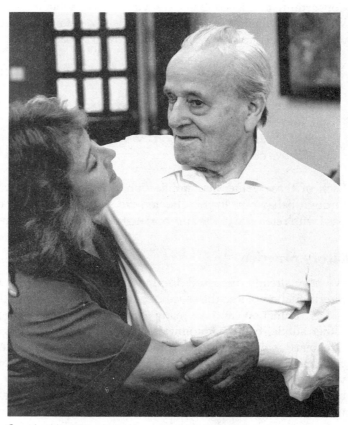

Considerable skill is required in emotional and psychological care, as well as in physical care

Surveys carried out in the United States on user satisfaction in care show that satisfaction with a care service is always measured in relation to the interpersonal skills of the staff. Recent publications from the Royal College of Nursing also recognise this, drawing attention to the differences between:

- **technical quality** (purely practical skills like taking blood pressure, or applying dressings) and
- **functional quality** (how the carer interacts with the patient in meeting their emotional needs).

In some businesses, functional quality is taught through 'customer care training'. However, this can be 'parrot-fashion', and can sound false if the **attitudes** of the staff are not also fundamentally changed. Attitudes result from values, and these are very difficult to learn or change (see Chapter 1).

Activity

Why do you think that attitudes are difficult to change? Give examples from your own experience.

It had been recognised from the beginning that the importance of values in care must be a major part of any qualification. All those working in caring services ideally should reflect the same values in how they do their work. For this reason, in 1992, the Care Sector Consortium published the Care Value Base, which now forms part of the National Vocational Qualifications in Care. It clearly details the principles of good practice on which all interactions with individuals are to be based.

> The Value Base of the NVQs in Care covers five major elements:
> - anti-discriminatory practice
> - maintenance of individual rights and choice
> - acknowledgement of personal beliefs and identity
> - confidentiality of information
> - effective communication.

Each of these values has implications for how we behave. After all, we infer values through behaviour. In this chapter, we will consider each of the elements of the Value Base with reference to the appropriate interpersonal behaviours.

Anti-discriminatory practice

We have already discussed discrimination in Chapter 2. In this chapter we shall discuss discrimination within the specific context of interpersonal skills.

Discrimination can take many forms and may not be immediately obvious. It can be rather subtle, being communicated through body language, tone of voice or humour. Organisational or personal practices in care may reflect assumptions which are discriminatory, for example a doctor who tells an elderly patient, 'What do you expect at your age?', or the manager of a residential home who disapproves of sex among residents. Perhaps there may be anxiety about employing gay men in children's homes or women with children as nurses.

Such discriminatory practices conspire to make us believe that those with such problems can make little contribution to an assessment of their own requirements.

Similarly, discriminatory practice has made some believe that those disadvantaged by health or social problems should not be accorded the same freedom in society as the rest of us. Much discrimination has it roots in history and, while people today do generally have more understanding of others, it does still exist in our society, albeit perhaps in a more subtle form.

There are, of course, policies and laws regarding discrimination, such as the Sex Discrimination Act, the Race Relations Act 1976 and the Disabled Persons Act 1986. However, legislation and organisational disciplinary procedures can never be wholly effective, especially against the more subtle forms of discrimination. To overcome discriminatory practice, efforts must be made to increase awareness. Many organisations now have publicised policies of anti-discriminatory practice, and some offer training courses to increase awareness among staff. Such training should target the fears that underpin intolerance, and involve modelling appropriate behaviours. These courses should be in an emotionally supportive environment, so that the fears of individuals may be safely expressed and dealt with. It should be emphasised that discrimination is not restricted to particular groups in society. Intolerance toward others may be demonstrated in every group.

> Anti-discriminatory practice is not just about written policies. It is about positive, demonstrable behaviour. A thorough understanding of the needs and feelings of people who differ from ourselves is the foundation of good care practice. This understanding is communicated through interpersonal interaction.

Maintenance of individual rights and choice

Essentially, clients should have the same choices and rights as afforded to all of us in everyday life. That means that the client's perception of his or her problems and preferred responses to those problems should be encouraged, listened to, acknowledged and recorded. This is very dependent on the effective communication skills of the care worker, which will be discussed later (see pages 43–59). Options, rather than solutions, should be presented to the client, and the differences among the options should be fully explained. Options should always be considered in respect of risk, but only in exceptional circumstances should the right to take risks be removed from the client. Most commonly, such a situation may arise when it is deemed that the client cannot make a reasonable assessment of the risk, such as in a case of mental illness or severe learning disabilities. In such a case, the client's rights would be legally protected by the Mental Health Act 1983.

We often talk of independence, but perhaps **interdependence** better describes the relationship that most clients would wish from a care service. For many, the care service becomes an important part of their lives, and the support offered should be emotional as well as practical. Care workers are often not allowed sufficient time to meet other than urgent practical needs. Therefore, it is important that clients are encouraged to develop relationships with their carers, and that these relationships are based on a mutual respect. Such relationships will be dependent on the carer's ability to promote and acknowledge the individual's rights and choices. This may entail sensitive areas, such as the right to have sexual feelings and to be able to express these in activities and relationships. Particular attention is drawn to this area, because in the past, many clients of care services have been denied such rights.

33

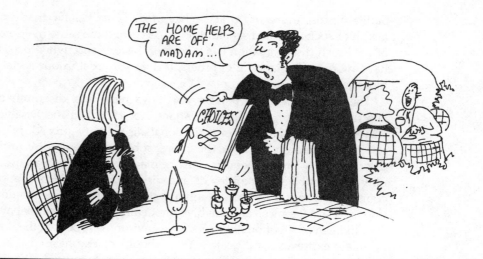

a In groups, discuss the ways in which you would support a client in making choices in an institutional setting, such as a hospital or a residential home.

b How might your activities create conflict within the work setting?

A client may not choose to be as independent as the professionals involved believe him to be capable. Moving individuals toward independence can only be done by encouragement, but the rights of the individual to choose their preferred level of independence is what is important. For example, an elderly person may wish more to be done for them because they choose not to push themselves. This process of disengagement is not unusual. Coercive pressure in this situation may be a consequence of the care worker's own feelings about the process of ageing.

> Carers must not only develop tolerance towards different types of individual, but they must also actively promote and support individual rights and choice. This requires good interpersonal skills.

Effective interpersonal skills are particularly important in dealing with challenging behaviour. Service users may be angry or aggressive, and the care worker will need good rapport and listening skills to calm the situation down. However, care workers need to be careful not to expose themselves to dangerous situations, and may need to call on the support of others, including the police, where necessary.

What if a client is not capable of exercising choice?

If a client is not capable of exercising choice, for example because of a mental disability, their rights to choice are not diminished. First, communication may be other than verbal. Choice may be determined by observing the client's behaviour toward different options. An individual's delight or dissatisfaction is often clearly observable. The techniques of checking for understanding are described later (page 48). Undoubtedly, an understanding of the options available should always be thoroughly attempted, using a variety of methods, if necessary. It may be necessary for the client to actually experience different options before making a choice. For example, a trial period in a residential home may be allowed before a decision about admission is reached.

When it is believed to be impossible for the client to comprehend, it is necessary to use a **client representative** or **advocate**. It is not accepted practice for the care worker, manager, or care agency to make decisions alone for such a client, because there may be a conflict of interests. The client's needs may be in conflict with the agency's or worker's needs. A suitable representative for the client in such a case may be a relative or a friend. Such an arrangement should be formal and recorded. Where a friend or relative is not available or willing, it may be necessary to use an advocate for the client. Advocates are non-professional volunteers, preferably trained, who will get to know the client very well, and advocate (advise) the opinions that they believe the client would express if they were capable of understanding the options open to them.

Advocacy schemes are formal, and advocates should be trained and supported. Hence, there are cost implications to the care organisation. Advocacy schemes have not generally been adopted by care organisations as widely as they should be, or would be expected to be by the Care NVQs Value Base.

Acknowledgement of personal beliefs and identity

Personal beliefs include views that the client holds in relation to areas of self, religion, culture, politics, ethics and sexual preference. The right to some personal beliefs are protected in law. The Race Relations Act 1976 and the Sex Discrimination Act are examples. The right to hold one's own views on virtually anything is a highly regarded aspect of a free society, as long as those views do not infringe or restrict the liberty of others.

Those who receive services from a care worker have the right to be addressed in their preferred manner. That means the choice of whether they are referred to by first name or more formally is theirs alone, and it is the responsibility of the care worker to find this out. Even the use of the term 'Christian name' may prove offensive to those not of the Christian faith, and should therefore be avoided.

We live in an age of political correctness, where the labelling of client groups has come under much scrutiny. Ultimately, an individual client should be referred to as they wish. For example, whether a client is referred to as 'deaf', 'hearing impaired' or 'hard of hearing' is solely a matter of the client's personal preference. Similarly, assumptions should not be made about the diet of a client from an ethnic minority. The client may, or may not, observe religious dietary laws. Every individual should be asked about their preferences at every opportunity.

If the care worker disagrees with particular views being expressed by a client, the worker must still respond in a way that is supportive of the client as an individual. The Value Base goes further than suggesting just tolerance of personal beliefs, it requires that **the personal beliefs of others should be positively encouraged, expressed, and listened to**. This would be the case even if the client was experiencing mental health problems, and their expressed beliefs appeared unusual to the care worker.

Activity

Identify situations in which you might find a client's beliefs in conflict with your own. How would you respond, and why?

Personal beliefs are important because they are an expression of the identity and uniqueness of the individual.

In seeking information, the care worker may find that he needs to focus the client's responses. An information-seeking interview can easily evolve into a social conversation, with little being disclosed. The care worker may need to bring the conversation back to the topic being discussed. This can also be done with the use of prompts. A simple reminder will often work, such as 'Does any of that affect your relationship with your son, Mrs Jones? I'd like to discuss that if it's OK.'

Active listening

Questioning, prompting, and self-disclosure are the ways in which we obtain information. However, it is important that the care worker shows the service user that he or she has been listened to and understood. This is called active listening. There are two types of active listening: **paraphrasing** and **reflective listening**. Some of the ground rules are:

- Avoid saying that you understand when you don't.
- Avoid jumping in with your own points of view.
- Use open questions.
- Pay attention to body language.

Paraphrasing

Paraphrasing is a simple and effective way to test understanding. A paraphrase is a repetition or a summary of what the client has said. It might begin with a phrase such as 'What you have been saying, if I've got it right, is...', and then repeating what the client has said. Paraphrasing checks for accuracy of understanding, and provides the client with an opportunity to correct any misunderstanding. Importantly, it communicates to the client that the care worker has been listening and trying to understand.

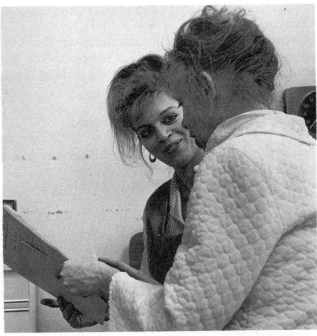

Good communication skills acknowledge the uniqueness of individuals

Activity

Work in groups of three. Two of the three will initially take an active part in the activity, while the third is an observer.

a Choose a subject for discussion (preferably one which can produce some heated debate or disagreement).

b One participant starts off with an opening statement.

c When the first participant concludes, the second has to respond. However, before doing so, he or she must summarise what the first person has said.

d The third person assesses whether the summary was correct. The second can then continue.

This process continues for as long as has been agreed.

The third person then takes the place of one of the first two, and the process repeats with a different subject, and then again, until each pair in the trio has had a discussion, and has practised paraphrasing.

A variation of this activity can be played with a larger group. The individual who initiates the discussion passes a stick on to a person of his or her choice. This second person must then paraphrase the first person's contribution before proceeding with their own. On concluding, the second contributor passes the stick on to another and so on until the agreed time for the activity has elapsed.

Reflective listening

Reflective listening is less concerned with the summarising of facts, and more involved with understanding the emotions and feelings that are being communicated. All interactions between people communicate only three basic things:

● emotions and feelings
● needs and wants
● facts or opinions.

In reflective listening, the listener sorts out the information received from the other person into these categories, and responds only in the order above. Emotions and feelings are the first and most important to respond to, using emotion and feeling words. Some examples of feeling words are:

happy	worried	sad	excited	concerned
angry	frustrated	frightened	depressed	disappointed.

How many more can you think of? Feeling words are important for identifying the emotions of those with whom we converse.

Examples

1 *Mrs Johnson:* Mike usually helps me with my bath. He will be here in an hour. Can you help me now instead?

Care worker: You seem worried about Mike giving you your bath.

Mrs Johnson might feel inclined to discuss what is worrying her because the care worker was able to label her emotion for her. If the care worker was mistaken, and Mrs Johnson was not worried, she had an opportunity to correct the care worker's mistaken perception.

2 *Bob (aged 8):*   The teacher caught me messing around, and kept me in during playtime.
   Care worker: You must have felt *embarrassed* in front of your friends.

The care worker invites Bob to talk about what happened at school by suggesting he might have felt embarrassed. To have been condemning of Bob would have shut him up.

Essentially, in reflective listening we are saying that how people feel is often more important than the facts or details of the situation. The care worker will use both verbal and non-verbal cues to determine how he believes the client is feeling. This is then checked with client. It does not matter if the care worker is mistaken. A feeling misread can give rise to many more improper responses.

Reflective listening is one of the major skills of childcare. Children need to have their feelings acknowledged. Much of our interaction with children is directive, prescriptive and factually based. Many of the problems we have with children are due to these forms of interaction. Telling a child that you can see when she is upset, happy or worried works wonders. By acknowledging the child's feelings, the child is likely to talk more. Perhaps it is because we often do not use reflective listening with children, that children grow up without learning this important skill themselves. All forms of interaction are learned by modelling. Those care workers who work with children will need to demonstrate desirable forms of behaviour.

Activity

Working in threes, start off with two participants and one observer. The two have a discussion about a topic of their choice, while the third scores them both for reflective listening. The observer will be watching each participant for the use of feeling words in checking out the other's emotions. This is repeated until all three have been observers.

All of the activities in this section are for you to experience the interaction techniques being described. Considerably more work would be required to master these techniques. At this stage it is important that you develop an understanding of what the techniques are.

Giving information

The skill of giving information has been covered in the discussion of the Value Base (see Chapter 3). Information has to be provided to clients in ways of their own choosing and subject to their capabilities. Barriers might include language, hearing, visual impairment or mental state. It is important that clients always have as much information as possible in order to exercise their right to choice.

Rapport

All of the interpersonal skills described above will be ineffective unless rapport (sometimes called 'meshing') is established. It has already been stated that care workers are most effective when they can match their outcomes with those of their clients.

Your outcomes, or goals, will not be achieved unless the other person also achieves theirs. The purpose of information seeking is to determine what outcomes the client desires. The care worker will then dovetail, or mesh, her own outcomes with the client's, so both achieve satisfaction. When a client's outcomes are not realised, the care worker's outcomes are not either, and the care worker experiences dissatisfaction with her work. An aim of all care workers is to finish the day's work knowing that something has been achieved, and feeling good about the part they have played in it.

So much of the care worker's effectiveness depends on the skill of rapport. Rapport is composed of a number of basic skills which take much knowledge and practice to master. For example, the following skills can be used:

- **Mirroring and matching** Both the verbal and non-verbal behaviour of the client can be mirrored by the care worker, including body movements and tone of voice. To mirror effectively, the care worker just hints at the client's movements or tone, but is careful not to mimic them. This skill is only used very subtly. For example, if the client is moving her head from side to side when talking, the care worker may only very slightly use the same movement. The care worker may adopt the same body posture as the client, such as crossing a leg or leaning forwards.

- **Pacing** The pace of speech or the breathing pattern of the client can also be mirrored, and then changed if necessary by the care worker. For example, if the client is anxious, he is likely to be breathing quickly. The care worker can pace his own breathing to match the client's, and then begin a process of slowing down, taking the client with him. The care worker can establish rapport with the client by matching the pace of speech. If the client speaks slowly, the care worker should adjust his tempo accordingly. Pacing can be particularly effective when faced with challenging behaviour.

Rapport is the process of developing a shared understanding with the client, and is therefore one of the core essential skills of health and social care. It is a process that we all engage in naturally up to a point. When brought into conscious control as a caring skill, its effect is powerful.

Activities

1 Work in groups of three. One person will be the observer. One of the other two engages in ordinary conversation about a topic of his or her choice. The other practises mirroring body movement.

   The observer's job is to ensure that the other two do not get carried away by the conversation. He will describe how effective the mirroring has been. The first student will also describe how it felt to be mirrored.

   The exercise is repeated until all three students have been the observer.

   Remember not to mimic. Mirroring is a minimised reflection of the other person's behaviour.

   This exercise can be repeated with pacing.

2 Repeat 1 above, but this time mismatch as many verbal and non-verbal cues as possible. For example, if one person is speaking slowly and low, the other speaks quickly and loudly.

Neuro-linguistic programming

The understanding of how we both give out and interpret even the minutest of physical cues has been enhanced through the on-going development of neuro-linguistic programming (NLP).

In spite of its unfortunate name, NLP is highly practical in its models, skills and techniques. NLP has studied what makes outstanding individuals so successful and presents the patterns and skills of success in a way that is learnable. The process is called modelling. For an excellent introduction to this developing and influential area of psychology, the book *Introducing Neuro-Linguistic Programming* by J. O'Connor and J. Seymour is recommended.

NLP was developed by Richard Bandler and John Grinder in the United States in the 1970s. The 'neuro' part of NLP refers to the fact that all behaviour results from the neurological processes of sight, hearing, smell, touch, taste and feeling. Our neurology is also responsible for the visible, physiological reactions we make to feelings and events. The 'linguistic' part of NLP emphasise the importance of language in ordering our thoughts and behaviour and in communicating with others.

NLP is based on three essential ideas:
- Know what you want – have a clear idea of your desired outcome.
- Rely on alert and sharp senses to notice what you are getting.
- Be flexible in changing your own behaviour until you get what you want.

Heightened sensory activity needs to be developed to be successful. You need to see, hear, and feel all that is happening around you, and have a sufficient number of responses to what you are experiencing. The more choices open to you, the more chances of success.

Communication is so much more than the words we say. It has been estimated that body language comprises 55 per cent of communication, tone of voice 38 per cent, and words only 7 per cent. NLP develops the ability to respond effectively to others, and to understand and respect their model of the world. There are many techniques for doing this, some even based on intricate observation of eye movements (Figure 4.1).

Eye movements can indicate the 'representational system' used by a person. Some individuals rely mostly on visual, auditory or kinaesthetic (feelings) senses in processing information. It is important to know which, so that we can present information to them that will be compatible with their information processing system. For example, we might refer to 'seeing what you mean' (visual), 'hearing what you are saying' (auditory), or 'being moved or touched by what you have said' (kinaesthetic). By matching an individual's representational system, it helps achieving rapport.

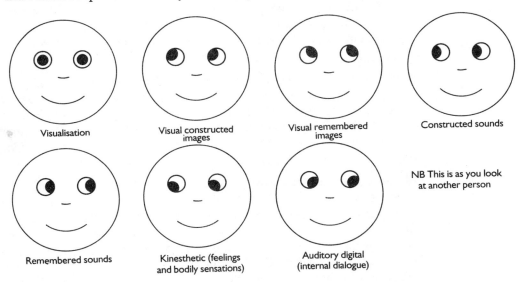

Visualisation   Visual constructed images   Visual remembered images   Constructed sounds

Remembered sounds   Kinesthetic (feelings and bodily sensations)   Auditory digital (internal dialogue)

NB This is as you look at another person

Figure 4.1

between society and the environment. None of them would be wrong but neither would they truly describe the interactions of a holistic model.

In this chapter we will consider some of the biological structures and show how they interrelate to contribute to health. In Chapter 6 we will look at ill-health and consider the importance of nutrition and health.

The initial concept: Gamete production

To understand the interactions in the adult it is important to have some understanding of how the body systems develop from a single cell. This cell, that becomes a potential new individual, is formed by the successful fusion of a male and female gamete (**sperm** and **ovum**).

The fusion of sperm and ovum is normally the consequence of sexual intercourse between a man and a woman. (Scientists have now developed successful ways of using syringes and petri dishes to bring about this fusion. It is not possible, however, to continue the process for any length of time outside the uterus.)

Pregestational factors relating to the health of the parents are important:

- There may be inherited, genetic factors.
- Environmental influences such as ionising radiation or harmful chemicals may damage the cells that form the sperm and ova.
- Also some lifestyles can affect the chances of conception. Stress and obesity are two factors that can affect an individual's fertility, and hence their ability to have children.

Activities

1 Find out what advice is available to couples wishing to conceive. This may include details of lifestyles or concern about inherited factors.
2 What advice is given about health for pregnant women, and where can it be obtained?

The origin of gametes

It could be said that a sexually mature organism is just a gamete's way of producing more gametes. In other words there is a natural cycle and as such the description of fertilisation and foetal development has to start earlier than the meeting of gametes.

Sperm production

The organs of the male reproductive system can be classified as:

- **essential organs** – the testes which produce the gametes
- **accessory organs** – the genital ducts, glands and supporting structure, the most obvious of which is the penis (see Figure 5.1).

The two primary functions of the testes are:

- the **production of sperm** (spermatogenesis) in the seminiferous tubules
- the **secretion of hormones**, chiefly testosterone by the Leydig (interstitial) cells.

Testosterone is the masculinising hormone that brings about the development and maintenance of the secondary sexual characteristics and the male accessory organs, including the prostate and the seminal vesicles. The hormone also has a stimulating effect on muscular development.

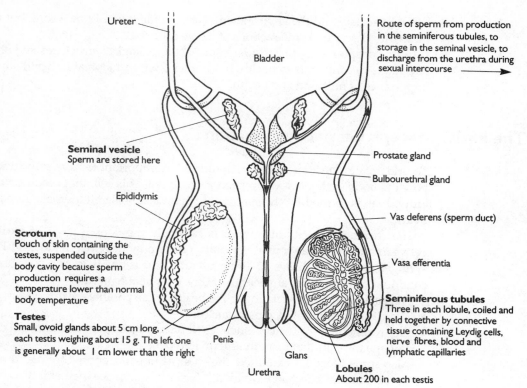

Figure 5.1 The male reproductive system

Within the seminiferous tubules is a layer of cells called the germinal epithelium from which the sperm develop. The cells of the germinal epithelium divide by mitosis to produce spermatogonia which then undergo meiosis to form four spermatids, each containing a half-set of chromosomes. These then differentiate into the familiar, tadpole-shaped spermatozoa. They pass through the various tubes (vasa efferentia, epididymis and vas deferens) out of the testes before being stored in the seminal vesicles.

During sexual intercourse the accessory organs have an important role. Sexual excitement causes the blood vessels taking blood away from the penis to become constricted and so the spongy, erectile tissue becomes engorged. This makes the penis erect which enables it to enter the vagina. Stimulation of the glans at the head of the penis eventually brings about muscular contractions during which the seminal vesicles discharge the sperm into the urethra. They are ejaculated in semen (secretions from the prostate gland, bulbo-urethral gland and the lining of the urethra) into the vagina.

Egg production

This process, technically known as **oogenesis**, starts as the ovaries are formed in the foetus but for practical purposes it is useful to follow the development through one of the monthly ovarian cycles that occur in a sexually mature woman.

The structure of the ovaries The ovaries develop during pregnancy from the same tissues as the testes do in a male foetus. Each ovary is attached to the uterus by an ovarian ligament. It is not, however, attached to the fallopian tube, the end of which forms a funnel embracing the ovary (see Figure 5.2). This gap between the tube and the ovary can, on very rare occasions, mean that fertilisation and implantation occur in the body cavity.

> At birth there are, within each ovary, up to 400,000 primary follicles, each of which contains a cell called an oogonium that has the potential to produce an ovum (egg). However, in a woman's normal reproductive life-span only about 400 of these ever mature and are released for possible fertilisation.

Activity

There are major differences in the number of ova actually released. Consider the effects of different contraceptive methods on the number of ova released by a woman. How many might have been released in earlier centuries when it was not unusual for women to be pregnant or breast feeding for most of their fertile lives?

The ovarian (menstrual) cycle This cycle of events, during which **ovulation** occurs, starts in a woman during puberty and ceases during the menopause. In the intervening years the cycle occurs roughly every 28 days in a healthy woman who is not pregnant. It is a cycle that is controlled by the interaction of several hormones which have the combined effect of causing the maturation and release of the ovum at a time when the uterus is able to support the development of an embryo (see Table 5.1).

Conception, pregnancy and birth

Fertilisation

The simple description of a sperm and egg fusing does not do justice to the very complex processes through which a female gamete is fertilised by a male gamete.

Ovulation involves the release of a cell called a **secondary oocyte** which is not the egg cell but is the penultimate stage of its production. Surrounding the oocyte are many smaller cells, which together are called the **corona radiata**. The actual day in the menstrual cycle that ovulation occurs can be calculated as 14 days before the expected onset of the next menstruation.

The oocyte is moved along the fallopian tube associated with the ovary by the combined actions of the thousands of microscopic hair-like cilia, which line the tube, and muscular, peristaltic movements of the tube wall. The passage down the fallopian tube takes about 3 days although the oocyte will only live for about 24 hours of this. It is clear from this that if successful fertilisation is to take place then it has to occur in the uppermost third of the fallopian tube.

Fertilisation requires many thousands of sperm although only one will carry out the penetration of the ovum. This need for many thousands of sperm is because the corona radiata provides a physical barrier to fertilisation. Each sperm releases an enzyme called hyaluronidase that breaks down the material that binds the cells of the corona radiata and it is the combined action of all the sperm that brings about its dispersal. Eventuallyone spermatozoon, leaving its tail behind, penetrates the zona pelucida that

Table 5.1 The ovarian (menstrual) cycle

Day	Hormone released	Source of hormone	Effect	State of uterus
I	Follitropin*	Anterior pituitary	Stimulates development of the primary follicles in the ovaries. One will eventually release the secondary oocyte. Stimulates oestrogen production	Breakdown of endometrium (start of menstruation)
I–14	Oestrogens (especially estradiol)	Ovaries	Stops production of follitropin and so only one follicle matures	Lining shed by day 6. New one starts to form.
12	Oestrogens	Ovaries	Level of oestrogens peaks, stimulating release of lutropin	
12 (peaks at day 14)	Lutropin **	Anterior pituitary	Causes release of secondary oocyte (ovulation) from follicle, leaving behind the corpus luteum (yellow body) which it stimulates to produce progesterone	
14	Progesterone	Corpus luteum	1 Stimulates the endometrium 2 Inhibits follitropin release 3 Inhibits lutropin release which causes corpus luteum to break down	Endometrium develops with increased blood supply to to receive fertilised ovum
20–28	Progesterone	Corpus luteum	1 As the corpus luteum breaks down progesterone levels drop until day 28 when menstruation starts 2 Inhibition of follitropin ceases so cycle restarts	Endometrial development ceases if implantation does not occur

*also known as follicle stimulating hormone (FSH)
**also known as luteinizing hormone (LH)

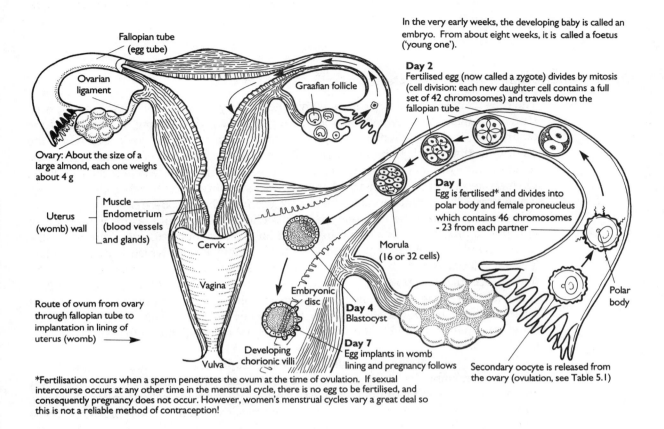

In the very early weeks, the developing baby is called an embryo. From about eight weeks, it is called a foetus ('young one').

Day 2
Fertilised egg (now called a zygote) divides by mitosis (cell division: each new daughter cell contains a full set of 42 chromosomes) and travels down the fallopian tube

Day 1
Egg is fertilised* and divides into polar body and female proneucleus which contains 46 chromosomes - 23 from each partner

Fallopian tube (egg tube)

Ovarian ligament

Graafian follicle

Ovary: About the size of a large almond, each one weighs about 4 g

Uterus (womb) wall

Muscle
Endometrium (blood vessels and glands)

Cervix

Vagina

Morula (16 or 32 cells)

Route of ovum from ovary through fallopian tube to implantation in lining of uterus (womb) ⟶

Embryonic disc

Day 4
Blastocyst

Developing chorionic villi

Day 7
Egg implants in womb lining and pregnancy follows

Vulva

Polar body

Secondary oocyte is released from the ovary (ovulation, see Table 5.1)

*Fertilisation occurs when a sperm penetrates the ovum at the time of ovulation. If sexual intercourse occurs at any other time in the menstrual cycle, there is no egg to be fertilised, and consequently pregnancy does not occur. However, women's menstrual cycles vary a great deal so this is not a reliable method of contraception!

Figure 5.2 The female reproductive system .

forms next barrier surrounding the oocyte. The effect of this is to make the zona pelucida impenetrable to any further sperm.

> An estimate of the concentration of sperm in semen is used as a measure of male fertility – between 300–500 million is considered normal.

The secondary oocyte undergoes a maturation division giving rise to a **polar body** and the **female pronucleus**. The latter provides the chromosomes which together with the chromosomes from the spermatozoon form the nucleus of the fertilised ovum, now called a **zygote**. It is from this cell that a new individual develops.

The zygote divides by mitosis (cell division) throughout its passage along the fallopian tube towards the uterus. Continued division leads to the formation of a hollow ball of cells called the **blastocyst** (see Figure 5.2).

If this ball of cells becomes implanted in the endometrial lining of the uterus, then the woman becomes pregnant. However, implantation does not always occur and in up to 75 per cent of potential pregnancies there is a failure of implantation. Failure can also occur where implantation occurs outside the uterus in the fallopian tube (ectopic pregnancy) or

Adolescence

Adolescence describes the period of time during which a person passes into adulthood. It encompasses physiological, emotional and social development. In western culture adolescence normally coincides with the growth spurt and physiological changes of puberty. In other cultures this rite of passage is determined by age and is not necessarily related to an individual's physical development.

During puberty the sex hormones (**gonadotropins**) are secreted and bring about the characteristic changes. Early signs in boys are axillary sweating in the armpits and groin, enlargement of the testes and growth of the penis. Later facial, under-arm and pubic hair develops and the voice deepens. In girls, breasts develop and axillary sweating commences. Later there is the onset of menstruation (menarche) although few if any eggs are released in the first year. As with boys, underarm and pubic hair grows, although the distribution pattern of pubic hair differs between the sexes.

Changes in the composition of sweat, together with changes in hormones can lead adolescent boys and girls to develop spots. While this is common and can develop into acne, it should not be seen as acceptable and is treatable. Acne has a second effect in that it often affects behaviour at a time when there is rapid psychological development.

Some of the issues related to adolescence are psycho-social in nature. It is a time when an individual's identity becomes established and moral, social and personal responsibilities are developed. Adolescent people often challenge accepted norms in order to test and establish their own mores. This is occurring at the same time as sexual awareness is developing and so establishment of intimate relationships, sometimes involving sexual experimentation, occurs. Unfortunately this can lead to unwanted pregnancy, the prevention of which may well reflect the quality of learning and support given to the person in the rite of passage to adulthood.

Adulthood and old age

During adulthood most people reach a peak of performance. Skeletal growth ends in the late teens or early twenties, and physiologically a person is at a peak at a similar time. Intellectually, this peak may occur later and social development may take longer too. From the age of 30 or so signs of ageing begin to show. As discussed earlier, physiological changes indicate a slowing down of many processes. This is often associated with increase in the bulk of adipose tissue and a loss of elasticity in connective tissues resulting in the development of a 'middle-age spread' and wrinkles. Skeletal changes mean that joint strength and flexibility are diminished. Cartilage becomes less resilient.

There is a clear stage of development in women (at anytime from their mid-thirties to late fifties) at which their natural ability to reproduce ends. During this period of time, called the **menopause**, the ovaries reduce production of the sex hormones. As a result egg release is reduced and menstruation becomes irregular. Eventually ovulation and menstruation cease. As we have already seen, these changes have significant effects on the skeleton. The reduction of oestrogen production also means that the balance between oestrogen and adrenal testosterone alters. An effect of this is often observed as increased facial hair.

Changes at the cellular level are also noticeable. Some cells, such as nerve cells, die and are not renewable. Others function less well and accumulate toxic metabolites and other substances. Environmental effects can lead to damage to chromosomes giving rise to gene mutations which occasionally lead to abnormal cell growth and cancers.

Physiological interactions

It will is clear from what you have read so far that for a human being to live and grow the various systems need to interact to maintain a balance. Having identified how the systems develop we will now look at structure and function.

Communication systems

There are four systems closely involved with internal communication:
- the nervous system
- the endocrine system
- the cardiovascular (circulatory) system
- the lymphatic system.

The first two have specific roles in monitoring and responding to stimuli, the latter two are both circulatory systems and act as carriers serving all areas of the body.

The nervous system

The nervous system and the endocrine system are very different in structure, although in part they have similar functions and rely on biochemical interactions with cell membranes to carry out their roles.

The nervous system matures at a very early stage in a person's life. As a proportion of the body size the head is very large in a new-born baby compared with an adult. This is because the brain is already at an advanced state of growth.

The nervous system consists of:
- the **central system** (brain and spinal cord)
- the **peripheral systems** (all other nerves).

Nerves act by transmitting electrochemical impulses along their length, normally in one direction only. Sensory neurons (nerve cells) transmit impulses to the central nervous system (CNS) whilst motor neurons transmit them from the CNS. In each case the neurons terminate close to the 'message recipient' cells. A chemical neurotransmitter is released from the neuron to pass across the gap to the recipient cells where they bring about a response. Thus the stimulus from a neuron is targeted at a cell or group of cells. As a result the same transmitter substance can be released by different nerves, the specificity of response coming from the initimacy of the neuron with its target cells.

Within the peripheral nervous system, the most common neurotransmitters are acetylcholine and nor-adrenalin whilst in the CNS, in particular the brain, serotonin, dopamine and gamma amino butyric acid are the most common. The ability to produce dopamine, for example, is defective in people with Parkinson's disease.

The major changes that can occur, from about age 25 onwards, are degenerative. To a large extent they are characterised by a slowing of the transmission of nerve impulses. After the age of 25 cells within the central nervous system die and are not replaced.

Diseases of the nervous system Two important diseases of the nervous system which have major impacts are:
- **multiple sclerosis** The fatty myelin sheath that electrically insulates individual neurons from each other breaks down. This causes short circuits in the nerve and either causes the impulse not to reach its target or for the impulse to spread to different receptors.
- **Alzheimer's disease** This is normally associated with older people but not exclusively so. In this disease fibrous plaques form in the brain. The effect depends upon the area

of brain being damaged but normally includes a level of confusion. Short-term memory loss is often exhibited with sufferers not recalling drinking a cup of tea ten minutes before but having accurate recall of more distant events in their life.

The endocrine system

Endocrine glands are found in a variety of places around the body (Figure 5.8). They produce hormones which are released into the blood stream and which control many bodily functions. Unlike the neurotransmitters, therefore, many different hormones have to be produced. Table 5.3 gives details of some of the major hormones and their actions.

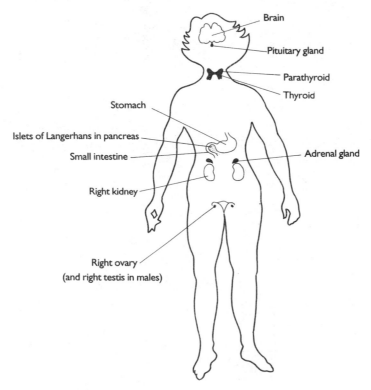

Figure 5.8 The main endocrine glands

The cardiovascular system

There are two circulatory systems:

- the **cardiovascular system** in which the **heart** pumps the blood around the body. The **arteries** and arterioles carry blood away from the heart, **capillaries** take the blood to individual cells or groups of cells whilst **veins** and venules carry it back towards the heart.

  The heart pumps blood from its right-hand side to the lungs where it releases carbon dioxide and picks up oxygen (**pulmonary circulation**). The blood then returns to the left-hand side of the heart from which it is pumped at pressure to the rest of the body (**systemic circulation**). By the time the blood reaches the veins it is at a very low pressure and so its return to the heart is aided by valves in the veins and the pumping action caused by body muscle movement.

- the **lymphatic system** (see page 87).

Table 5.3 Major endocrine organs

Endocrine organ	Hormone	Action	Excess (+) and deficiency (-)
Pituitary: anterior lobe	Somatotropin	Promotes growth and protein anabolism	+ Gigantism in children − Dwarfism in children
	Thyrotropin	Stimulates thyroid gland	As for thyroid
	Adrenocorticotropin	Stimulates adrenal cortex	As for adrenal cortex
	Follitropin	Stimulates ovarian follicle development	As for ovary
	Lutropin	Promotes growth of corpus luteum	As for ovary
	Prolactin	Promotes milk production	− Reduced ability to breast feed
posterior lobe	Oxytocin	Parturition, milk let-down and orgasm	− Can require assistance during birth, e.g. the use of artificial hormone
	Antidiuretic hormone	Increases water reabsorbtion	− Diabetes insipidus (excess urine production)
Thyroid gland	Thyroxine	Regulates growth and metabolic rate	+ Grave's disease; increased metabolic rate − Cretinism (children); Myxoedema (adults)
Parathyroid glands	Parathormone	Controls phosphate and hence calcium levels	− Low blood calcium leading to tetany − Bone decalcification
Pancreas: beta cells alpha cells	Insulin Glucagon	Decreases blood glucose Increases blood glucose	− Diabetes mellitus
Adrenal glands: adrenal cortex	Aldosterone	Controls sodium reabsorbtion	− Weak muscle action nerve transmission

continued

Table 5.3 *continued*

Endocrine organ	Hormone	Action	Excess (+) and deficiency (−)
	Cortisol	Controls conversion of fats and proteins to glucose	+ Excessive protein breakdown; Cushing's disease
adrenal medulla	Adrenalin	General response to stress	+ Stress-related illness
Ovaries (see Table 5.1)	Oestrogens (esp. estradiol)	Development of secondary sexual characteristics; important in ovarian cycle	− Masculinisation; infertility
	Progesterone	Maintains corpus luteum	− Infertility; spontaneous abortion
Testes	Testosterone	Development of secondary sexual characteristics	+ Potential violence − Infertility; low sperm production

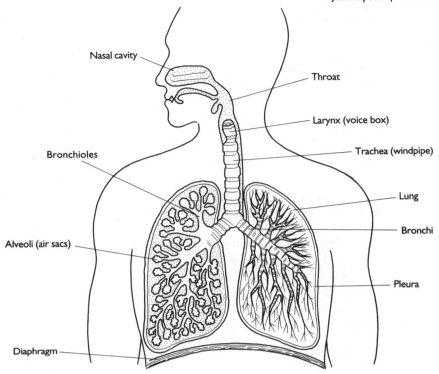

Figure 5.12 The respiratory system

mucus trap larger particles before they even reach the trachea. The eddies in the air currents set up by the shape of the nose also mean that bacteria and viruses can also be trapped in the mucus.

> **The nose also has the important function of warming the air before it passes to the lungs. You will notice this on cold days when your nose is significantly colder than the rest of your face. This role is important as thermal shock would damage the alveoli.**

The alveoli look in many ways like bunches of grapes at the end of the branches of bronchioles. There is a very thin layer, one cell thick dividing the air space inside each alveolus from the blood flowing alongside. The inner wall (air side) of the alveolus is covered with a layer of water in which the oxygen dissolves before diffusing through the cells into the blood stream.

This water also has dissolved in it a **surfactant**. This is a detergent like substance which reduces the surface tension. It is important because it means that when the lungs expand during breathing in there is little effort expended in overcoming the surface tension.

> **In premature babies the lungs are not completely developed and there is often little or no surfactant and so the babies have difficulty in breathing. This is now being overcome with artificially-produced surfactant which is given to the babies immediately after birth, and so more premature babies are now surviving.**

Breathing Breathing describes the passage of air into the lungs which is brought about by a sequence of movements that increase the volume of the **thorax** (chest cavity) so reducing the internal pressure. Normal atmospheric pressure forces the air from the outside into the lungs. It involves the piston like movement of the diaphragm up and down, and the movement of the rib cage.

During inspiration the diaphragm moves down and the external intercostal muscles move the rib cage upwards and outwards. During expiration the diaphragm moves upwards and the ribs return to their resting position. Forced expiration involves the internal intercostal muscles pulling the rib cage down and inwards. This rapidly increases pressure in the thorax and forces the air out.

The control of breathing is normally undertaken by the respiratory centre in the medulla oblongata of the brain. This sends motor neuron impulses to cause the diaphragm and ribs to move and monitors the expansion of the lungs. Thus there is a rhythmical inspiration and expiration without conscious thought. Higher brain centres in the cortex allow voluntary control of this movement to enable speech and other controlled breathing movements. However, it is not possible to totally over-ride the control of the medulla oblongata.

The rate and depth of breathing alters, for example, with exercise. This is controlled by the level of carbon dioxide (also acidity) in the blood. As energy use increases, so carbon dioxide levels increase and the demand for oxygen increases. Small rises in the level of carbon dioxide cause a large increase in the rate and depth of breathing. It is interesting to note that the body responds to these small changes in carbon dioxide levels, while a drop in oxygen levels is not so effective. Oxygen starvation does not trigger increased breathing until levels are critical and a person loses consciousness.

Inside the lungs, oxygen diffuses through the walls of the alveoli into the intimately connected capillaries and reacts with haemoglobin in the red blood cells to form oxyhaemoglobin. In this form it passes to the tissues where the reduced pH caused by the presence of the carbon dioxide brings about the release of oxygen. Thus active tissues, using energy, produce carbon dioxide that triggers oxygen release.

Carbon dioxide from the tissues is carried in the blood, both attached to haemoglobin and also as bicarbonate ions. At the lungs it is released and diffuses in the alveoli and is breathed out.

Health and the respiratory system

- Your lungs are capable of a biggest breath (vital capacity) of over 4 litres.
- Normal resting breathing means that you take in about 0.6 litres of air in each breath (tidal volume).

Exercise It is clear to see that only about one eighth of the gas exchange surface is used in resting breathing. Exercise increases the demand for oxygen and so the rate of breathing increases, as does the size of each breath. Regular exercise increases the reserve capacity (the difference between normal breathing and large breaths) making gas transfer with the blood much more efficient. This also means that oxygen can more readily pass to working muscles so that they can continue working aerobically. **Aerobic** exercise regimes develop the muscles and lungs in harmony so that there is always a balance between oxygen intake and oxygen use. Exercise should not be so strenuous that the muscles actually have to work without oxygen (**anaerobic** respiration). In this situation the muscles use glucose inefficiently and produce lactic acid.

One way of determining the type of exercise is to monitor how long it takes for breathing to return to normal:

- Aerobic exercise, because of the balance between oxygen supply and usage, should show up as a rapid return to resting breathing.
- Anaerobic exercise, on the other hand, is characterised by the need to continue breathing deeply after exercise, and the return to resting breathing is slow. This is because the body has built up an oxygen debt whilst respiring glucose to produce lactic acid. The lactic acid requires some oxygen and energy to be reconverted to glucose or fully respired. The oxygen required to clear the lactic acid makes up the oxygen debt.

Asthma There are several ways in which breathing efficiency and effectiveness can be reduced. The most common of these is with asthma. People suffering from asthma can breath normally most of the time. However, sometimes the smooth muscles in the bronchi and bronchioles contract making it much harder to pass air in and out. At the same time the production of mucus can increase, again reducing air flow. The trigger from asthma attacks varies, and can be related to stress, atmospheric pollution, infections, sensitivities and allergies. Most asthma is controllable with drugs and should not stop the 'sufferer' from participating in normal activities.

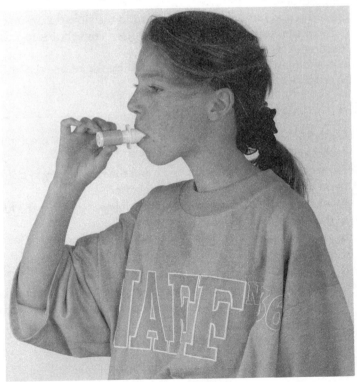

Drugs can assist asthmatics to lead normal healthy lives

Smoking More severe problems come when the respiratory system is damaged. A clear cause of this is smoking. Smoking has several damaging effects:

- The first, very rapid effect, is to damage and destroy the cilia lining the trachea and bronchi. This means that mucus is not cleared from the trachea but passes back into the lungs. Attempts to clear the mucus as it builds up in the trachea leads to the classic 'smoker's cough'.

- The loss of cilia means that the lungs are not so well protected from dust particles and bacteria. They are therefore more open to mechanical damage and infection. The build up of mucus also contributes to the mechanical damage, destroying alveoli walls reducing the surface area available for gas exchange. There is also an immediate physical effect of mucus build up in the reduction of vital capacity. As resting breathing only uses about 15 per cent of the lung capacity, this filling up with mucus is not noticed until exercise is taken and demands for oxygen increase. At this point parts of the lungs are found to be unavailable for gas exchange and the coughing reflex is used to attempt to clear the blockage.

- A third and much more serious effect of smoking is the promotion of lung cancer. This is thought to be brought about by the potent carcinogens in tobacco tar being trapped in intimate contact with the lung tissues. The cancers so caused have the effect of reducing respiratory efficiency and eventually, if untreated, causing death. The treatment often involves major surgery with the removal of part or all of an affected lung.

Ageing The effect of ageing on the respiratory system is two-fold:
- the natural loss of elasticity caused by the replacement of elastic fibres by collagen
- the reduction in vital capacity related to the slow accumulation of mucus in the lower parts of the lungs. Atmospheric pollution contributes to this and can be seen as dark staining of the lower regions.

These two features are often exacerbated by the reduced exercise levels often associated with older people.

Review questions

1 Describe two key functions of the cardiovascular system and two key functions of the respiratory system.
2 How do the cardiovascular system and the respiratory system interrelate and depend upon the correct functioning of each other?
3 How does the structure of each of the following reflect the function:
   a the heart?
   b arteries?
   c veins?
   d capillaries?
4 Describe the main functions of the pulmonary artery and pulmonary vein.
5 Give four examples of valves that are present in the heart and explain the functions of at least two.
6 What are the effects of ageing on:
   a lung function?
   b cardiac function?
   c the blood vessels?
7 What effect does smoking have on the heart?
8 What are the benefits of exercise on the cardiovascular system?
9 How is a thrombosis produced and what are its possible effects?

10 How does smoking affect the structure and function of the respiratory system?

11 Describe how the body co-ordinates response to changes in the external and internal environment. Give two examples.

12 Give examples of ways that maternal lifestyle and activities can affect a developing foetus.

Assignment 5
The physical effects of exercise

This assignment develops knowledge and understanding of the following element:
3.1 Examine how body systems inter-relate

It supports development of the following core skills:
Application of number 3.1, 3.3
Information technology 3.1, 3.2, 3.3

This assignment is designed to support your understanding of the inter-relationships between the circulatory and respiratory systems. It allows you to gain personal experience of the effects of mild exercise on both the circulatory and respiratory systems.

WARNING You should not attempt these exercises if you suffer from any cardio-vascular or respiratory disease without first obtaining medical advice. The exercises are not dangerous, but it is always better to err on the side of safety.

Your tasks

For all of these activities it is useful to work with a partner who should take all the readings.

1 In pairs, determine what you would consider to constitute mild exercise. This will depend upon your own assessment of your physical fitness. It may vary from walking gently up stairs to carrying out the normal warm-up exercises before undertaking more physically demanding activity.

2 Whilst lying down, at rest, measure your pulse rate, blood-pressure, breathing rate and tidal volume. For the blood pressure readings you will need access to a sphygmomanometer and for the tidal volume you will need to use a spirometer.

3 Carry out your mild exercise for periods of 1, 2, 5 and 10 minutes, each time monitoring the effects on the four parameters previously measured. After each time interval record the time needed for the measured parameters to return to the resting figure

4 Devise an experiment which enables you to monitor the effects of different levels of exercise on the four parameters you have measured. You will need to ensure that the amounts of exercise are timed and repeatable.

5 Plot the results of your experiments as graphs (using computers if you wish) and

series of doses of the vaccine. The first dose causes the body to produce antibodies and B–memory cells. Subsequent doses cause an increases in the number of memory cells and the amount of circulating antibody which enables the body to respond rapidly before an infection causes ill-health.

Chemical and drug therapies differ significantly between bacterial and viral diseases. Bacterial diseases can often be treated with antibiotics which interfere with the ability of the bacteria to grow and reproduce themselves. The first of this class of drugs, penicillin was only discovered in the middle of the twentieth century and was originally extracted from a fungal toxin.

Viruses on the other hand rely on the body's own cells to reproduce and are unaffected by antibiotics. In fact the difficulty is that to stop a virus reproducing, the host cell has to stop its normal functions. Any drug therapy is likely therefore to destroy the host cells as well as the virus. The body does produce a protein called interferon in response to viral infection and this has now been manufactured and is being used to attempt to control viral diseases. However, with most viral diseases prevention is easier than cure and there are many vaccines available against the viral diseases.

Activities

1 During your lifetime it is most likely that you have been vaccinated against a variety of diseases. It is also likely that you have suffered a bacterial or viral illness.

Use your own experience, health education material and books to identify diseases and the vaccines that are available. Compile a table containing the following information
- disease
- method of spread
- availability of vaccine and to whom it is normally given
- the recommended frequency of booster vaccination
- whether you need to have the vaccination or a booster.

Include in the table not only vaccinations routinely given to growing children in the UK, but also identify those offered to people with specific occupations or to people travelling abroad.

2 Use old records of your locality or talk to people over 60 years old and try to identify causes of ill-health that were common 60 or more years ago. Use mortality statistics to identify the number of people who died of diseases such as whooping cough, polio and smallpox. Compare the common causes of death today with those of 60+ years ago.

Ill-health without a causative organism

There are many causes of ill-health that do not have an infective cause. In this category are:
- inherited gene disorders
- occupational diseases and disorders
- degenerative illnesses
- deficiency diseases
- psychiatric illness.

With some of these there is a clear indicator of the cause. With many, however, the causes are not well understood but include an interaction of the person with the environment (including social condition). The list is not mutually exclusive; Alzheimer's disease, for example, is degenerative and leads to mental disability.

Activity

a In this section a variety of diseases and disorders will be mentioned. Draw up a table identifying the different classes (from the list in the opening paragraph) and indicate into which catagories the ill-health can be placed. Include other illnesses in the list, such as multiple sclerosis and muscular dystrophy, and any others that you think of.

b It is easy for a health service to deal with specific illnesses with a simple cause and a known cure. What effects do you think these multi-factor illnesses have on planning treatment and seeking cures?

Inherited gene disorders

Just as we inherit characteristics such as eye colour from our parents, and a tendancy to diseases such as asthma and heart disease, so we can also inherit defective genes from our parents that give rise to ill-health. Included in this category are single gene disorders such as:

- phenylketonuria
- cystic fibrosis
- Huntington's chorea
- sickle cell anaemia
- colour blindness.

Other inherited disorders involve whole chromosomes and cannot always be traced in families, such as

- Down's syndrome
- Turner's syndrome
- Kleinfelter's syndrome.

Single gene disorders

A person inherits two copies of most genes; one from the mother and one from the father. (In sex-linked disorders, such as red-green colour blindness, a male child inherits a copy from his mother only.) If one of the genes is defective, it is likely that the second is 'normal' and so normal function is achieved. However if two 'abnormal' genes are inherited, then the function of the 'normal' gene is lost. With phenylketonuria (see page 111) the lack of normal copy means the metabolism of the amino acid phenylalanine, controlled by the gene, does not occur and so the disorder develops. The 'abnormal' gene is masked by the 'normal' gene and so people can carry the defective gene and pass it on without showing any effects themselves. In this way so-called recessive disorders can skip generations in families.

With some disorders, the presence of the 'abnormal' gene always has an effect. If the gene is sufficiently dominant just one copy brings about the full abnormality, an example of this is in the relatively rare bone disorder, inherited multiple exostoses. This gene, if present, must express itself and so the disorder cannot skip generations.

Some genes do not exhibit full dominance and so the presence of one copy brings about a reduced effect compared with the full effect from two copies. A disorder in this category is sickle cell anaemia. A person with 'normal' and 'abnormal' copies of the gene exhibits sickle cell trait. The trait creates problems for the person during times of physiological stress because of the abnormal haemoglobin produced by the gene. A double dose of the gene is normally a lethal condition with children not surviving to adulthood. Again, this disorder does not skip generations.

Sickle cell disorder is interesting. In some cases, the disorder has a positive advantage. People with the sickle trait are less susceptible to some forms of malaria and so natural selection has favoured the gene in areas where malaria is endemic.

Chromosome abnormalities

Occasionally the meiotic cell division to produce gametes goes wrong and a gamete receives too much or too little chromosome material.

Case study ──

Down's syndrome

In the case of Down's syndrome, a gamete from either the mother or the father contains an extra chromosome number 21 as a result of a genetic 'accident' either when the gamete was made or during the intial cell division following fertilisation. The child produced as a result has three copies of the chromosome 21, and therefore 47 in all, rather than 46. Ninety-five per cent of cases of Down's syndrome are a result of this 'accident'. The effect is to produce characteristic features and a level of mental incapacity. Most people with Down's syndrome have a reduced life expectancy and a reduced level of fertility.

It is not fully understood why the abnormal gametes are produced but it is known that the older a woman is the greater the chance that a pregnancy will result in a child with Down's syndrome. However, the majority of babies with Down's syndrome are still born to younger women, simply because the overall birthrate is higher in that group.

Approximately 1 in 100 people with Down's syndrome have inherited the condition from their mother or father because of a genetic abnormality called Translocation. There is a third, equally rare type of Down's syndrome known as Mosaic Down's syndrome.

Source: Information supplied by the Down's Syndrome Association

Control and cure for inherited disease

Should we say that people from families with genetic disorders should not have children? Should we test for genetic disorders in the womb and then abort the foetus?

It is easy to identify simple ways in which people with genetic disorders could ensure they do not pass on the genes. Some extreme regimes have even tried to cleanse the population of people they consider to be genetically inferior. Nazi Germany was an extreme example of this. It has not been, and never can be, a viable way of 'controlling' inherited disorders. Apart from the very clear moral issues, biology is also against any such programme. A simple example in the case study of phenylketonuria can identify the weakness.

Case study ──

Phenylketonuria

Phenylketonuria is controlled by a single gene, the defective one being recessive. A test is available for babies born in the UK, soon after birth, to identify if they have inherited two defective genes and have the disorder. About 1 in 25,000 babies have the disorder. Surely if people carrying the gene could be persuaded not to have children, then the disorder could be eliminated and the cost of 24,999 wasted tests could be saved? The question then arises, 'How many people would be asked not to have children?'

The Hardy–Weinberg equation can be used to calculate the number of people carrying the gene in the population. It relies on several issues but at its simplest it can be expressed thus:

Assume that there are two versions of a gene that occur with the frequency p and q, where p + q = 1. Any person can have a double dose of either gene or one of each. The frequencies of these is related by the formula:

$$p^2 + 2pq + q^2 = 1$$

So, for the gene controlling phenylketonuria we can say that the normal version K has a frequency of p, while the abnormal one k has a frequency of q. The frequencies of each combination of genes are expressed thus:

$$
\begin{aligned}
KK &= p^2 \\
Kk &= 2pq \\
kk &= q^2 \\
\text{We know that} \quad q^2 &= 1/25{,}000 \\
\text{Thus} \quad q &= \sqrt{1/25{,}000} \\
&= 0.0063
\end{aligned}
$$

As we know p + q = 1 and also that q is very small, we can say that for easier calculation p = 1.

By putting these figures into the Hardy–Weinberg equation we calculate the frequency of people carrying the abnormal gene:

$$
\begin{aligned}
2pq &= 2 \times 1 \times 0.0063 \\
&= 0.0126
\end{aligned}
$$

This means that the frequency of 'carriers' in the population is 0.0126 or 1 in 80.

So to get rid of phenylketonuria, 1 in 80 people would have to give up having children. This may seem almost possible but everyone carries at least five versions of genes that could give rise to inherited disorders. To follow this to its logical conclusion; to eliminate all genetic disorders everybody should stop having children. There would then be no problem of inherited disorders in the next generation. But who would form the next generation?

Obviously from this case study it can be seen that eliminating defective versions of genes is not easy. However, the understanding of inherited disorders does mean that people can be counselled by trained counsellors about the risks and can make informed decisions about having or not having children.

Is cure possible?

It has long been the dream of some geneticists to be able to manipulate genes to correct defective versions. Currently this is not being practised although in theory it may be possible. It is possible, in a limited way, to introduce normal copies of genes into cells with defective copies and so allow effects of the abnormal versions to be overcome. The genes are introduced using specially modified viruses in droplets that can pass across cell membranes. In the next few years such techniques may be used to treat cystic fibrosis. As more genes become identified and isolated the technique may spread to other disorders.

Currently the technique is not proposed to alter the genes passed into gametes and so the person would still pass on the defective versions. In your lifetime it will be possible to alter defective genes in gametes. There is already a debate about the ethics of such practice and it may prove useful for you to consider some of the issues.

Activity

Gene therapy

Ever since the science of sexual reproduction became known and, more recently, the ability to manipulate genes became possible, people have talked about using the science of gene therapy to eliminate genetic disorders and thus improve the genetic status of humankind. Such techniques would not only be able to 'cure' genetic disorders but also enable choices about specific inherited traits such as hair and eye colour to be made.

a Make your own list of pro's and con's for gene therapy.
b What rules would you impose on gene therapy?

Occupational diseases and disorders

There are several causes of ill-health related to specific occupations. These can have a causative organism, such as the thermophilic bacterias and fungi, which cause **farmer's lung**. They can also be brought about by inhalation of dust particles related to specific industries, such as the inhalation of coal and stone dust by miners causing **pneumoconiosis** and the inhalation of asbestos fibres causing **asbestosis** and **lung cancer**.

A more modern industrial disease is that caused by the repetition of a small range of movements. It has recently been noticed that people using word processors develop very painful wrists. This is caused by the strain and friction generated by the rapid repeated movement of the tendons controlling the movement of the fingers during typing. The friction causes swelling of the sleeves through which the tendons slide and causes great pain. These **repetitive strain injuries** (RSIs) have been identified, and health and safety legislation aims to promote good working practice to avoid this.

Before the invention of the word processor, typists did not suffer from the disease because the mechanics of the typewriter reduced the speed at which a person could type. So the movements were less frequent and injury was less likely to occur. It is interesting to note that the familiar QWERTY keyboard was originally designed to be difficult to use and so stop efficient typists from working faster than the mechanical typewriters were able to work. This built-in difficulty is now contributing to the development of repetitive strain injuries.

Personal situations and ill-health

There are many facets of ill-health that have no causative organism or that are made worse by the situations in which people find themselves. In this brief section we will try to tease out some of the factors related to ill-health where the environment contributes to the nature of the health.

The constituents of a balanced diet

You will have noticed that we have not given you the recommended daily allowances (RDAs) of nutrients. This is because they are subject to change, and are currently the subject of debate. Find the most up-to-date copy of the RDA tables that you can and compare them with one issued more than 20 years ago.

a What are the differences?
b Try to account for the changes.

Ideas about what constitutes a balanced diet have changed significantly. In the past it was perfectly acceptable for a baby to be overweight. Eggs and butter were seen as desirable daily elements of a good diet and white bread was more acceptable than wholemeal.

There is now a greater consciousness about the food we eat, often about the levels of vitamins and minerals as well as the major nutrients. Several diseases of malnutrition have been identified. Heart disease and high blood pressure are variously linked to too much sodium in the diet and too much saturated fat. Saturated fat has also been linked to increased blood cholesterol levels in some people. It is important to recognise that sodium is important as part of a balanced diet and that saturated fats are not cholesterol, nor is dietary cholesterol a significant factor in blood cholesterol levels. It is also important to know that cholesterol is manufactured in the body from similar precursors to other steroids such as estradiol and testosterone. A diet that so reduces the production of cholesterol could also interfere with production of other steroids.

The basic message is that a balanced diet contains a range of foodstuffs in sufficient quantities to meet needs. Excess of anything may be malnutrition. The recent trend towards identifying specific nutrients as healthy or unhealthy and so devising diets to reflect this does not reflect a balanced diet and may cause problems.

Case study

Vitamin C

The recommended daily allowances (RDAs) for vitamins were initially established as about double the amount below which symptoms of deficiency diseases would occur. In the 1970s Linus Pauling, an internationally renowned biological chemist, argued that the RDA figure of 50 mg for Vitamin C was too low and postulated that our ancestors probably consumed at least a gramme a day. Ascorbic acid (Vitamin C) is a powerful antioxidant and it has been argued that high doses may well prevent damage from potential carcinogens. The arguments seemed promising and so many people consumed gramme quantities of Vitamin C, often as effervescent tablets.

Vitamin C is not stored in the body and excess amounts are excreted in the urine. Also the effervescent tablets contain a high concentration of sodium which has been linked to high blood pressure. The reasonable hypothesis that over a day of gathering and eating fresh fruit and vegetables early man may well have consumed large quantities of Vitamin C was distorted and turned into a fad diet, the major effect of which was to make the manufacturers and retailers of ascorbic acid tablets richer.

The NACNE Report, 1983

In 1983 there was a discussion paper on 'Proposals for Nutritional Guide-lines for Health Education in Britain', prepared for the National Advisory Committee on Nutrition Education (NACNE).

The paper was wide-ranging in its coverage but concentrated on areas on body weight and health together with issues relating to carbohydrate, fat and coronary heart disease, salt and blood pressure and alcohol.

Body weight

The report concluded that even being mildly overweight increased health risks. They used the table below (Table 6.4) as the benchmark for acceptable weight ranges.

Table 6.5 summarises the report's guidelines for Health Education in Britain.

Table 6.4 Acceptable weights as recommended by the Fogarty Conference, USA 1979 and the Royal   College of Physicians, 1983

Height without shoes (m)	MEN Weight without clothes (Kg)			WOMEN Weight without clothes (kg)		
	Acceptable average	Acceptable weight range	Obese	Acceptable average	Acceptable weight range	Obese
1.45				46.0	42–53	64
1.48				46.5	42–54	65
1.50				47.0	43–55	66
1.52				48.5	44–57	68
1.54				49.5	44–58	70
1.56				50.4	45–58	70
1.58	55.8	51–64	77	51.3	46–59	71
1.60	57.6	52–65	78	52.6	48–61	73
1.62	58.6	53–66	79	54.0	49–62	74
1.64	59.6	54–67	80	55.4	50–64	77
1.66	60.6	55–69	83	56.8	51–65	78
1.68	61.7	56–71	85	58.1	52–66	79
1.70	63.5	58–73	88	60.0	53–67	80
1.72	65.0	59–74	89	61.3	55–69	83
1.74	66.5	60–75	90	62.6	56–70	84
1.76	68.0	62–77	92	64.0	58–72	86
1.78	69.4	64–79	95	65.3	59–74	89
1.80	71.0	65–80	96			
1.82	72.6	66–82	98			
1.84	74.2	67–84	101			
1.86	75.8	69–86	103			
1.88	77.6	71–88	106			
1.90	79.3	73–90	108			
1.92	81.0	75–93	112			
BMI* 22.0	20.1–25.0	30.0	20.8	18.7	23.8	28.6

*Body mass index = weight in kg/height in metres

Table 6.5 National Guidelines for Health Education in Britain (NACNE, 1983)

Dietary component intake	Current estimated	Proposals Long-term	Short-term
Energy	–	Recommended adjustments of types of food eaten and an increase in exercise output so that adult body weight is maintained within the optimal limits of weight for height.	
Total fat	38% of total energy (128 g)	30% of total energy (101 g) 10% reduction	34% of total energy (115 g)
Saturated fatty acidenergy (59 g)	18% of total energy (33 g)	10% of total energy (50 g)	15% of total energy
Polyunsaturated fatty acid	–	No specific recommendations – if total fat intake is reduced to 30% then this will automatically tend to increase the P:S ratio	
Cholesterol	–	No recommendations	
Sucrose	38 kg/head/year	20 kg/head/year (approx. 50% reduction)	34 kg/head/year (approx. 10% reduction)
Fibre	20 g/head/day	30 g/head/day (50% increase)	25 g/head/day (25% increase)
Salt	8.1–12 g/head/day	reduce by 3 g/head/day	reduce by 1 g/head/day
Alcohol	4–9% of total energy	4% of total energy	5% of total energy
Protein	11% of total energy	No recommendations	

Why did NACNE reach these conclusions?

Fats

Given that their first recommendation was to maintain adult body weight within the optimal limits, then a reduction in fat intake would do this. There had also been evidence from the medical profession that death rates from cardiovascular disease in the UK are amongst the highest in the world and that this is related to fat intake.

The recommendation was two-fold:

- to reduce the total fat intake
- to look at ways at increasing the ratio of polyunsaturated fatty acids to saturated fatty acids.

This followed evidence that a diet with a high proportion in polyunsaturated fatty acids could reduce the incidence of cardiovascular disease. Part of this has been linked to the synthesis of cholestrol-rich atheromatous plaques and their association with thrombosis.

Further research has identified certain types of polyunsaturated fatty acids as being specifically beneficial. Epidemiological studies identified a very low incidence of heart disease with people who consume a large quantity of fish. Analysis of this fish found the fats to be high in long-chain polyunsaturated fatty acids with a double bond in the 3 position (omega 3 fatty acids). These fatty acids lead to the formation of high density lipoprotein in the blood stream and reduces the amount of low-density and very low-density lipoproteins. These last two are linked to blood cholesterol related to atheroma. It has been demonstrated that fish oil dietary supplements can reduce serum triglyceride by up to 70 per cent. These triglycerides appear to reduce the level of clot-digesting enzymes in the blood. Omega-3 fatty acids therefore help in two ways by reducing atheroma production and decreasing the risk of thrombosis.

Carbohydrates

The recommendation was:
- to reduce sucrose (sugar) intake
- to increase the intake of complex carbohydrates as fibre.

The reduction in sugars is part of the drive to reduce overweight. There is also a link with dental caries (tooth decay), although it is thought that the proposed reduction would have little effect on the incidence.

There is an argument that carbohydrate should be in a complex form. This has the effect of slowing down absorption and reducing the swings in blood sugar levels, thus affecting the physiological response to hunger. There is also the point that most complex carbohydrate is also associated with vitamins, minerals and indigestible fibre.

Fibre

The recommendation was to increase this by 50 per cent. There is a strong suggestion that low levels of dietary fibre are associated with large bowel disease including irritable bowel syndrome, constipation, diverticulosis and colon cancer. It is known that the effect of the dietary fibre is to increase the bulk of faeces and reduce the time material stays in the colon. It is also thought to adsorb carcinogens and toxic materials such as bile salts, giving them less chance to come in contact with and damage the intestinal lining.

There is some evidence that soluble fibre has an effect of lowering blood cholesterol and that cereal fibre is protective against coronary heart disease.

Salt

The recommendation was to reduce salt intake. Experiments have shown that very high intakes of sodium lead to high blood pressure (hypertension) and that above average levels of intake can have a similar effect on those with a genetic predisposition to hypertension. The recommendation to reduce salt intake takes account of these results, especially as any genetic predisposition may not be known to the individual.

Alcohol

The aspects of alcohol and diet were not studied in detail but, in line with energy reduction, the recommendation was to reduce the intake. Alcohol is associated with liver damage and so is seen as something to be reduced. However, there is evidence that total abstainers have a low blood concentration of high density lipoprotein. Moderate alcohol consumption, 140–170 g per week increases the level of these lipoproteins. The links with cholesterol and coronary heart disease have already been discussed.

Protein
No recommendations were made about protein intake although a suggestion was noted that people eat a little less protein as current intake was greater than required.

Summary of NACNE recommendations

It is important to recognise that the NACNE report concentrated on health education aspects of nutrition and so set targets for health education to meet in terms of changing people's attitudes and diets. Table 6.6 summaries the recommendations.

The types of fat and carbohydrate were recommended to be changed. This would translate into a change in the types of food consumed leading to an increase in minerals, vitamins and essential fatty acids.

Table 6.6 Summary of energy intake recommended by NACNE, 1983

Dietary component	Recommended intake (as % of total energy)	Reduction/increase
Protein	11%	No change
Fat	34%	Reduction
Carbohydrate	50%	Increase
Alcohol	5%	Reduction
Total	100%	

Activity

Look at your diet for one day. How well does your energy intake meet the NACNE recommendations?

Specialist diets

In spite of all the previous information, there are people who either for medical need or personal preference eat a specialist diet. This can be because of a need to lose or gain weight, reactions to goods, or because of ethical or religious requirements.

Diets for weight loss and weight gain

Weight loss
Most people equate the word diet with losing weight. To do this, the diet needs to be balanced in terms of meeting the requirements for protein, vitamins and minerals but provide less energy than is used. In doing this the shortfall of energy is made up from stored fat.

smoking or nail-biting in adult life as evidence of frustration or over-indulgence during these very early years. A child who is frustrated by too little stimulation at this stage may become aggressive, depressed and often unable to develop personal relationships. Too much stimulation may lead to people having a high opinion of themselves and being dependent on others.

The anal phase

During the second and third years of life, the child becomes more capable of control over its bowels and is said to obtain pleasure from the retention and expulsion of faeces. Potty training starts during this period and if parents approach this training in too strict a manner, Freud argued, it could result in the formation of what he called the 'anal personality' in adulthood. People with an 'anal personality' may become excessively concerned with order and cleanliness and unable to bear unpredictability or untidiness. They become over-possessive, obsessive, sadistic and generally miserable.

The phallic phase

This is the last of the important phases in child development in Freudian theory. During this phase, between 3 and 5 years, the genitals become the area of the body from which the child gets most pleasure. Freud saw this stage as the most important stage in personality development. During this stage, children will be socialised into learning what is right or wrong and learning sex roles. Girls unconsciously want their father (what Freud called the 'Electra complex') and boys their mother (what Freud called the 'Oedipus complex'). It is at this stage that the sex role develops, masculine behaviour in boys and feminine behaviour in the case of girls, through the process of identification that involves the adoption of the father's or mother's whole range of attitudes, values and beliefs. After this stage, a child may act as they think their mother or father would in a given situation.

Freud's theories have been criticised, because he worked as a therapist and gained most of his experience and insights from the behaviour of his patients. It is argued that his experience was limited and his sample biased because it was middle-aged, middle-class and mostly women. His theory is said to be unscientific, cannot be repeated and has too many hypothetical notions that are not directly observable.

Summary of psychoanalytic theory

- **Oral stage 0–2 years** According to Freud this is the first stage of personality development. The baby has the instinct to take pleasure from feeding. Fixation at this stage can occur because of too little or too much stimuli.
- **Anal stage 1–3 years** The stages may overlap and at this stage the child continues to derives pleasure from his mouth. During the anal phase the child starts to learn to control its body, arms and trunk and anus. Fixation at this stage may be caused by lax or too strict potty training.
- **Phallic stage 3–6 years** Freud argued that at about 3 years of age the child begins to experience sexual feelings about its parents. Boys develop such feeling for their mother and girls towards their father. Children begin to develop feelings of guilt because of these feelings and so begin to 'identify' with the respective parent to solve these feelings. Boys begin to act like their father and girls like their mother. If this stage is not successfully negotiated then problems may develop later with sexual relationships.

Cognitive development approach to socialisation

This focuses on the cognitive aspect of morality and, hence, on moral development. This approach offers a progressive view of morality. It differs from Freud's approach because it views morality as developing gradually throughout childhood and adolescence into adulthood.

During the last half century Piaget (1954) developed a theory of how children learn about things. His theory is concerned with how the child's knowledge and understanding change with age. He did not believe that intelligence was fixed at birth. His theory is concerned with how our senses take in information from our environment that we store in our brain and as we process this information our behaviour changes as a result. His theory emphasises the importance of imitation, imaging and symbolic representation during the period 2–7 years. He claimed that human thinking develops in a fixed sequence of stages, and it is not possible to skip a stage. He stressed that children think in a different way to adults. Over a number of years and numerous experiments, he came to the conclusion that the morality of the 5–9-year-old is subject to another's laws or rules, and that the child of 10 years or over is subject to their own law or rules.

Piaget was particularly interested in how children understand the world. The child's development takes place through the development of what he calls 'schemata', mental representations or ideas about what things are and how we deal with them, that can be likened to a set of rules about how to interact with the environment. The first schematas are for reflexes: thinking in the young child is only concerned with the information it picks through its senses that are mostly concerned with the child's needs and wants. These 'reflexes' allow a young child to survive during the few months of life. The reflexes are stimulated by any stimuli, for example if a child touches a hot object it will pull its hand away. It is not until about the age of 7 that the child begins to think about its own actions and their effect upon other people.

As the child reaches 10–15 years, it starts to develop logic and reasoning and starts to thing about what things 'ought' to be like. Piaget stresses self-motivation, emphasises self-regulation, which he calls the 'process of equilibration'. This process has two aspects:

- **assimilation** – children absorb experiences into structures that they already possess through the process of 'assimilation'.
- **accommodation** – structures within the child have to be modified and adjusted to take in experiences that do not fit into the structures already in existence. For example, John a 2-year-old has established that wheels are round. When he was given a wooden truck with squared wheels that moved when pulled by a string, he had to adjust his thinking to take in this new fact.

Essentially Piaget shows that the child's thinking moves from a stage of egocentricity in early childhood to that of reversible reaction in early adolescence. Although he was primarily concerned with intellectual development, his theory has important implications for socialisation. A child in the egocentric stage is intellectually only able to see the world from his or her own point of view. For example, a mother told her 6-year-old daughter off for wandering away while playing on the swings and getting 'lost'. The child was quite unable to understand mother's anxiety and said 'but I knew where I was'. In other words, the child could not see or appreciate that the situation could look different from the mother's point of view.

One could argue, that the primary consequence of socialisation, is to be able see a situation from another person's point of view. According to Piaget, this is quite a late development and it is not until adolescence in many cases when logical ability to 'go back to the beginning (i.e. reversible reactions) develop, that a child can look at the same situation from different view points. Piaget devised many simple but elegant experiments to illustrate this progression. For example, he had a piece of cardboard that was blue on one side and red on the other. He sat opposite the child and showed both sides of the cardboard to the child so they could see each side was a different colour. He then placed the cardboard vertically between himself and the child. He would ask the child, 'What colour can you see?' The child would answer 'Red'. He then asked, 'What colour can I see?' and the younger children would answer, 'Red'. They were unable to see that the piece of cardboard looked different from his point of view, even though they had been shown both colours beforehand.

In this way Piaget shows that the process of socialisation is inextricably linked with the developing brain and intellect of the child and that at different ages, the thinking of the child operates according to different rules to those of the adult.

Piaget claimed that children tend to spend their first ten years not able to use the rules of logic that most adults would use. He argued this logical thought develops from about puberty. One criticism of Piaget's work was that he was always looking for what the average child could do at various stages. By doing this, he ignored the great variations in the ways individuals think. Others argue that Piaget under-estimated the ability of younger children.

Summary of the cognitive development theory

- **Adaptive stage 0–1 year** This is often referred to as the 'sensory motor stage'. Piaget believed that children were born with reflexes that helped the baby to survive and adapt to their environment. As the child adapts to the environment it has different kinds of experience and cognition. This cognition in Piaget's terms is not something that can be measured as it is individual to each child.

  Piaget calls this process of organisation and adapting 'invariant' functions. These functions are individual to each child, as are the 'schematas' (mental representations about how to deal with things, i.e. cross the road, or eat bread), and 'operations' that allow the child to order 'schematas' in a logical way. This allows children to imagine what might happen if they take a particular course of action.

- **Pre-operations stage 2–7 years** During this stage the child only sees the world from their own point of view (egocentric), and also believes that everyone else holds the same view. The child also believes that everyone holds the same way of thinking about right or wrong (moral realism). Seeing things from other people's point of view can begin when the child develops the ability to imagine so – decentring. During this stage the child also believes that all objects have consciousness and feel emotions (animism).

- **The concrete operational stage 7–12 years** During this period the child begins to think logically. They can think about objects without the object being present. The egocentric stage declines as does the belief in animism. Children begin to see situations from other people's point of view.

- **The formal operations stage 12–16 years** The teenager begins to think in an abstract manner, to work things out in their heads. Young people begin also to consider moral and philosophical matters.

Activity

What explanation would you give to a parent to explain why their child always seems to get lost if not watched every moment.

The role of culture in the development of individual identity

Construction of meaning in language

Language is an organised system of symbols which humans use to communicate with one another. Every known human society has a language. This ability to use language is one of the main things that separates humans from the animal kingdom. Humans are the only species that have the ability to use language. However, not every human brain is adequate for the acquisition of language.

There is no society in the world where the newborn baby immediately begins to imitate speech it hears. It is argued that in the first year the baby is maturing and developing some of the ideas that it may want to communicate in language in later years. Before a child can produce recognisable words, it will produce sounds that will become steadily more varied and deliberate. Many children, before speaking recognisable words, pass through a stage of jargon. This is the stage that an adult may feel sure that a child has said words but they cannot make out what the words could be.

Activity

Talk to a mother with a very young child. Find out what sounds the child produces and ask the mother how she knows what the child is trying to communicate.

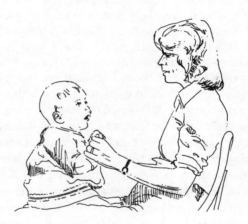

By the time a baby is about 3 months old, if its attempts at communication are positively reinforced by adults, it will be producing a variety of sounds. It will vocalise – make sounds in response to others. The sounds that are reinforced are likely to continue to be used by the child, while those that are not are less likely to be repeated. By the time a baby is 6 months old, it has begun to listen and can distinguish familiar and unfamiliar voices, and also begin to understand some of emotional tones in it the speech it hears. By 9 months, there are usually clear signs that the baby has grasped that making sound can bring some action from others and by the time it is 1 year old, it will often show by its behaviour that it understands a few familiar words in context. From around the first birthday, the words used are likely to be for people or things the child is most familiar with such as 'mama', 'dada', 'cat' or 'teddy'.

Early in the second year, the child begins to produce words and by the middle of the second year it starts to make two-word sentences. By the end of the third year, it is able to use a large part of the basic grammatical apparatus of the local language. Some psychologists argue that the first ten to eleven years are critical period for language development. However, some studies indicate that the first ten years may not be so important, as illustrated by the following case.

Case study

Genie was confined to a small bedroom, harnessed to a potty seat and left, unable to move. She heard no sounds, saw no daylight, was force-fed, deprived of all stimulation until she was discovered when she was 13 years old. She then had essentially to learn her first language, which was constrained and lacked the spontaneity of normal speech. She had to be taught the rules of language long after a normal child would have picked them up, although it was more difficult for her than a younger child.

However, the fact was that she *did* learn a language which tends to contradict the argument of those who say that the first ten years are critical in language development.

Biology is critical for language acquisition, but a number of situations have made it quite clear that learning opportunities and environment also are important. There are a number of sad cases of children being deprived of stimulation that illustrate this. For example, Isabelle was found in America in the 1930s, hidden away, with no contact with anyone but her mother who could neither hear nor speak. Isabelle was just over 6 years old when she was found, and she could not talk. After care and training she began to vocalise and two years later her speech could not easily be distinguished from the speech of other children of the same age.

Certain groups of children lag behind others in their speech development. Middle-class children have been shown to talk more and produce a greater variety of vowels and consonants than children from working-class backgrounds. Children also seem to have a tendency to develop language in some form or other. This is illustrated by the case of four children, deaf from birth. They developed sign language, including grammar, even though their parents had no knowledge of sign language.

Activity

How important do you think contact with other humans is for the development of language?

Temperament and self-concept

As a community we negotiate the meaning of words, this makes 'self' a difficult term to define. Much of its meaning will derive from personal experiences that are difficult to communicate and agree upon. The term refers to the way we would *like* to describe ourselves, the kind of person we *think* we are.

One way of finding out how people see themselves is to ask 'Who am I?' This question usually produces two main categories of response:
- social roles
- personality traits.

of the spectrum, the elderly suffer almost worse than any other group when they are bereaved.

Obviously, the elderly are not an homogeneous group and as individuals they may come anywhere in the spectrum, but there is some evidence to suggest that as a group they do badly, in particular they are more likely to die. The mortality of elderly widowers is some 40 per cent above that expected for age-matched unmarried men, and deaths from physical diseases such as arteriosclerosis and heart disease are some two-thirds above that expected. The elderly survivor is likely to be seriously at risk from depression and even death. There is increased risk that the bereaved may die within six to twelve months after the death of their partner.

Activity

List the reasons why you think that the morality rate for widowers is so high compared to married men of the same age.

Loss can occur at any age, but we are only now beginning to appreciate the effect of loss in old age. Many people remain remarkably fit into extreme old age and stay strong and mentally agile. However, there are many losses that affect the elderly, including:

- loss of status and defined role, as a result of retirement
- loss of income, as a result of retirement
- loss of health and bodily function, leading to loss of mobility and independence
- loss of sexual function
- loss of company, for example spouse, friends. pets
- loss of independence and home by admission to residential home or hospital
- loss of life.

Changes in employment

Some groups are particularly vulnerable to become unemployed, such as those on low wages. A survey in 1980 of over 2,000 registered unemployed men found that as many as 50 per cent had been receiving the lowest earnings in the national earning distribution. There is clear evidence that there is a high rate of unemployment among young people, older workers, those in poor health and women.

Researchers suggest that the loss of a job is comparable to bereavement. Many unemployed men, for example, experience feelings of hopelessness, self-blame, sadness, lack of energy, loss of self-esteem and self-confidence, insomnia, suicidal thoughts and an increase use of tobacco and alcohol. People react to unemployment in different ways depending on:

- the availability of work in the future
- the individual's feelings about the circumstances surrounding his or her loss of job – for example, does the unemployed person feel the victim of circumstances and not personally responsible?
- the response of wife, husband, children and relatives
- the sense of 'loss of face' or respect in the community
- the financial implications
- the extent of supportive networks in the community.

Many unemployed people experience significantly fewer positive feelings, and more strain, anxiety and depression, becoming employed again very quickly restores well-being.

155

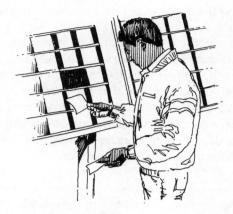

Researchers suggest that loss of job is comparable to bereavement

The effects of unemployment upon health, however, are not at all clear. Some American studies have found little correlation between unemployment and ill-health but British studies indicate that it may be a factor in poor health, finding high levels of stress among the unemployed. Unskilled persons (social class V) and those who have been unemployed for long periods tend to have higher blood pressure and also tend to be fatter than those people in the professional class (social class I – remember social class was defined in Chapter 2). They are also more likely to suffer from arthritis, angina, respiratory problems, alcohol-related disease and mental illness.

Activity

What do you think the effect of job loss could be upon an individual?

Coping with change

Despite the possibility of positive outcomes, change is often resisted by individuals. Resistance to change, or the thought of the implications of change, appears to be a common phenomenon. People seem to be naturally wary of change.

Resistance to change

Resistance to change may take a number of forms:

- **Selective perception** An individual's own perception of stimuli presents a unique picture of the 'real' world and can result in selective perception. This can lead to a biased view of a particular situation, which fits comfortably into the individual's own perception of reality. For example, lecturers may have a view of students as irresponsible and therefore oppose any attempts to involve them in decision-making about their own learning or course organisation.
- **Habit** Individuals tend to respond to situations in an established and accustomed manner. Habits may serve as a means of comfort and security. Proposed changes to habits may be resisted.

- **Inconvenience or loss of freedom** People will resist change if it is perceived as likely to directly or indirectly make life more difficult or reduce their freedom.
- **Security in the past** People tend to find a sense of security in the past. In times of frustration or difficulty, individuals may reflect on the past. They may wish to retain old and comfortable ways.
- **Fear of the unknown** Situations which confront people with the unknown tend to cause anxiety. People may resist a job change because of the uncertainties over changes in responsibilities.

People attempt to adapt to change by adopting what are commonly called **defence mechanisms**, which they are unaware of. People will react to change in individual ways. For example, some will become depressed, while others may see it as a challenge.

Defence mechanisms

It is always important to remember that defence mechanisms are defences against anxiety and are always unconscious, which means that the individual is not aware that they are using such mechanisms. If a person is aware of what they are doing, then it cannot be a defence mechanism.

Defence mechanisms are sometimes seen as protection against the pain of traumatic life experiences. Some of the most common forms of defence mechanisms are:

- **Identification** This occurs when an individual unconsciously copies the dress, behaviour, mannerisms of the person he or she admires or envies.
- **Repression** People may repress from their consciousness any thought of a situation which may cause anxiety. They may, therefore, refuse to come to terms with the change in their lives. For example, you may forget a dental appointment or some other unpleasant appointment.
- **Denial** People often deny that some change in their lifestyle has happened. For example, after bereavement a person may carry on as if the dead person is still around the home.
- **Regression** This involves a return to earlier modes of functioning. The most extreme form may manifest itself in the individual reacting to a traumatic shock by regression to childhood behaviour. For example, a previously toilet-trained child may revert to incontinence on the birth of a new brother or sister.
- **Projection** A person uses this defence mechanism when they attribute their own feelings to another person. This is the most common form of defence mechanism. It may be as 'normal' as blaming someone else for some everyday incident, such as seeing all the problems on a ward or in a residential home as due to the shortcomings of the other shift, or more seriously in the individual who is suffering from paranoid delusions.
- **Introjection** This is the global taking-in of attitudes. The individual will tend to internalise the attitudes of those who may be creating a threat. For example, a child might pretend to be a ghost to cope with his or her fear of ghosts.
- **Reversal or reaction formation** This is the transformation of feelings into their opposite. For example, a person tempted by unacceptable feeling of love may instead hate the object of such love.
- **Sublimation** This is also one of the common forms of defence mechanism. To keep their mind off a situation, a person may throw themselves into their work or take up some sport.

- **Displacement** This is particularly applicable to people in institutions. Emotions stirred up by one situation are displaced and expressed in an inappropriate situation. For example, a senior member of staff shouts at junior staff who, instead of shouting back, shouts at a more junior member of staff.

Activity

Mary, a residential care worker, has just experienced a serious telling off by her senior manager. On returning to the main day room she see a resident spill some tea on the carpet. Mary shouts at the resident who then goes into the garden and tries to take out her frustration on the establishment's cat.

What defence mechanisms have Mary and the resident exhibited?

Stress

One of the most common causes of illness and disease is stress. It is a major part of our everyday lives. Most of us realise that too much stress can be harmful, it can lead to acute or chronic ill-health. The term 'stress' is used in two distinct ways:

- **external stressors** – conditions in the world around us that induce feelings of discomfort, tension and pressure
- **internal stressors** – internally induced reactions.

> ### Stress: A definition
> 'There is a potential for stress when an environmental situation is perceived as presenting a demand that threatens to exceed the person's capabilities and resources for meeting it.'

In the last century, the emphasis of research into the causes of disease was on 'science'. Causes were sought in agents such as germs and pathological processes. As a result, social or psychological explanations for the causes of disease (such as stress) were ignored because they were unscientific.

Freud was the first to argue that certain illnesses could be explained in terms of the individual's response to internal psychological conflict. This anxiety is an emotional state that involves feelings of uneasiness, fear or apprehension. According to Freud, we develop a number of defence mechanisms to counteract this anxiety. These defence mechanisms have already been discussed. Stress-related diseases such as ulcers, skin diseases and asthma began to be seen as the body's expression of unconscious tensions that the individual could not deal with in any other manner. We now know that psychological stress produces vulnerability to a wide range of diseases.

Measuring stress

Estimating stress is one approach to the examination of the impact of key life events and the extent to which stress may contribute to subsequent illness. In 1967, T.H. Holmes and R.H. Rahe published a table of stress factors (see Table 8.1). It attempted to express in quantitative terms the amount of stress involved in a range of specified key life events. Events near the top of the list are highly stressful and often seem to produce adverse effects upon health. Those events near the bottom of the list are only mildly stressful and have less impact upon personal health. A score of 300 points or more accumulated over a 12-month period, is considered high and a strong indication of ill-health. Most people can cope with up to 150 points over a 12-month period.

Table 8.1 Stress scale

Key life events	Points	Key life events	Points
Death of husband or wife	100	Major change of work	39
Divorce	73	Large mortgage taken on	31
Marital separation	65	Starting a new school	26
Jail sentence	63	Leaving school	26
Illness or injury	53	Change in residence	20
Marriage	50	Change in sleeping habits	16
Loss of job	47	Major change in eating pattern	15
Retirement	45	Holiday	13
Pregnancy	40	Christmas	12
Sex problem	39	Minor violation of law	11

Job-related stress

Many jobs are more stressful than others.
The most stressful occupations are:
- advertising
- journalism
- acting
- dentistry
- doctor
- social worker
- pilot
- police
- nursing
- mining
- construction.

The least stressful occupations include:
- banking
- nature conservancy
- nursery nurse
- beauty therapy
- biologist
- linguist.

Student nurses, for example, find certain aspects of their job more strestop of their list is care of the dying, conflict with other nurses, insecurity about competence and fear of failure. Engineers, on the other hand, put wasting time and interpersonal conflict as the top stressors.

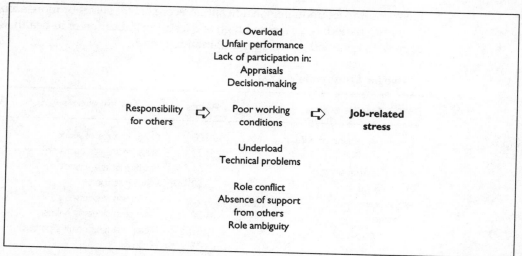

Figure 8.1 Job-related stress

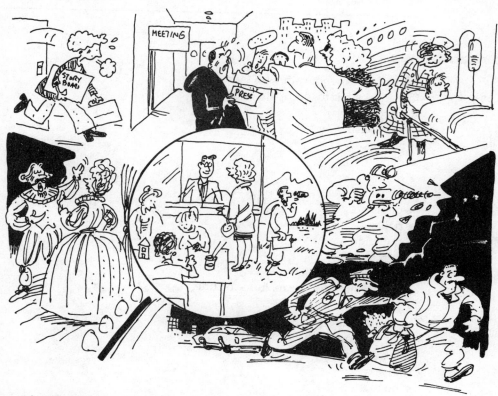

Some jobs are more stressful than others

Reaction to stress

Events have different effects on different people. Certain changes in life, such as divorce, leaving school, change in residence may ultimately reduce stress, as those events may improve the quality of our lives. Why do some people readily succumb to the stress produced by traumatic life events? Why are some people quite resistant to this factor and continue to function effectively in the face of one personal disaster after another? What factors account for these differences in susceptibility? People who believe that they are in control of their lives and those with a sense of purpose and meaningfulness seem not to let themselves be affected by stress factors. Those who perceive change as a challenge or an opportunity for development rather than a threatening burden are also less likely to suffer from stress.

Activity

Taking into account what you now know about the process of socialisation, why do you think that people react differently to stressful situations?

Burnout

Some people who experience stress in their job develop a stress-related condition known as 'burnout'. Over time some individuals are gradually worn down by stress, they become exhausted. Burnout is a syndrome of emotional, physical and mental exhaustion resulting from prolonged exposure to stress. It is not uncommon in health and social care workers. Burnout sufferers may be physically run-down, suffer headaches, feel bored, guilt, confused and may be rigid in their outlook (Figure 8.2).

Recovery from burnout is possible using the steps shown in Table 8.2.

The body's reaction to stress

- Physiologically – the heart rate, blood pressure and respiration all increase and the flow of blood to the skeletal muscles rises sharply.
- Psychologically – we experience feelings such as fear, anxiety and tension as the body seeks to evaluate or appraise the current situation to determine just how dangerous or threatening it really is.

Coping behaviours range from attempting to deal directly with sources of stress through to actions simply designed to make us feel better.

Some people are capable of dealing with intense levels of strain or pressure, while others seem to fall apart at even the slightest sign of stress. When individuals undergo stressful changes in their lives, their personal health does indeed suffer.

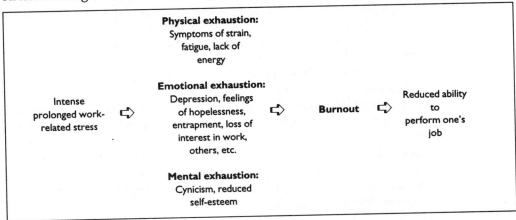

Figure 8.2 Burnout

Table 8.2 Recovery from burnout

Step	Value in countering burnout
Admit there is a problem	Unless individuals are aware that they are suffering from burnout they will fail to take any actions to overcome it.
Reorder priorities	Individuals should recognise that they cannot do everything and scale down their goals accordingly
Establish a network of social support	Friends who appreciate one's work and understand one's problems can be helpful in overcoming negative feelings
Divide life into work and non-working segment	By learning to leave problems at work, individuals can gain the time needed to recover from stress
Cultivate hobbies and outside interests	Such activities can help individuals avoid going stale and prevent them from becoming totally wrapped up in their work

Activity

a List as many situations or activities that cause you, as a student, stress.
b What are the signs that tell you may be under stress? Look at Figures 8.3 and 8.4.
c What factors in a person's lifestyle would lead you to believe that they are capable of dealing with intense levels of stress or pressure?

Stress-related illness

Studies over the last 20 years have found a relationship between life change and subsequent illness. The greater the number and intensity of stressful life events endured by an individual in a given period of time, the greater is their likelihood of developing serious illness.

Some researchers have found that life events relate to disturbance of control of symptoms, in people managing diabetes with insulin, for example. It is thought that hormonal changes, brought on by stress, upset the physiological balance maintained by insulin. Others have found a relationship between life events and a range of physical illnesses, such as duodenal ulcer and urticaria.

Many studies have identified both psychological and physical causes of coronary artery disease, angina, heart attacks and sudden death. About half the deaths as a result of coronary artery disease can be attributed to physical causes such as family history of coronary heart disease, cigarette smoking, high blood pressure, obesity, diabetes mellitus, high blood cholesterol and a sedentary life style. Of the other half, psycho–social factors associated with stress are prominent causes. Some individuals react more strongly to certain circumstances than others – their blood pressure rises more acutely and they also suffer more from coronary heart disease. It seems that there is a link between stressed personalities and heart disease.

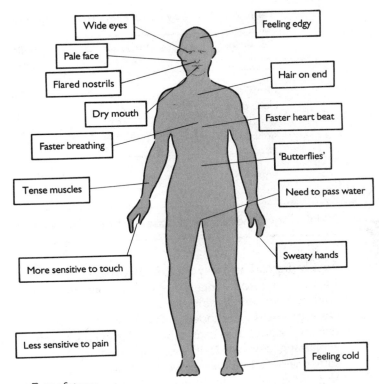

Figure 8.3 Short-term effects of stress

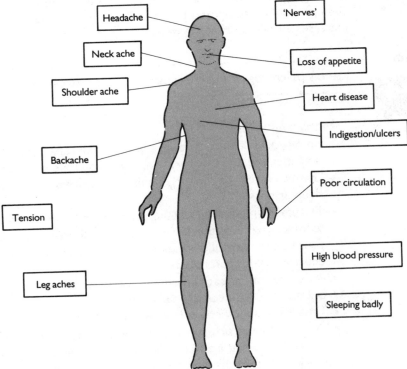

Figure 8.4 Long-term effects of stress

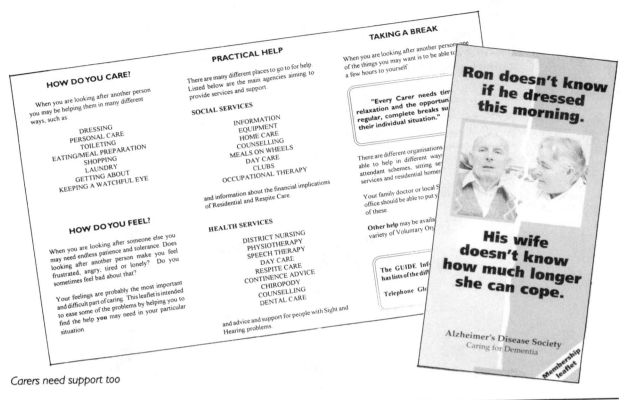

HOW DO YOU CARE?

When you are looking after another person you may be helping them in many different ways, such as:

DRESSING
PERSONAL CARE
TOILETING
EATING/MEAL PREPARATION
SHOPPING
LAUNDRY
GETTING ABOUT
KEEPING A WATCHFUL EYE

HOW DO YOU FEEL?

When you are looking after someone else you may need endless patience and tolerance. Does looking after another person make you feel frustrated, angry, tired or lonely? Do you sometimes feel bad about that?

Your feelings are probably the most important and difficult part of caring. This leaflet is intended to ease some of the problems by helping you to find the help **you** may need in your particular situation.

PRACTICAL HELP

There are many different places to go to for help. Listed below are the main agencies aiming to provide services and support.

SOCIAL SERVICES

INFORMATION
EQUIPMENT
HOME CARE
COUNSELLING
MEALS ON WHEELS
DAY CARE
CLUBS
OCCUPATIONAL THERAPY

and information about the financial implications of Residential and Respite Care.

HEALTH SERVICES

DISTRICT NURSING
PHYSIOTHERAPY
SPEECH THERAPY
DAY CARE
RESPITE CARE
CONTINENCE ADVICE
CHIROPODY
COUNSELLING
DENTAL CARE

and advice and support for people with Sight and Hearing problems.

TAKING A BREAK

When you are looking after another person one of the things you may want is to be able to get a few hours to yourself.

"Every Carer needs tim relaxation and the opportun regular, complete breaks su their individual situation."

There are different organisations able to help in different way attendant schemes, sitting se services and residential homes

Your family doctor or local S office should be able to put y of these.

Other help may be availa variety of Voluntary Or

The GUIDE Inf has lists of the diff

Telephone Gl

Ron doesn't know if he dressed this morning.

His wife doesn't know how much longer she can cope.

Alzheimer's Disease Society
Caring for Dementia

Membership leaflet

Carers need support too

Example

Carers and Alzheimer's disease

Carers of people with Alzheimer's disease, particularly close relatives, often feel a sense of bereavement and loss for the person 'they once knew'. As the disease develops, the sufferer will have increasing difficulty communicating and making him or herself understood. They lose the ability to remember, learn, think and reason. They may forget recent events (things they have only just done) but still remember things that happened years ago — they may even forget who their carer is. The symptoms of this disease can be particularly difficult and distressing for a carer to deal with alone — it can almost be like looking after a child, but a child who was once a 'normal' adult!

Read the case study 'Alice's tale' on page 260, Chapter 12.

Social support groups

One of the most important social support groups is the family. Recent changes in society have highlighted the role of the family. Recent policy has emphasised a diminishing role for the state and an increasing role for self-help and care by the family. Professional services are changing and a greater burden of responsibility for the sick has shifted back to the family from the state. Some families, however, do not have the resources (capital, financial or psychological) to provide support for the long-term sick. Unemployment, poverty, the increase in one-parent families and the necessity for women to work outside the home have rendered many families incapable of looking after their dependent members. Families with young children, the unemployed and the elderly living alone are less likely to the have these resources.

However, the family still plays a major role in the support of its dependent members. It provides for health by means of maintaining a home, provision of housing, proper diet, teaching standards of hygiene and health care, facilitating professional help and also caring for those who fall ill.

Activity

a How does the family provide support for its dependent members?
b What services exist in your area to help families to look after their members?

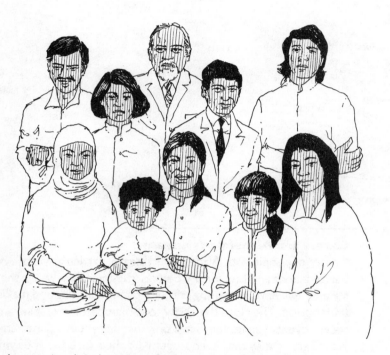

The family still plays a major role in the support of its independent members

There is a body of knowledge that suggests that a lack of social support, such as practical assistance, financial help, information and advice, psychological support, and close social or emotional relationships can increase vulnerability to illness and disease. In one study, those who were classed as socially isolated were two to three times more likely to die than those who were part of an extensive social network. Other studies show that disabled people with few social contacts were more likely to deteriorate in physical functioning than people with high levels of contact with others (Patrick and Scambler 1986). The main contribution of social support would seem to be that of a buffer particularly when people are experiencing adverse life events.

Activity

a Make a list of reasons why the socially isolated are more likely to die than those with an extensive social network.
b Compare and discuss your list with those of your class colleagues.

Access to information and health maintenance services

Who uses the health services? Table 8.8 shows the uneven use of health services by children under seven from different social classes.

Table 8.8 Social class and use of health facilities (percentage of under 7s)

Social class	Visited dentist	Smallpox	Immunised against Polio	Diphtheria
I	16	6	1	
II	20	14	3	3
III	21	21	3	5
IV	27	29	6	8
V	31	33	10	11

Source: Adapted from OPCS, 1978 and *Occupational Mortality Decennial Supplement 1970–2* (HMSO)

The Black Report strongly argues the need to improve the distribution of health service resources in order to match the greatest need with most effective care. It argues that there is unequal access to health services because there is less provision in some localities, such as inner cities, and the ways in which existing services are organised are not always appropriate for the nature of the population they serve. Class differentials in the use of various services derive from the interaction of social and ecological factors. Also the structure of the services is organised in accordance with the values, assumptions of the middle-class patient. Less attention has been paid to the less well-off and less able who are unable to express themselves in acceptable terms and who suffer from lack of command over resources in terms of time and money.

Activity

Visit your local social services department or your GP's surgery. Examine the information, publicity, leaflets, etc. produced by these organisations. Do they invite communication from users? Could they be improved?

People in different social classes seem to behave differently when confronted by a medical problem, because of the different levels of knowledge they may have. Those who understand the nature of illness, the services available and the procedures for using them will get better support than those who lack such knowledge. Middle-class people are more likely to have access to this knowledge than working-class people. On the whole, middle-class people will question and be critical of any shortcomings in services than working-class people. It is suggested that different social classes perceive health services in the same way but the working class are more diffident about expressing their views. Because a particular group of people (a social class or ethnic group) does not make full use of a service as expected, attention is often focused on what's wrong with members of that group, rather than what may be wrong with the service or its delivery.

Activity

Why do you think that middle-class people are more likely to criticise shortcomings in services compared to working-class people?

Just as individuals react differently to available medical facilities, so do the providers of these facilities react differently to differing groups in the community. Middle-class patients are given longer consultations by doctors and more problems are discussed during these consultations. Doctors are most frequently drawn from the middle class so they may find it difficult to empathise with other groups.

Difficulties of access to health care may be compounded for black people by direct or indirect discrimination, and by lack of knowledge and awareness among health care staff of their way of life and economic circumstances. Different ethnic groups are susceptible to different illnesses, for example:

- Cystic fibrosis is more likely to occur in white groups than in other ethnic groups.
- People of Afro–Caribbean origin are more susceptible to high blood pressure than any other ethnic group.
- Babies with dark skin may suffer from jaundice more than white children.
- Children from the Asian culture suffer from a higher incidence of rickets. (Thought at first to be a problem that lay in the Asian culture because of the diet that may Asians follow, recent studies have now shown that the traditional vegetarian diet is not in itself a significant factor.)

Activity

Why is it necessary to have an understanding of the lifestyle of people from different ethnic groups?

Review questions

1 a What is meant by the term 'key life event'?
  b List as many as you can think of and prioritise them in order of their effect upon an individual.
  c What would you do to support a client experiencing such a life event?
2 a What is a defence mechanism?
  b Explain how at least four of them work.
3 How important is the possession of income and capital in a person or family's ability to cope with life changes?
4 Suggest two ways in which diet may influence individual health maintenance.
5 Give three examples of how access to information on health may influence individual health maintenance.
6 Explain how important social support networks are to the individual. Give examples of what might happen to the identity of an individual if these support networks are not available.
7 How can social support networks provided by the family support an individual experiencing bereavement?
8 How can social support networks provided by self-help groups help an individual coping with redundancy?

9 Give an example of how possessing capital assets can affect an individual's ability to cope with loss of job.

10 Suggest two examples of how possessing an income can affect an individual's ability cope with loss of health.

11 Give an example of a psychiatric disorder linked with stressful life events.

12 Which skin disorders may be caused by stress?

13 Suggest a method of protecting or supporting adults in respect to changes in housing.

14 Illustrate a threat to an elderly person's individual identity that can be posed by emotional abuse.

Assignment 8
An investigation into the relationship between social and economic factors to health

This assignment develops knowledge and understanding of the following element:
4.3 Investigate the relationship of social and economic factors to health

It supports development of the following core skills:
Communication 3.1, 3.2

This assignment will allow you to examine the role of economic and social factors in assisting individuals to cope with threats from key life events.

Consider the situations of the following individuals:

- **Individual 1** is a bank official who lives in a large private house in a small village on the outskirts of a large city. He/she has capital assets, health insurance and his/her employers will pay salary for the first year of sickness. No close family live nearby and most friends live in the city.

- **Individual 2** is a gardener for a local authority and lives in a council high-rise flat in the centre of a city. The area has been earmarked for redevelopment for many years. He/she is paid a weekly wage and is entitled to two months' pay when sick, after which they must obtain state entitlements. He/she has lived all their life in this part of the city and has many close members of their extended family living nearby.

Both of these individuals are suffering from heart conditions requiring by-pass surgery for which there is usually a long waiting period. Both are also in the middle of divorce proceedings and may also have to leave their present accommodation.

Your tasks

1 Find out what facilities are available in your health authority for providing heart by-pass surgery and how long the waiting list is.
   This information will be available from managers of appropriate hospitals, but you may also get relevant information from the local Community Health Council.

2 **a** What social support networks are available to help each individual?

    b Investigate how desirable it is to have the support of family members at a time of stress.

3 **a** What facilities might be available from the local authority to support each individual?

    b Find out from your local Social Services department what the charging policies might be in relation to these two cases.

4 **a** Research the local facilities that are available to offer information on health to people in the community.

    b Which services should these two individuals seek information from?

5 Write up your findings in report form and make a recommendation to each of the individuals as to the best course of action, bearing in mind all the data you have gathered.

9 Health and social well-being

What is covered in this chapter

- Investigating health risks
- Smoking and health
- Other forms of drug abuse
- HIV and AIDS
- Acceptability of risk
- Lifestyle risks
- Personal safety

These are the resources you will need for your Health Promotion portfolio:

- health education leaflets on drug and solvent abuse, sexual practices: HIV and STDs, and smoking
- tobacco and alcohol advertisements
- current statistics for drug and solvent abuse, HIV, STDs and smoking
- your individual health promotion plan
- your written answers to each of the activities in Chapter 9
- your written answers to the review questions in Chapter 9
- your report for Assignment 9.

Investigating health risks

You have a right to know as much as possible about the causes of ill-health and social problems, and to know what you as an individual may be able to do to reduce the risks. This basic human right was affirmed by the World Health Organisation in 1978. The provision of information on health, health and safety, and social issues enables individuals both to influence political decision-making on a broad scale and to make personal decisions about their own health and lifestyles. Knowledge is power, and knowledge is the basis of people being able to make informed choices.

The prevention of ill-health, accidents in the workplace and social problems would directly result in less personal intervention by doctors, nurses and social workers. For example, we shall see later in the chapter the role that employees play in creating a safer workplace. Intervention by professionals is comparatively expensive and time-consuming.

The process of promoting health and social well-being is a highly skilled activity, which differs little from activities more commonly referred to as education marketing and public relations. In the past, health and social care organisations have put little effort into promotion. Policies and budgets were targeted more directly to treatment and care rather than to prevention. More recently, however, the arguments in favour of applying marketing and public relations skills to health and social care have become more apparent. This can be seen in the present government's policies relating to Community Care, the purchaser – provider split, and the mixed economy of care discussed in Chapter 11.

Risks to health

Most accidents occur in the home. About 6,000 people a year die on roads in the UK. Many others are injured and die because of accidents at work. We all take risks: we smoke, drive cars, drink alcohol and work in situations which cause ill-health. All these activities present health risks of varying degrees; all have been the subject of media attention; all have been related to health promotional activities. Modern health and social well-being promotion is not just about saying what is good for people, it is also about assessing risk.

Activities

I **a** List as many risks to health and social well-being as you can.

   b From this list select and rank in order of importance the five risks that concern *you* most and the five risks that you feel are most worrying in society in general. Keep these lists as we will refer to them again.

2 Use your personal list to begin to develop an individual action plan for your own health and well-being. Discuss this action plan with your class colleagues.

Continue to develop your action plan as you work through this chapter.

It is likely that your list will have included concerns about specific diseases, accidents, assault, drug abuse, cancers, heart disease and poverty. The precise nature of your five main concerns will vary according to your current circumstances and issues currently being highlighted by the media. They will reflect some of your perceptions of risk. Other people would have different priorities; for example, with many elderly people the fear of assault ranks high because of stories in newspapers and on TV about elderly people being mugged, while people from some parts of the world would have more pressing concerns about obtaining sufficient water and food.

It is clear that promotion of health and social well-being is not an absolute, but is based on the perceived needs of the individual within the wider contexts of the needs of society. We all see risks in different ways. There is a massive industry gathering information to support decision-making; to provide the facts which contribute to the assessment of risk. In this chapter we will help you to identify factors that affect health and social well-being and give you the opportunity to assess risks using as much evidence as possible.

Children at risk: Accidents in the home
As children develop they become more capable of injuring themselves.

Table 9.1 Developmental stages and potential risks

Developmental age and abilities	Risk
3 months: wriggles and waves limbs	Can move sufficiently to fall from raised surfaces Head can be trapped in badly-designed cot
5 months: puts objects in mouth	Choking from small objects, e.g. buttons and pins
8 months: crawling	Falling down steps Cuts from contact with and grasping sharp objects Climbing/falling out of buggies and high chairs
12 months: opens lids	Choking and poisoning from things put in boxes and tins
18 months: imitates, climbs and explores	Climbing onto window sills May be able to open medicines without child resistant containers May be able to undo child restraint in cars
2 years: turns on taps	Risk of scalding from hot water system

The changes are rapid and need to be planned for in order to avoid putting the child at risk. What seemed impossible one day becomes easy the next, as the skills develop and the risks increase.

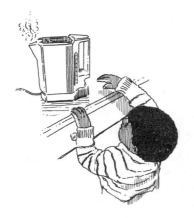
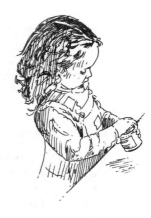

There are many areas of potential risk to young children in the home

Why look at risks?
To talk of risk is to talk of the chance that something will happen. When flipping a coin, probability theory tells us that half the time a coin will land showing tails and half the time it will show heads. To gamble £5 on heads, yet have to pay £10 if it turns up tails entails a high financial risk.

Assessing risk
There is a massive industry based on taking risks related to health – life insurance. The insurance industry makes use of statistics to judge the chance of almost any occurrence and uses this to determine the premium to be paid. Data gathered from millions of individuals is used to predict the potential risks associated with insuring the life of, for example a 30-year-old non-smoking man with those of a 30-year-old woman who smokes.

Activity

The figures in Table 9.2 show, for example, that the premium per £10,000 of insurance for a man wanting insurance for a 25-year term varies from £0.73 to £3.64 according to his age, if he is a non smoker, and £0.96 and £5.73 if he is a smoker.
What would be the figures for a woman wanting a 10-year term?

Table 9.2 Life insurance premiums, monthly contributions (in £s) per £10,000 insurance

		Age next birthday					
	Term	19		30		40	
Women	(yr)	Non-S	Smoker	Non-S	Smoker	Non-S	Smoker
	5	0.28	0.46	0.36	0.46	0.65	0.98
	10	0.28	0.46	0.44	0.56	0.86	1.36
	15	0.34	0.53	0.44	0.67	1.17	1.89
	25	0.55	0.65	0.75	1.09	1.97	3.08
Men							
	5	0.51	0.77	0.66	0.88	1.26	1.82
	10	0.63	0.87	1.32	1.36	2.74	3.92
	20	0.65	0.88	1.50	2.03	3.17	4.76
	25	0.73	0.96	1.57	2.26	3.64	5.73

Source: Figures adapted from Allied Dunbar tables

Government involvement in health statistics gathering

The study of patterns of ill-health, mortality and the causes of disease is not a new science. You may think that the link between tobacco and cancer has only recently been established. In fact, the link between snuff-taking (inhaled powdered tobacco) and cancer of the nasal lining was described in the early 1900s. Another chemically induced cancer known in the nineteenth century was cancer of the scrotum, in child chimney sweeps, caused by the soot. Links between sunlight and skin cancer have also been known since the last century.

When John Snow identified source of a cholera outbreak as the water from a pump in Broad Street, London in 1844, the organism that caused it, Vibrio cholera, was not known. His later work, using data gathered by William Farr about the source of water supplies to houses of cholera victims relative to a sewage outflow, led to the identification of sewage pollution as the source of cholera infections.

It is easy, with hindsight, to say that the link is logical and that pathogens (disease-causing organisms) and drinking water should not be allowed to mix. What in many ways is more important is to recognise that the results were an almost immediate success for the new science of epidemiology.

Gathering statistics

Both Snow and Farr had a powerful friend in Edwin Chadwick the Secretary of the Poor Law Board. In the mid-nineteenth century, he instigated the legislation that required the gathering of statistics relating to birth and death which helped in Snow's analysis. This work still continues and much of the data used today has its origins in statistics gathered by the Office of Population Censuses and Surveys.

Activity

Table 9.3 Live births in the UK
(All figures in thousands with earlier ones representing an annual average from a three-year period)

Year	Total	Male	Female
1900	1,095	558	537
1920	1,018	522	496
1940	723	372	351
1950	803	413	390
1960	946	487	459
1970	880	453	427
1978	687	353	334
1979	735	378	356
1980	754	386	368
1981	731	375	356
1982	719	369	350
1983	721	371	357
1984	730	371	351
1985	751	385	366
1986	755	387	368
1987	776	398	378
1988	788	403	384
1989	777	398	379
1990	799	409	390

Source: OPCS

a Using Table 9.3, plot a graph with the birth rate on the y-axis and the year on the x-axis.
b What trends do you notice?

c Try to predict how many births there will be in the next decade. Remember that the number of births will relate in some way to the birth figures of 25 years previously. Save the graph to help you in a later activity related to life expectancy.

From such data health risks can be analysed and health promotion developed. There is an increasing knowledge and understanding of people from not only sociological but also biological and psychological points of view. Putting all of these together it is possible to assess risk and propose actions taking into account the broader context within which the risk is based.

What are life tables?

These tables provide information about statistical life expectancy, and are produced and used by insurance companies when they determine the risk for life insurance. In this crude form they give no indication of cause of death and so cannot be used to show increased risk factors.

Table 9.4 Life expectancy

Age	Males		Females	
	I	ex	I	ex
0	100,000	72.4	100,000	78.0
10	98,710	63.4	99,086	68.8
20	98,238	53.6	98,786	58.9
30	97,396	44.1	98,442	49.1
40	96,240	34.5	97,723	39.4
50	93,451	25.4	95,858	30.1
60	85,361	17.2	90,828	21.4
65	77,087	13.8	85,705	17.6
70	65,369	10.8	78,242	14.0
75	50,075	8.3	67,536	10.8
80	32,993	6.3	53,154	8.0
85	17,410	4.7	35,317	5.8

Key

I = the number of people out of 100,000 who would survive to the exact age stated if the death rates do not change over their lifetime.

ex = the average future lifetime of a person of the age stated if the death rates do not change over their lifetime.

Source: OPCS. Figures based on the interim life tables for 1987–9 produced by the Government Actuaries Department

Example

- Of every 100,000 men born in the years 1987–9, 96,240 will live to their fortieth birthday at least.
- A woman at birth has an average future lifetime of 76.4 years. However, if she were already 75, she would have an average life expectancy of 10.4 years.

Activity

It is important in planning provision for health and social care to be able to predict the demand for services. In this activity you will have to use the data from the birth tables and the life tables to predict some of the market need for care.

a Using data from Tables 9.3 and 9.4, plot graphs of the number of people born in the years 1978 to 1990 who will live to be 20. (To do this you will need to assume that the life table data in column 1 can be applied throughout the range of years 1978–90.)
   This graph represents the potential number of people entering the work-force.
b What use do you think these data might have in terms of planning care services?
c Using the birth data from Table 9.3 for 1980, 1985 and 1990 together with the life table data in Table 9.4, predict the number of 75, 80 and 85-year-old men and women there will be alive in 2065. (Assume the life table data apply to all of these birth years.)
d If it is assumed that these people will be in need of some level of social care use the figures you have calculated to make predictions about possible demand.

Smoking and health

'If smoking is so bad for people why does the Government not ban it?' – this would seem to be a legitimate question to consider in a discussion of health promotion.

As stated earlier, the links between tobacco and ill-health were known in the nineteenth century. Further links with lung cancer and circulatory disorders have been established this century. There has been more recent evidence that the pollution of the air by tobacco smoke can induce cancers in non-smokers by so-called 'passive smoking'. Whether it is chewed, inhaled or smoked tobacco is a health risk. But should its use be banned? Let's consider some of the issues:

- Do smokers have the right to smoke – after all it's their health they are damaging?
- Do non-smokers have the right to breath smoke-free air?
- Doesn't it have addictive properties and kill people?
- What is the real risk of smoking? Look back at the life insurance data in Table 9.2.

It is possible to find out the mortality figures for cigarette smokers, but an easy exercise is to look at some of the 'junk mail' that is delivered to your home. Insurance companies often send out details of insurance policies and quote premiums for both smokers and non-smokers.

It is interesting to note that life insurance companies do not usually 'load' premiums for those who drink alcohol or who are overweight in relation to height. (On the other hand, car insurance companies will give reductions for non-drinkers.) The figures indicate that insurance companies rate a non-smoker as having a significantly better chance of living for longer than a smoker. Between 13 and 24 per cent of all deaths are smoking-related.

183

reduce the spread but is often seen as an encouragement to drug use and so needle issue and exchange schemes are not seen as priorities and are sometimes positively opposed.

An interesting point when considering health promotion is in a knock-on effect from the message that barrier methods (condoms) should be used during sexual intercourse to prevent the spread of HIV. There was a marked decrease in the reported cases of sexually-transmitted diseases, such as gonorrhoea and syphilis (Table 9.6). This was particularly true with homosexual men although it was noted with all groups.

The campaign had therefore reached people who were likely to be the vectors of the disease in the heterosexual population. People who become infected with a sexually transmitted disease (STD) normally do so through sexual intercourse with an infected partner. The greater the number of partners the greater the risk of infection and of passing it on. The decrease in the reported cases of STDs meant that either people were having fewer partners (unlikely) or that they were using condoms. The more partners a person has the greater the risk that one of them will be infected with HIV so an increased use of condoms in this group would decrease the rate of transmission into the general population.

The limited lifetime for behaviour modification

The downward trend in reported STDs in the mid-1980s has not been maintained and the numbers are now increasing (Table 9.6). The evidence is also indicating that these increases are in relatively few clinics in urban areas. This suggests that groups who modified there behaviour as a result of the threat of HIV infection may now be reverting to previous patterns with associated increased risk.

This is an example of a well-known phenomenon associated with many health education campaigns. The initial response is one in which behaviour is modified and then, either because the campaign ends or because people become de-sensitised to the message, there is a move back towards old behaviours. However, the campaign may have been successful, the disease rates reduced, leading to a belief that risk is also reduced.

In the mid-1970s reports started to appear that some children had reacted to whooping cough vaccine and as a result were brain damaged. Some parents responded by refusing to have their children immunised because they felt the risk of brain damage was too great, however small the risk. Whooping cough is a disease which does not have a steady background level in the population but which has an irregular cycle of epidemics. The reduced number of infants immunised meant that the next 'outbreak' was likely to be of a greater size than previously. There was a drop in vaccination in 1976 which would be reflected in later years in the increase of reported cases. The irregular cycle can be seen with peaks in 1978, 1981 and 1986 which appear to be getting successively lower as the uptake of vaccination increases (Table 9.7).

The reaction of the population can be interpreted as initial fright at the thought of brain damage followed by a realisation of the greater risk of lung damage caused by the disease. The greater evil (brain damage) was risked compared with the more common but lesser risk of lung damage. Other factors that contributed to this increased uptake were a re-examination of the vaccine to ensure its safety and a constant reminder to parents of the risks of whooping cough.

Table 9.7 Whooping cough reported cases and vaccination statistics 1971–89

Year	Per cent vaccinated (of 2 year olds)	Cases reported (x 1,000)
1971	78	
1976	39	
1978	70	5
1979	30	8
1980	20	1
1981	46	18.3
1982	52	62.5
1983	81	8.3
1984	64	5.2
1985	64	20.2
1986	66	34.4
1987		14.3
1988		4.8
1989		11.0

Source: Adapted from government statistics

Acceptability of risk

The acceptability of a risk can be determined by:

- an individual – for example, climbing stairs, for most people, presents an acceptable risk
- legislation – for example, the risk of food poisoning by cross-contamination means that there is legislation requiring uncooked meats and cooked meats to be stored in ways to prevent cross-contamination. The legislation in this case does not apply in non-commercial kitchens. The risk of food poisoning in your own home is seen as something that legislation cannot affect (it would be impossible to monitor) whereas the risk of food poisoning in a public eating place is deemed to be such that there is legislation to try to reduce the risk as greater numbers of people are likely to be at risk of infection.

The difficulty in trying to teach about safety is that there are no absolutes other than in specific areas where safety standards are defined. The skill is to be able to assess the risks in terms of the people involved. To leave a toddler in a room with an open bottle of bleach is unacceptable, whereas if the bottle has a 'child-proof' cap on it then it may be more acceptable. But at what age can you expect a child to be able to open the bottle and make the risk unacceptable once again?

These examples illustrate some of the issues around health promotion related to specific illness where certain actions can help to reduce the risks. They also show how decision-making and actions may have a variety of influences on them and may explain why people don't always do what the 'health professionals' think is best for them. Later on we will look at the environment and illustrate some ways to investigate and evaluate safety risks in different contexts. The Thirteenth Annual Report of the Home Accident Surveillance System highlights the fact that:

'There is no such thing as "absolute safety". To say that something is safe effectively means that the risks are known and deemed to be acceptable for the benefits conferred.'

Life-style risks

There are many risks to well-being that come from the way that we live. They arise from aspects of a person's life that include: work roles or lack of work, the food that a person eats and the physical activity that is undertaken. In short, they relate to the day-to-day habits and philosophies that make up a person's lifestyle.

Diet

It would seem odd to talk of malnutrition in the western world or of people in the UK dying of malnutrition. There are, however, regular reports that say that this is happening. The reports tend not to talk of starvation and deficiency diseases, but of excessive consumption and heart disease.

The composition of a balanced diet has already been discussed in Chapter 6. Here we will look at some of the information that is commonly available and its impact on health and social well-being. As such we will consider two specific issues of malnutrition: excessive eating and dietary lack of specific nutrients.

Is being overweight really bad?

The simple answer to this, if insurance premiums are a guide, is no. Tables of ideal weights with respect to height have been published. These normally show an area representing ideal weight range with other bands for overweight and obese people – the implication being that people should strive to maintain their weight in the 'ideal' band. Insurance companies do not load premiums for people who are outside the ideal weight band unless they are well into the obese band. In other words, there is limited statistical evidence that being mildly overweight is life-threatening.

Research in America and the UK has indicated that there are greater dangers involved in the typical cycles of dieting followed by weight gain than in maintaining a constant 'overweight' figure. There are, however, indications that being overweight can exacerbate some skeletal problems and affect quality of life.

The level of saturated fat (where the fatty acids have no carbon–carbon double bonds) in the diet, especially where energy intake is in excess, contributes to the manufacture of cholesterol in the body. Studies have indicated that the level of cholesterol in the blood stream may be one of the contributory factors in heart disease and the narrowing of the arteries in aterosclerosis (see page 88).

From these simple examples, it can be seen that malnutrition from excessive intake of food can affect health. Health promotion must, however, take into consideration a range of factors and the simple advice to go on a weight-reducing diet may be more dangerous than accepting a steady level of overweight.

What causes overweight?

Where a person takes in more food energy than can be used at that time the excess is stored in the body as a high energy storage material, namely fat, the bulk of which is in the form of triacylglycerol. Eating fats only contributes to these fat reserves if the dietary fat is in excess of the immediate need. The figures are that for every extra 38 kJ of energy taken in then 1 g of fat can be stored.

With some medical exceptions the basic cause of overweight is taking in too much energy in the diet. This is unfortunately all to easy in the UK as high energy foods are relatively cheap and food processing often involves adding high energy fats to lower energy foods. For a simple example, look up in food tables the energy value of potato crisps compared with boiled potatoes.

Dietary lack of specific nutrients

It is difficult to see how a person in the UK could suffer from dietary insufficiencies. We can easily obtain food and health education about diet has been available in schools for many years. However, there is still a level of such malnutrition that falls into three broad areas:

- **malnutrition through social deprivation** where the welfare state has failed in its support of a person who therefore has a general insufficiency. This can also be seen with addicts to alcohol or other drugs who fail to maintain a balanced diet.

- **malnutrition caused by change** A common example is with young girls at puberty who have their iron reserves depleted during menstruation and do not adequately replace them, thus leading to iron-deficiency anaemia. A second example can be where a person has changed to a vegetarian or vegan diet and has not ensured a sufficient balance of protein to supply all of the essential amino acids. This is often compounded by a move to vegetarianism during adolescence when there is a considerable amount of growth occurring.

- **malnutrition by default** It is possible to be eating a balanced diet according to the published tables but still be malnourished. This usually occurs when research has shown that recommended daily intakes of micro-nutrients do not meet the needs for those nutrients. In the UK the RDAs for vitamins were once based on a figure that was twice the amount below which a person developed the deficiency disease. It is now thought that some vitamins, in particular vitamins C and E have important roles as anti-oxidants in preventing some diseases. It may be that the RDAs will be increased in the future. (One eminent biochemist, Linus Pauling did recommend up to 6 g per day of vitamin C compared with the RDA of 50 mg.)

It is thought that the antioxidant vitamins help to mop up free radicals formed in the body. These highly reactive chemicals can cause significant amounts of damage at the biochemical level within cells. Links have been postulated to cancer and atherosclerosis

What constitutes an ideal diet?

The key term to remember is a 'balanced' diet. The diet is balanced to an individual's needs. These needs are met by sufficient of the seven classes of nutrient in proportions to maintain the person.

In reality, most people think of the word diet in relation to weight reduction. In this case the skill is to make an imbalance between the energy intake and that required for metabolism. If the balance shows a deficiency of energy intake than the extra requirements come from reserves of fat. It is not easy to determine the metabolic requirements as they vary from individual to individual.

The requirements are based on a person's:
- size (surface area)
- sex
- age
- amount of thyroid hormone
- state of well-being; fever, drug regime, emotional state.

All of the above contribute to the basal metabolic rate (see page 129). On top of this there are other factors, such as:
- level of exercise
- food intake (it takes energy to digest food)
- the environmental temperature.

The total metabolic rate consists of the sum of the basal metabolic rate and all of the other factors. Guidance on weight reduction must take all these things into account and ensure that reducing energy intake does not remove other specific nutrients that are essential in a balanced diet. A simple diet is to reduce on high fat and carbohydrate items and increase exercise: but it shoudl be done slowly and with advice from a doctor.

Exercise

The knowledge that exercise can help in weight reduction is useful but it also has other beneficial side effects. In particular exercise increases cardiac output, improves muscle tone and improves the efficiency of the respiratory system. There is also a psychological benefit in being physically fit. That does not mean, however, that everyone should take up running marathon races.

In improving the various systems, the effect is to make them work more efficiently. The resting heart rate drops along with the respiratory surfaces becoming more effective for gas exchange. This means that the heart and lungs do not become stressed under exercise and that exercise can be sustained for longer periods.

The more efficient supply of oxygen to muscles means that they can work aerobically and so make a better use of stored glycogen (the carbohydrate energy stores in muscle). Muscles that are poorly supplied with oxygen work anaerobically producing lactic acid as a by-product which causes cramp.

Specific exercise can also have an effect in remodelling bone and joints to cope with the extra stresses. This is used by physiotherapists in their work.

As with diet, any new exercise programme needs to be monitored and, where there may be some risk, checked with an appropriate professional. Most regimes advise starting slowly and building up the exercise over a period of time. A measure of what level of exercise is appropriate can be made by monitoring the pulse before, during and after exercise to ensure that the rate does not rise too much and that it returns to normal reasonably soon after stopping. The success of the regime would be shown with the ability to work at the same level for longer or to work with increased loads (for example, to run at the same speed for longer or run faster over a fixed time period.

Stress

(See also Chapter 8.)

A biological indication of stress is an increased level of the hormone adrenalin in the blood. This hormone is naturally released in preparation for fight or flight. It prepares the body by increasing the heart rate, breathing rate and increasing the production of muscle glycogen. The muscles are made ready for action. There is a heightened awareness as the

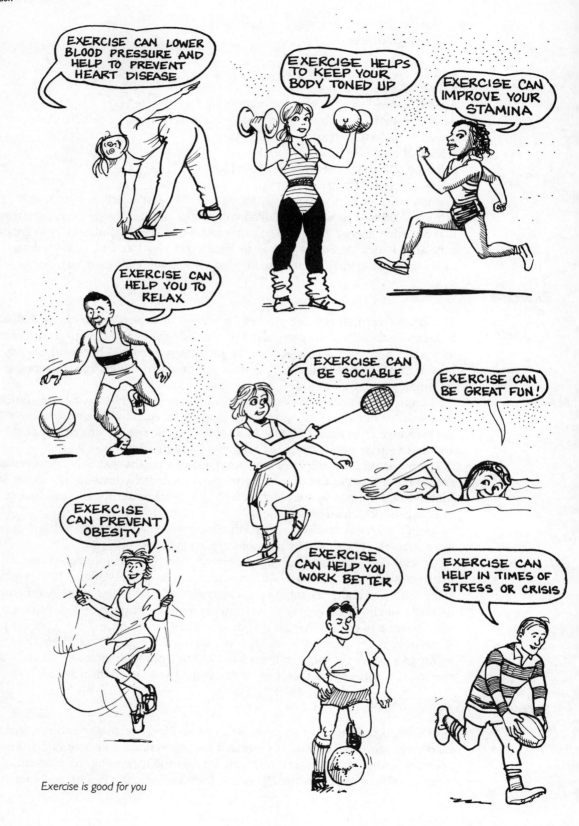

Exercise is good for you

body by increasing the heart rate, breathing rate and increasing the production of muscle glycogen. The muscles are made ready for action. There is a heightened awareness as the senses are made more acute.

These reactions are natural and help in times of major emergency. However many lifestyles now involve a constant background level of stress. There is a constant release of adrenalin at low levels which keeps the muscles in a state of readiness without allowing them to actually make use of the heightened levels. Over time this affects the heart muscles and also the psychological well-being. A second, less well understood effect is the weakening of the immune system. People suffering from stress have decreased resistance to infection and take longer to recover from infections and other traumas.

There are now many people teaching stress-management to employers, employees and the general public. They teach strategies for relaxation and reducing the current physiological stress, as well as techniques to prevent the stress levels developing. In supporting well-being promotion, it becomes important to identify the causes and develop strategies to deal with them.

It must be emphasised that some level of stress can be useful. It would be difficult to imagine an examination without the pre-exam nerves which can help performance. It is the long-term effects of a constant drip feed of adrenalin as a result prolonged stress that is physiologically and psychologically damaging.

Case study

Stress in the health service

In the latter half of the 1980s there was a dispute between two factions in a mental health unit in the Midlands. The dispute was over the setting up of community-based mental health care. One group was very strongly in favour of moving patients away from the hospital environment, whilst the other wished to establish mental health units within general hospitals. The former group was advocating the development of care in the community sometime before the ideas were put forward in the NHS and Community Care Act.

There were two consultants on the anti-community-based care side, and one consultant, a head of psychology and the head of social work on the pro-community side. Acting as a neutral referee was the unit general manager. There then ensued a battle of wills that went on both in and outside meetings. The different factions were constantly pushing forward their own views and trying to 'sabotage' the other position.

As a result of all of this, the participants were under a great deal of stress for over two years. The final decision was to set up a mental health team in the district general hospital and another in the community. Thus neither viewpoint had prevailed and the original mental health unit had been split into two.

The effects on the personnel were more marked. Of the three consultants, one had a heart attack and two had nervous breakdowns. The head of psychology had a heart attack and the head of social work developed myalgic encephalomyelitis (ME). The neutral unit general manager also suffered a cerebro-vascular accident (stroke).

While none of these incidents can be proved to be a direct result of the conflict, all of them have been identified as linked to persistent, high stress levels. It is reasonable to assume that the constant stress of the conflict contributed to the ill-health described.

Activity

How might the participants have attempted to reduce their stress levels, given that their individual views were strongly held and, in their eyes, professionally justified?

Personal safety

It is difficult to talk of personal safety without referring to health and safety legislation. This lays down various requirements of both employers and employees to ensure the safety of themselves and others. In this book, we must assume that you have a reasonable understanding of the dangers of overloading electrical sockets or using equipment with bare or trailing flexes. We must also assume that you know of the risks of drinking poisonous liquids! We will concentrate on the health and safety legislation that is important in your working environment and that, as you will see, provides more general standards for you to maintain.

It is important to understand the definitions of risk and hazard that are used.

> **What is a hazard?**
> The hazard presented by a substance is its potential to cause harm.
>
> **What is a risk?**
> The risk from a substance is the likelihood that it will harm you when you use it. This will depend on:
> * the hazard presented by a substance
> * how you use it
> * how it is controlled
> * who is exposed, to how much and for how long
> * what you are doing
> * how you are doing it.
>
> Poor use or control can create a risk but with proper precautions the risk by even the most hazardous substance can be adequately controlled.

Health and Safety at Work

The protection of workers' health and safety is not just a matter that concerns the workers as individuals: it is not a question of their following rules of good and healthy living. The protection of workers is a social question concerning the conditions in which they work. This is an issue that must be seen within the context of the relations between employers and their employees, and of the legal framework that structures these relationships.

Many aspects of a work situation can actually be bad for you. We have come a long way from the conditions in factories and coal mines of the Industrial Revolution that we find it hard to perceive the hazards that may await the worker in a modern hospital, old people's home or office. Many of the modern hazards cannot be seen – they are invisible risks, such as stress, radiation or inadequate information as to the handling and lifting of clients. Health hazards may often affect workers slowly over many years.

The first attempt by the state to legislate in the cause of health and safety dates from the Health and Morals of Apprentices Act of 1802, which was designed to protect young children working in cotton and woollen mills. It was common practice to put four children in a bed during the day and four more in the same bed at night, while the day time occupants were working. The 1802 Act aimed to eliminate this type of abuse. Since then a number of Acts to protect workers have been enacted, as have various pieces of legislation to protect specific groups of workers such as coal miners, shop workers, railway workers and children. The motives of some of the protagonists were not particularly altruistic, sometimes the legislation was designed to restrict the hours of work of women and young children in order to benefit adult male labour (albeit indirectly).

The original intention of much of this legislation was that the Health and Safety laws would be enforced through the use of criminal sanctions. The emphasis has changed over the years because of a gradual realisation that a rigorous enforcement of this policy would probably lead to the closure of large sections of industry. Individual workers could always bring civil actions in respect of injuries suffered as a result of their employees failure to observe their statutory duty.

Why Health and Safety at Work?

Before 1970 many workers were not protected by any legislation and to remedy this the Labour government established a Royal Commission under Lord Robens to consider the whole field of occupational health and safety legislation and to make recommendations.

This committee reached some fundamental conclusions:

- The legislation in operation did not prevent the 'annual carnage' which took place each year, evidenced by the numbers killed or injured.
- Much of the law was obscure and unintelligible to employers and employees.
- Enforcement authorities overlapped which caused confusion.

The main conclusion of the committee as to why accidents happened was apathy by employers and employees at all levels. The report stated:

'Our present system encourages too much reliance on State Regulation and on personal responsibility and voluntary self generating effort.'

The publication of the Report in 1972 led to the **Health and Safety at Work Act 1974**.

What are healthy and safe systems at work?

Healthy and safe systems cover procedures for the control of infection, the wearing of protective clothing, using correct lifting techniques and training in the use of equipment.

What is a healthy and safe working environment?

- Good standards of hygiene, safe disposal of waste, adequate ventilation when working with hazardous fumes, proper heating and lighting
- Healthy and safe premises with adequate amenities; safe plant, machinery, equipment and appliances, maintained in good order
- Equipment should conform to safety standards and be properly maintained and procedures supplied for those who work equipment
- Safe methods for handling, storing and transporting materials – for example, drugs must be stored and used in such a way as to minimise risk to health. If a new cleaning agent is introduced, an employer is obliged to tell safety representatives and employees of any possible harmful effects
- Adequate instruction and training for employees
- Employers must provide training in safety precautions – for example, in lifting techniques

- Adequate supervision by competent personnel
- Information available to employees to ensure their health and safety at work

Safety policy

Employers must keep employees informed of what they need to ensure their health and safety. They must draw up a safety policy, which should detail what the employer intends to do to protect the health and safety of employees and identify the key managers responsible at various levels. This policy should be prepared in consultation with safety representatives and trade unions. The document should be translated to make it accessible to the work-force if English is not their first language.

What are your responsibilities under the Health and Safety at Work Act?

- You have a duty to take 'reasonable care' to avoid injury to yourself or to others. For example, a care worker whose health was affected by not using the correct lifting procedures, when aware of them and having been taught the correct method, would probably not be successful in claiming any compensation.
- If by your action you cause harm to others at work, you may be liable for prosecution. For example, if you injure client by not using the correct lifting procedure or adaptions. The employee **must** also report any hazards or accidents to their employers.

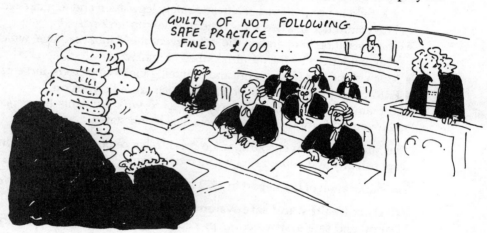

Hazardous substances

The Health and Safety at Work Act clearly covers roles and responsibilities in respect of hazardous substances. However, a second piece of legislation was introduced in 1988 to specify more clearly the responsibilities of employers – the **Control of Substances Hazardous to Health Regulations (COSHH)**.

Some substance used by carers are obviously dangerous – drugs, cleaners, etc. However, many materials used are not obviously hazardous, but they do sometimes unexpectedly exhibit hazardous qualities. At work people can encounter a wide range of substances capable of damaging their health. Many are used in service functions such as cleaning or decorating. The health of many carers can be at risk from hazardous substances they encounter if the right precautions are not taken. Hazards may be biological, chemical or physical.

The COSHH regulation lays down the essential requirements and a sensible step-by-step approach for the control of hazardous substances and for protecting people exposed to them. In particular, empoyers must audit all the materials they use and identify their contents to employees along with details of the safety procedures to be used.

What is a substance hazardous to health?

Substances labelled as dangerous under other statutory requirements are hazardous to health, i.e.those that are:

- very toxic
- toxic
- harmful
- irritant
- corrosive
- any materials, mixture or compound used at work which can harm a person's health.

Case study

Health authority in breach of Health and Safety at Work Act

A health authority which ignored its responsibility to provide proper protection for a worker exposed to a commonplace toxic chemical was found to have been in breach of the Health and Safety at Work Act.

The authority was censured for its failure to supply rubber gloves for staff to use when they were cleaning hospital corridors. One woman who had worked at the hospital for two years part-time had an unpleasant attack of irritant dermatitis, a skin disease. Her duties included cleaning mop heads with a carbolic soap. The attack coincided with the introduction of a new brand. She experienced tingling and itching, and her hand blistered. She had only been given overalls – no gloves, glove liners or barrier cream.

The Health and Safety at Work Act 1974

Checklist of your responsibilities

It is your duty:

- to take care of yourself and anyone else, that means the clients, customers, their families, who may be affected by your working activities
- to co-operate with your employer, helping in any way that you can to carry out their duties under the Act
- not to tamper with or misuse anything provided in the interests of the health and safety of you or others. For example, it would be your duty as a care worker looking after people in their own homes to take care of yourself and anyone else, the clients, their families and friends, who may be affected by your working activities. You would have a responsibility not to tamper with or use and equipment that you may feel is faulty or may cause harm to anyone.

As a care worker you should be prepared:

- by being dressed appropriately for work. Wear any protective clothing you have been given by your employer such as overalls and rubber gloves. Also remember to wear well-fitting, comfortable shoes
- by being always on the look-out for safety hazards
- by reporting any hazards or accidents to your supervisor immediately
- by using only safe methods of working.

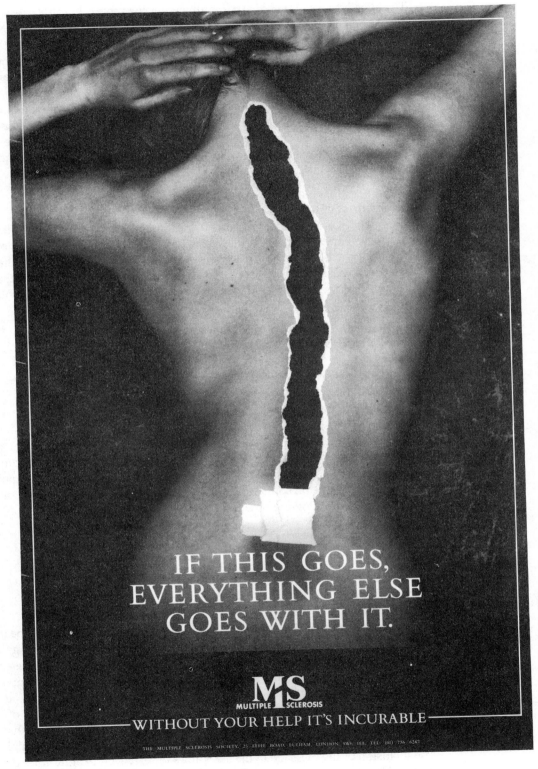

A moral appeal on behalf of multiple sclerosis sufferers

The effectiveness of personal communication channels is highly dependent on how the audience perceives the persons selected to deliver the message. Highly credible sources are the most effective, provided that they are perceived as having expertise, and as being trustworthy and likeable. Such individuals may be perceived as role models. Personal communication channels may be useful in primary prevention, for example, by establishing effective education programmes in schools, but they are particularly effective in secondary prevention, where networks of social workers, nurses and doctors working in the community may be mobilised as communication resources. The use of peers may also be effective. For example, ex-drug addicts have been highly effective in both getting the anti-drug message across, and in working directly with addicts in order to get them off drugs.

Non-personal communication

Non-personal communication uses no personal contact or feedback. It relies on print media (newspapers and magazines), electronic media (radio and television) and display media (billboards, signs and posters). Non-personal communication channels may be directed at a mass audience (large and undifferentiated) or at specialised audiences. It is important that the differences between advertising and publicity (or public relations) be understood.

Advertising and the media Advertising includes:
- print and broadcast advertisements
- mailings
- producing magazines
- videos and films
- brochures and leaflets
- billboards
- symbols and logos.

The advantages of advertising lie in its being a highly public mode of communication. It is pervasive, with the message being repeated many times. It is also dramatic, making the most artful use of print, sound and colour. However, advertising carries on a monologue with the audience, allowing no opportunity for response.

Publicity Publicity includes:
- press releases and information kits
- speeches
- seminars
- annual reports
- public relations.

An important part of the publicity and public relations approach to health and social well-being promotion is to keep the message in the news. Media coverage of events and human-interest stories may be more effective than directly pitching messages, especially when well-known personalities become involved. An example is the campaign to get ME (Myalgic encephalomyelitis) accepted as a genuine illness. Both television and newspapers carried stories about how the illness had changed the lives of sufferers, and the campaign used personalities such as Clare Francis in order to establish credibility.

News stories are not perceived as obvious advertising, and have a higher credibility. The inclusion of the message in the story-lines of television programmes and films is also highly effective. It is far less expensive than advertising campaigns.

Childhood diseases haven't died. Children have.

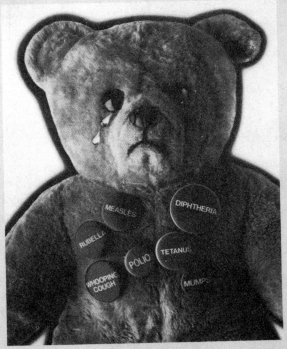

It's sad, but true.

Childhood diseases like Mumps, Measles, Rubella, Diphtheria, Tetanus, Polio and Whooping Cough can all have very serious consequences.

They can lead to blindness, deafness, paralysis, brain damage and even death.

Rubella can be especially serious for a pregnant woman, whose unborn child may be born deaf, blind or even brain damaged.

However, children don't have to be at risk.

Immunisation can protect against all these diseases and help to wipe them out.

So parents who don't immunise their children are taking needless risks.

The time to start your child's Immunisation programme is at the age of two months.

For more information and advice see your doctor or health visitor or just pop down to your local clinic.

They're there to help.

Remember, it's better for you to see your doctor before your child has to.

IMMUNISATION The safest way to protect your child.

Issued by The Health Education Authority and The Department of Health

A magazine advertisement used as part of a campaign for immunisation by the Health Education Authority and the Department of Health

Clare's still in the swim

FORMER round-the-world yachts woman Clare Francis, 42, who has become a best selling adventure novelist, would like to reassure her public that she is still alive and kicking.

Because it has been well documented that she is one of an estimated 100,000 suffering from Myalgic Encephalomyelitis (a viral attack on the nervous system which causes intense tiredness and muscular weakness). Clare fears that people think she has sunk forever into a life of terminal inertia.

'Half the world think I'm at death's door, but I'm out doing things and leading a 95 per cent normal life. It takes a long time, but I'm nearly fully recovered,' says the petite, blonde former Royal ballet School pupil.

Indeed, at the five-storey Kensington home she shares with her 10-year-old son Tom, Clare is working on a fourth novel — which she says has an environmental theme — and celebrating the fact that her last novel, Wolf Winter, has just topped the best-seller list in Australia.

Since a specialist first diagnosed M.E. (her doctor had wrongly thought it was depression), Clare has been helping fellow sufferers through her presidency of the M.E. Action Campaign. David Puttnam has just joined as patron of the group, which has been lobbying to get the illness recognised and for more research into it.

But coping with the viral disease has not helped as far as relationships for the beautiful novelist, who was divorced in 1985 from her French husband Jacques Redon. Clare tells me: 'M.E. is a wrecker of marriages and I thought I was better off on my own. I severed a relationship when I got M.E. — it wasn't fair.'

Source: *The Daily Mail*, 28 February 1989

News stories are not perceived as obvious advertising

Using a promotion mix

Few campaigns of health or social well-being promotion would rely on only one means of communicating a message. Many campaigns would also seek to establish their influence in all three types of prevention. Therefore, a promotional campaign would develop a promotion mix. A strategy for a promotion mix would look like this:

Table 10.1 Health promotion campaign mix

	Primary promotion	Secondary promotion	Tertiary promotion
Target audiences	General public	People who smoke	Victims of smoke-related diseases
Response sought	Don't start smoking	Give up smoking	Co-operate with treatment
Type of appeal	Rational	Emotional/fear	Emotional/rational
Communication	Ads/publicity	Ads/publicity/personal	Personal
Channel/ Choice of media	Print, broadcast, video press, billboards	As Primary plus warnings on packets	Leaflets, information kits, counselling

Attitudes

Before concluding this discussion, some understanding of the concept of attitudes would be helpful. Essentially, health and social well-being promotion is about attitude change. An attitude always has a focus. This focus may be a person, an ethnic group, a nation – almost anything!

Attitudes are a means by which we form impressions in order to generalise in comparing one thing to another. They are characterised from favourable, through neutral to unfavourable. Attitudes are not directly visible. They may only be inferred from interpersonal behaviour. Therefore, it is important that those engaged in health and social well-being promotion have some expertise in measuring attitudes before and after the promotional effort, in order to determine the degree of attitude change. This is easier said than done, as attitudes are difficult to assess. The right questions must be asked in the right way. In addition, people may be less than truthful when their attitudes are being assessed. For example, Sarason (1977) reports that professional people like doctors and lawyers are less than truthful when being questioned about job-satisfaction.

Social psychologists believe that attitudes and values change because of the introduction of inconsistency. The human mind has a strong need to remain consistent in its beliefs. This consistency is necessary in order to form a sensible view of the world around us. When ideas are presented which are inconsistent with present beliefs, there will be some adjustment. It is the responsibility of the health and social well-being promoters to carefully introduce the inconsistency, and to manage the message so that the adjustment is in the desired direction. For example, smokers damage their health. This is inconsistent with survival. The desired direction for the smoker is to give up smoking, in order to survive.

Although attitudes tend toward stability, they in fact change all of the time. Therefore, attempts at attitude change need to be sustained. Among the most effective ways to sustain attitudes changed in the desired direction, is the association of the message with credible, respected personalities, and the identification of the message with a positive perception that individuals hold of themselves or aspire to.

Politics of health and social well-being promotion

Health and social well-being promotional messages are not themselves value-free. They represent the beliefs of the people who promote the message, and these beliefs may not be universally shared. Messages may prove to be contentious, and provoke alternative messages to enter the marketplace. Some of these alternative messages may be financed by powerful lobbies and/or commercial organisations, such as sugar manufacturers, breweries or tobacco companies. The anti-smoking campaign of ASH has been countered by organisations who believe that the right to smoke is an individual choice, and that our civil liberties are being threatened by the anti-smoking lobby. In addition, the targeting and presentation of certain messages may be coloured by prevailing politics. For example, messages , which might best be targeted at particular groups, may not be due to sensitivities surrounding issues of equality. The AIDS awareness campaign had to be careful about targeting the homosexual community, so as not to portray homosexuals as being any more vulnerable to the disease than anyone else.

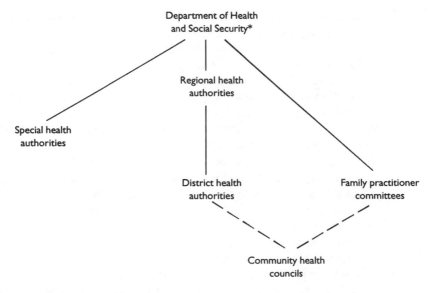

*The DHSS became the Department of Health in 1988

Figure 11.3 The structure of the NHS, 1982-90

It is these units (hospital or community-based) that have more recently become self-governing trusts (see page 224).

Activity

a What different units cover your health area?
b What services does each offer?

The move towards a mixed economy for care

The Griffiths Report (1983) highlighted weaknesses in the general management of the NHS and a major concern was that the process of devolving responsibility to the units was far too slow. Accordingly the report recommended that general managers should be appointed at all levels in the NHS to provide leadership, introduce a continual search for change and cost improvement, motivate staff and develop a dynamic management approach.

There was also a recommendation that management be streamlined at the centre with the establishment of a Health Services Supervisory Board and an NHS Management Board within the then Department of Health and Social Security (DHSS), with the chairperson of the Management Board being drawn from outside the NHS and civil service.

Further change was instigated with the government white paper 'Working for change' in 1989 which proposed the creation of competition between hospitals and other service providers:

• It introduced the concept of a distinction between **purchasers** and **providers** of health care. District health authorities (DHAs) would have the responsibility for purchasing

223

services for patients, using funds based on the population (taking into account factors such as age, sex, etc.). Hospitals would then have to contract to provide services. The aim was to make the providers more responsive and more efficient as money would follow patients. DHAs could purchase services from public, private and voluntary providers. An example might be for a DHA to purchase one hundred tonsillectomy operations from a local hospital. The money for these would be paid to the hospital, be it NHS or in the private sector.

- Hospitals (and any other units) would be able to opt out of health authority control and become **self-governing NHS trusts**.
- Family practitioner committees (FPCs) were to become **family health service authorities** (FHSAs) which would be accountable to the regional health authorities rather than directly to the Ministry of Health. An FSHA would have a general manager together with four health professionals, five non-executives and a chairperson.
- At the same time as trusts were able to move towards direct control of their own affairs, there was also a move to take some of the purchaser roles from the DHAs. GP practices with a large number of patients were to be able to receive funding directly from the regional health authorities to purchase a defined range of services for their patients (known as **fund-holder GP practices**). These services include outpatient services, diagnostic tests and in-patient and day-care treatments for which it was possible to choose the time and place of treatments. Part of the funding also formed a budget for prescriptions.

National Health Service and Community Care Act 1990

There had been an earlier white paper in 1988 called 'Caring for people', that had proposed that local authorities be given the lead in planning community care. They would be required to prepare community care plans with the DHAs/trusts. Thus, areas of personal social services were becoming linked more strongly to health issues. The NHS and Community Care Bill 1989 received Royal Assent in 1990. As with most legislation relating to care, there was a phased introduction with one of the earliest effects being the formation of 56 hospital trusts in April 1991, with a further 95 hospital and service trusts in 1992. Also in April 1991 300 fund-holding GP practices were established.

The local authority responsibilities were phased in more slowly with planning for 'community care' being required in 1992 and responsibility being taken from April 1993.

> ### Summary of the NHS and Community Care Act 1990
> The principal areas covered by the Act are:
> - community care plans
> - assessment and care management
> - purchasing and contracting
> - complaints procedures
> - inspection units
> - specific grant for mental illness.
>
> The implementation targets to be completed by April 1991 were:
> - complaints procedures in place
> - inspection units set up to evaluate public, private and voluntary care provision, to ensure a consistency of approach and to improve quality control

- the specific grants for mental illness and drug and alcohol services to be available – these were to ring-fence money for these areas so that it could not be diverted to other services
- community care plans to be written
- contracting procedures to be in place – bringing in the purchaser–provider relationships
- assessment procedures to be set up
- case management procedures to be in place.

By April 1992, the developments of 1991 were to be continued, with the following additional targets:
- community care plans and planning agreements between local authorities and District Health Authorities and Family Health Service Authorities to be in place.

By April 1993:
- assessment procedures for all clients looking to local authorities for support to be working
- payments and charging mechanisms to be in place
- funds for 'Care in the Community' to be transferred to local authorities
- contracting arrangements to be implemented.

Source and further reading: *Community Care in the Next Decade and Beyond: Policy Guidance* (HMSO 1990)

The structure of the Health Services from April 1991 is shown in Figure 11.4. Similar structures are planned, or are in place, in Wales and Northern Ireland.

Case study

Fund-holder GPs and access to care

Early experience of the implementation of the has meant that several hospitals have completed their contracts before they have completed the financial year. Newspapers have highlighted the fact that in some hospitals routine surgery was only available to patients of fund-holding GPs.

What has happened is that the hospitals have contracted with the district health authority to carry out a certain number of the routine surgical operations. Once that number has been achieved, there is no more funding available to carry out more.

This means that people still requiring such operations will have to wait until the next financial year. It may well be a problem at the district level where the original number was determined. It may also be that the hospital had charged more than others and so was allocated fewer operations.

The situation is complicated by the fact that the hospital can still accept contracts to fill the empty places but the only funds available are from fund-holding GPs. These doctors contract with hospitals to carry out routine procedures for their patients and have some control over with whom and when the contract will be carried out. This explains the newspaper headlines highlighting queue jumping by the patients of fund-holding GPs.

Activity

In your own area, establish who delivers health care. Identify where they fit within the structure of the NHS and whether they are part of a trust.

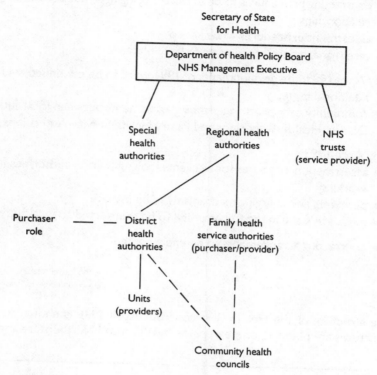

Figure 11.4

Personal social services

The origins of personal social services are in many ways more diverse than the National Health Service. The legislative origins are in the . This was based on the idea that people were poor largely through their own fault, and that to provide care would only encourage idleness. The law stated that those able to work would not receive financial assistance in their own homes. They would have to leave home, with their families and enter a workhouse. There the families would be split up and work provided at wages lower than the lowest agricultural work. The Poor Law guardians provided basic welfare and so could be described as the first state social workers.

Activity

In groups, consider how the Poor Law met only some basic needs of clients. What rights did it deny clients? How did it disempower them?

The mid-nineteenth century saw the formation of several important charities. In 1861 there were 600 charities with overlapping services in what can be described as social care. The predominant image of the charities was that of rich people distributing money to those less fortunate with the belief that the misfortune was often the person's own making and so charity was reserved for the 'deserving poor'. The origins of the charities were often within religious organisations and most had a very strong moral imperative.

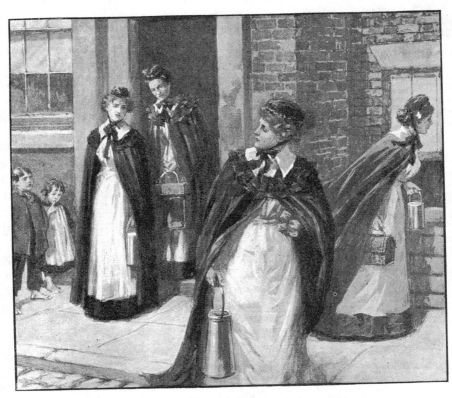

Voluntary lady assistants taking out food to the sick poor, 1899

Several important charities that still play an important part in social care were formed at this time, including Dr Barnado's, the NSPCC and the Church of England Children's Society. All three were founded to support children who clearly were, and still are, a very vulnerable group.

There was a rapid growth in the number of charities in the mid to late nineteenth century, many of which were working in overlapping areas. In 1869 co-ordination of these charities started with the Charity Organisation Society, which established an administrative and academic base in the East End of London. From this, some of the early social work theory in group work and community work was developed.

The development of social work and investigation into the causes of poverty continued into the twentieth century. In particular there was significant work in the late nineteenth and early twentieth centuries by Charles Booth and William Beveridge in London and Seebohm Rowntree in York.

This body of research into poverty began to form the basis for pressure on government to take some responsibility for social reform. The Liberal government of the first decade

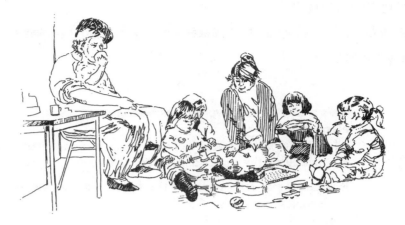

A nursery nurse at work

Review questions

1 The principals of health and social care subsume a number of related functions. Give six examples of the principal functions of health and social care services.

2 Many professional people such as doctors or social workers are perceived as having 'power' in society. Why may such people be perceived as having 'power'.

3 How many avenues of complaint exist for people who are dissatisfied with either the service of a social services department or a health authority? List the organisations they might complain to and the organisation' functions.

4 Explain how National Health Service hospitals are funded and explain how they differ from National Health Service Trust organisations.

5 How do social services structures differ between England, Wales and Northern Ireland?

6 How does the relationship between GP fund-holders and hospitals differ from that of non-fund-holders and hospitals?

7 List as many agencies or organisations as you can think of that are engaged in the provision and development of community health services. Explain the function of two such organisations in detail.

8 Explain the differences between the role of those who provide services and those who purchase services in a social service department under the National Health Service and Community Care Act 1990.

9 a Give two examples of services provided by social service   departments under enabling legislation.

   b Name two services which are mandatory to provide under legislation.

10 Give two examples of the role of health and social care professionals who are employed by:

   a the Health Service

   b a local authority.

Explain what their job is.

Assignment 11
Investigate the structure of a local health or social care provision

This assignment develops knowledge and understanding of the following elements:
6.1 Investigate the structure of health and social care provision
6.2 Investigate the impact of legislation and funding on provision and priorities

It supports development of the following core skills:
Communication 3.1, 3.2, 3.3
Information technology 3.1, 3.2, 3.3

This assignment is designed to allow you to:
- examine a particular social care or health agency and how well it satisfies the needs of local people
- to provide an opportunity to investigate the interlocking roles of workers from the agencies or agency you have decided to investigate.

Your tasks

1 Decide which service or agency you are going to investigate. Read relevant documentation on the role and objectives of the agency. Reference all sources in the text of your report (see 4 below).
2 Decide how your are going to collect the relevant data on such areas as:
   - the legislation that influences the provision of the service
   - how the service is funded
   - how the agency priotises its services
   - key personnel
   - the referral process
   - how users gain access to the service
   - the services that are provided
   - how well the service is used
   - advantages and disadvantages of the service for users.
3 Decide on a system for recording information you will receive from individuals you are intending to interview. Draw up an interview schedule (or several) to make sure you make the most appropriate use of your time and that of the people you interview. (Use a computer for recording information, if you have access to one.)
4 Write a report in an appropriate format covering all the areas mentioned in 2 above.
   - Use appropriate charts, diagrams or graphs to illustrate and highlight the points you make.

- Give your conclusion on how effective and efficient the organisation is, support your conclusions with facts and figures.
- Give realistic recommendations on how the service might improve its efficiency and effectiveness.
- Provide a list of books and other sources you have used, and a bibliography.
- Use a word processor or computer, if you can.

12   Systems of health and social service

What is covered in this chapter

- Access to care
- Funding health and social care
- The role of the voluntary sector
- Constraints on care delivery
  - Preventative care
  - Interventionist care
  - Remedial care
  - Multi-disciplinary care
  - Therapeutic care
  - Holistic care

These are the resources you will need for your Structure and Practices of Health and Social Care portfolio:

- copies of charters, both local and national
- newspaper articles on the funding of health and social care
- your written answers to each of the activities in Chapter 12
- your written answers to the review questions in Chapter 12
- your report for Assignment 12.

Access to care

Having established something of the organisation, structure and staffing of the caring services, it is important to look at how people can make use of the services offered. There are basically three ways that a person can be referred to the care services:

- **self referral** – where people seek help themselves, which may involve support from family members
- **referral through professionals** – in this case a doctor, social worker, nurse, teacher or other professional may assist the person to request care
- **compulsory referral** – where the person in need of care is taken into care by an authorised care worker for their own (or others') protection.

These are dealt with in more detail below.

Self referral

This is often the first route for most people receiving health and social care. Within the health service this may be by simply turning up at the GP's or dentist's surgery. The first point of contact can also be through a health visitor. Within social care, referral may be to an area office, a patch office or direct to a care facility, such as a day care centre or a nursery.

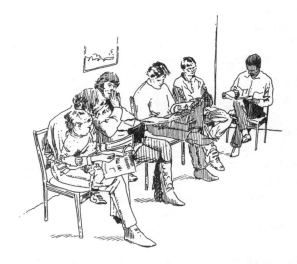

In all cases, the initiative is with the person requiring care or a friend or relative making the initial contact, for example, a spouse of a person who is behaving oddly seeking professional help.

Referral through a professional

Unless admitted to hospital as an accident or emergency case, the only way that a person may voluntarily receive hospital treatment is by referral from another professional, normally a GP. Where a GP diagnoses, or suspects, ill-health that requires specialist treatment, the patient is referred to an out-patient clinic, or admitted direct to a ward if the case is urgent.

In social care, an example of referral by professionals might be when a teacher in a school suspects child abuse and refers the case through to the duty social worker. Under the 1989 Children Act, all schools should have a named person who makes this referral. Another example might be referral through the police who have given a 'warning' to a child who has committed an offence and they feel should be referred to social services.

Activity

Discuss with colleagues the different scenarios that can lead to people seeking care and identify the people who might assist them.

Compulsory referral

Compulsory referral may be made under three Acts of Parliament:
- the National Assistance Act 1948
- the Mental Health Act 1983
- the Children Act 1989.

The National Assistance Act 1948
This Act placed a duty on local authorities to provide residential accommodation for

older people who were unable to look after themselves. It also gave them power to compulsorily admit these people to residential care on the recommendation of a named medical officer. Because this power appears in Part III of the Act the accommodation is known as **Part III accommodation**.

The Mental Health Act 1983

Section 2 of this Act lays down procedures by which a person, unwilling to receive treatment for a mental disorder, may be compulsorily admitted to a suitable hospital for assessment. Application can be made by either the patient's nearest relative or a social worker who has been authorised to act as an approved social worker. The application must be supported by two doctors, one of whom has previous acquaintance with the patient. The detention can last for up to 28 days.

An emergency admission for up to 72 hours can be made on an application supported by only one doctor. Within this 72 hours a second medical opinion can be added and the detention extended to 28 days.

There is provision within the Act for courts to hear objections to compulsory admittance from nearest relatives. There is also the option for courts to refer people convicted of a criminal offence to be admitted and detained in a specified hospital such as Broadmoor Special Hospital. Crown courts can also impose restrictions on discharge.

The Children Act 1989

Clearly the idea of compulsory admission to care is to protect people unable to protect themselves. One of the most vulnerable groups in society is children, and so there has been much legislation relating to children in need of care. This has been brought into some sort of logical order with the 1989 Children Act. In summary, compulsory care and supervision can come about as a result of:

- a **care order** which places the child in the care of the local authority to safeguard and promote the child's welfare. The authority shares parental responsibility and must work with the parents. The order lasts until discharged by the court or when the child reaches the age of 18 years or marries.

    Where the care is in dispute courts are required to make or approve arrangements, taking the child's needs as paramount. To safeguard the needs of the child the court appoints an independent social worker to act as Guardian Ad Litem (GAL). The GAL prepares a report based on local authority records, interviews with carers, parents and other to assist the court in reaching a decision

- a **supervision order**, where the child stays with parents but is supervised by a social worker or probation officer. The parents retain parental responsibility. Orders last for one year and may be extended for up to three years.

- an **emergency protection order** (EPO). Where a child is likely to suffer significant harm a court may grant an EPO which lasts for a maximum of eight days (extendible by a further seven). Care is passed to the local suthority. The child, parent or carer can apply to the court for the order to be discharged after 72 hours.

    The police can also remove a child into protection for a maximum of 72 hours but they must allow reasonable contact with parents/carers in the child's best interests.

- a **child assessment order** which requires a child to attend for medical, psychiatric or other assessment. This remains in force for seven days

- an **education supervision order** is made where a child of compulsory school age is not being properly educated. Supervision is by the education authority and the order lasts for one year.

It must be emphasised that all of these orders are made as a result of placing evidence before a court and the order is made by the court.

Case study

The story of John: A child in need of care

There has often been a view that children are placed in care at birth for the purpose of adoption. There is always a flood of offers to adopt an abandoned baby. The reality of care under the Children Act is very different and many decisions have to be made to enable the children to access care. John's story is typical of many cases and is based on a real case, though modified sufficiently to protect the people involved. The case gives an indication of some of the people and agencies involved in assisting young people to access care.

John was the youngest of six children. His mother had been diagnosed as schizophrenic. Her first husband, and father of four of the children, had died of a heart attack. At the time of John's birth his mother was living with her third husband.

The neighbours had noticed that the children appeared to be well cared for, although they did not always go to school and at times appeared to be left for up to an hour in the care of the oldest child (a 12-year-old). The school had also reported the sporadic attendance to the Education Welfare Officer.

On visiting the home, the Welfare Officer noticed that the mother's drugs were left on the kitchen work-surface and that her level of anxiety and actions gave cause for concern. With the mother's permission, he contacted the family GP who arranged for her admission to a psychiatric hospital.

John's father refused any help and insisted that he could cope with the children. However, after a week a neighbour contacted the NSPCC because he had heard one of the children crying for over an hour during the Saturday evening and when he called round discovered that John's father was working overtime to earn enough money to support his children. He had impressed on the oldest child that nobody should know that he was out or they would all be taken away to children's homes.

The NSPCC social worker called and worked hard to find ways in which the family could stay together and support be provided. This included setting up regular after-school care for the children, along with counselling and guidance. It was during the after school care that the carers noticed disturbed behaviour from three of the younger children. Observing them and listening to them convinced the carer that the children may have been either physically or sexually abused by one or other parent. This was reported to the social worker.

The evidence was significant enough for the social worker to call a case conference and seek an emergency protection order as it was thought that all of the children were in danger. A care order was later sought and granted. After many weeks of work with the family in care, and with both parents, it was decided that in the best interests of the children they should be placed for adoption. This decision had come about as a result of the father's prosecution and conviction for assault and the mother's requirement for long-term permanent mental health care.

At this point the care of the children was transferred to the local authority social services. This was no reflection on the NSPCC, but shows the way in which the various organisations co-operate. Under the Children Act the needs of the children are paramount and one of those needs was thought to be to stay together, but another need was for them to be taken away from institutional care and placed with a family or families.

It was not possible to find one family prepared to adopt all of the children and so the decision was made to split the children. At the same the arrangements for the care had to be agreed with the court. The judge agreed the details and made a recommendation that the children should meet up on at least two occasions a year.

Eventually all of the children were adopted. John, being the youngest, was easiest to place and eventually ended up with his 12-year-old sister who, after a long search for adoptive parents, was placed with John's new family.

Who receives care?

Access to health and social care is not simply about the procedures of achieving treatment or care. There is the very important issue of who receives care and whether access is equal to all groups in society. The introduction of the welfare state hoped to remove the inequalities of access to care. One of the tenets was access to all, free at the point of delivery. If access to care is equal for all who need it then there should be no inequalities and the health of the general population should improve.

The Black Report in 1980, which looked at inequalities in health, highlighted issues of differing mortality and morbidity levels related to social class. It emphasised the significance of broad social, economic and environmental influences on health. It argued that attention needed to be paid to factors such as housing, income support and nutrition if class differences in health were to be reduced. The issues are discussed in more detail in Chapter 8.

These issues were at the heart of the development of the welfare state and the legislation that went before it. The three prongs of health care, social care and welfare benefits were intended to reduce the differences between social classes in terms of access to health and social well-being. The evidence is that in many ways the divide is just as great today as it was in 1946.

Funding health and social care

Health care funding

When the NHS was first formed one of the important aims was to improve the health of the nation. One of the tenets of the provision was that while initial costs would be high there would be a reduction in costs later as health improved and demand for health care decreased.

Activity

a Table 12.1 details the cost of the National Health Service. Use these figures to plot a graph of NHS costs in actual and inflation-adjusted terms.

b Why have the costs in real terms increased? Consider issues such as life expectancy and advances in medical techniques, amongst others.

In 1992–3 the total gross expenditure of the NHS in the UK was 29.3 billion and was funded as follows:

• 80.8 per cent from general taxation

Table 12.1 The cost of the National Health Service

Year	Total (£m)	Total (at 1949 prices £m)	Year	Total (£m)	Total (at 1949 prices £m)
1949	437	437	1969	1,791	875
1950	477	477	1970	2,040	929
1951	503	466	1971	2,325	950
1952	526	499	1972	2,682	997
1953	546	452	1973	3,054	1,054
1954	564	459	1974	3,970	1,171
1955	609	477	1975	5,298	1,229
1956	664	489	1976	6,281	1,271
1957	720	509	1977	6,971	1,258
1958	764	515	1978	7,997	1,288
1959	826	549	1979	9,283	1,324
1960	981	623	1980	11,914	1,434
1962	1,025	628	1981	13,720	1,498
1963	1,092	655	1982	14,483	1,479
1964	1,190	695	1983	16,381	1,584
1965	1,306	728	1984	17,241	1,581
1966	1,433	769	1985	18,412	1,602
1967	1,556	816	1986	19,690	1,670
1968	1,702	861	1987	21,488	1,737
			1988	23,627	1,797

Source: OHE (1989) and C. Hamm, *Health Policy in Britain*, 3rd Edn. (Macmillan, 1992)

- 13.9 per cent from National Insurance contributions
- 3.9 per cent from charges to patients
- 1.4 per cent from capital sales.

The major charges to patients include:

- attending a person involved in a road traffic accident and for their initial out-patient treatment
- accommodation and services for private patients
- non-emergency NHS treatment of overseas visitors
- for drugs and appliances on prescription by a doctor or dentist
- dental treatment.

Initially health services funding was provided to hospitals directly from central government through the structures then in place. The way funds were allocated was not controlled directly by demand. While there were constraints on spending and demands for planning of provision, the provision was controlled by the individual units in consultation with district and regional authorities.

More recently the NHS and Community Care Act has divided the functions of providing funds for health care from the provision of care. The purchaser–provider relationship was introduced with the idea of freeing up the market place and introducing a level of competition. The aim , of course, being to reduce the costs of health care.

The purchasers are able to purchase health care from any provider, whether NHS,

Constraints on care delivery

To explain constraints on care delivery, it is important to identify more clearly the ways in which care can be made available.

Preventative care

Clearly in your early life, from conception, you have made use of the caring services. Even as a foetus care has been given to you. Much of this has been linked to the prevention of your need for future care, for example immunisation in your early life prevents the need for medical care related to the disease for which immunity is achieved. Similarly early health education provides strategies for preventing ill-health in later life. This model targets a large population at low cost in an attempt to prevent a later more expensive need for care.

Interventionist care

There are also times when the carer has to intervene to deliver care. In health this is easily identified in the prescription of drugs to support the body's own defence mechanisms in fighting disease. The extreme in social care would be the compulsory admission to care. The interventionist model empowers an outside agency to become involved when the need for care is evident. As such care is defined where and when it is seen to be needed. This model can induce dependency, relying on care givers to intervene, and take over. It can also impose a level of social control, with the need for intervention being determined by the care providers.

Remedial care

If dependency after intervention is to be avoided, then there is likely to be a need for remedial care. This is a time for enabling the client to work towards a situation requiring the minimum of care. The client's need for care is reduced. An example occurs where the NSPCC works with a family. The initial care may be an interventionist act to deal with the immediate needs. However the NSPCC's aims are to work with the family members and enable them to progress together away from the need for care. This second stage represents the remedial stage for care.

Multi-disciplinary care

Approaches to care delivery can also involve a variety of agencies. This has been legislated for in the NHS and Community Care Act in which there is a requirement for health and social services to work together in assessing the need for care.

Such an approach has the benefit of reducing the risk of people being discharged from one form of care without another agency continuing to monitor and provide care. A multi-disciplinary approach also allows the various professionals involved to deliver to their strengths and reduces overlap in provision.

Therapeutic care

Areas of care that aim to bring about change by looking at activities and lifestyles are often described as therapeutic care. Therapies can range from those commonly employed in the health services (occupational, speech and physiotherapy) to those employed by therapeutic communities based on philosophical or religious standpoints.

The principles behind the latter types of therapy all tend to involve the people participating in the work of the community; developing their skills and confidence from the mutually supportive atmosphere. Many communities have been set up for people who for many reasons are unable to cope with living in modern society, or for whom modern society sees no role. The ultimate aim of most of them is to enable the members to develop their own self-worth and eventually re-enter mainstream society wherever possible.

Examples of therapeutic communities include Rudolph Steiner Homes (for mentally handicapped people), Phoenix House (for drug misusers), the Richmond Fellowship (for mentally ill people) and the Langley House Trust (for people, especially offenders, with behavioural problems). Each community adopts its own strategies for assisting the client group involved and some of the regimes may appear harsh and involve strict discipline, but they all have good evidence of the success of their work.

Holistic care

So far we have focused on care delivery for specific needs. Another approach which builds on the multi-disciplinary is to turn the focus on the total mental and physical state of the client not just the presenting problem. This approach recognises the inter-relationships of body systems, the psychological and social states of a person. This was touched on in the case study of the Starlight Foundation in Chapter 8.

What determines the strategies to be adopted?

Ideally the strategy adopted should be the one that meets a client's needs totally. However, many issues, funding being a major one, mean that the ideal cannot be met. Other constraints include management, organisational and decision-making processes.

Funding

All care has to be paid for and there must be a limit on the money available. All care agencies have to predict expenditure, and do so, rather like insurance agencies predict risk. However, there is never enough money available to provide all the services people would like. In social care this tends to mean that statutory services are provided and decisions are made to provide only some of the 'optional' services defined in enabling legislation. In health care it is often the non-urgent treatment that is delayed. Advances in medical care mean that funding decisions become even more complex. Is it better to provide kidney transplants and save life, or carry out plastic surgery on burns victims and improve quality of life?

Case study

Controlling access to care: Shepherding the resources

There are many demands on resources in the NHS. One of the ways in which these demands can be managed is to consider the value added to a patient's quality of life. This can lead to a purely numerical system for determining the benefit of carrying out an operation.

It would be clear to say that it would not benefit the patient greatly if a kidney transplant were carried out on an 87-year-old man with terminal cancer and an estimated month to live. The improved quality of life and the risk of dying under the anaesthetic would indicate the unreasonableness of carrying out the operation.

More difficult decisions need to be made where the risk of the operation means that life expectancy is not improved although quality of life may be.

There have been cases where access to care has been conditional on the patient changing his or her lifestyle in some way. An orthopaedic surgeon may insist that a patient lose weight before carrying out a hip replacement. The logic for this being that the reduced weight will make the operation easier and will improve its long-term success. It is not an unreasonable request.

Of more concern is the insistence that a person give up smoking before being treated for an unrelated illness. There was a case of a person who was refused access to an investigation for heart by-pass surgery unless he gave up smoking. He subsequently died of a heart attack. In this case the argument was almost the same as the one put forward at the start of this study: the operation had a reduced chance of success; continued smoking would recreate the problem, thus making the original cost a waste of money!

The difficulty with all of these decisions is that it is easy to theorise and make pronouncements about general situations, but the needs of individual patients are real, not theoretical.

In the end, to be efficient, funding has to look at cost benefits. In terms if immunisation it is cheaper in the long run to provide rubella vaccine to all women before they have a chance of getting pregnant than it is to provide care to a damaged child for its lifetime. Similarly, the cost of providing domiciliary support for an Alzheimer's disease sufferer and his or her carer is less than providing full-time residential care. It could be argued that in the latter case the cost is in the carer's loss of quality of life.

Activity

Read the article on page 260.
a What are your views on the issues?
b How might medical decisions be affected by funding issues?

The population changes in the UK over the next half century mean that, as people live longer, the cost of care will increase, whilst the work-force is decreasing. Legislation already recognises this problem as the NHS and Community Care Act requires local authorities to assess need, but does not require them to meet all of the assessed need. Greater demands are now being made on the relatives of people needing care. The cost of caring for these carers has yet to enter the equation.

Old should be spared 'inhumane' treatment, says study

Call to curb surgery on terminally ill

Chris Mihill
Medical Correspondent

SOME old and sick patients are suffering needlessly because operations are carried out without a realistic hope of success, a report published yesterday says.

The report, produced by the royal medical colleges, says of such operations: "Surgery should be avoided for those whose death is inevitable and imminent. A more humane approach to the care of these patients should be considered."

It also blames a shortage of facilities, unsupervised surgery by junior doctors and a lack of research, for causing post-operative deaths.

The inquiry, which looked at 1,400 of the 18,000 adult deaths within 30 days of surgery from April 1991 to March 1992 in England, Wales, Northern Ireland and the Channel Islands, identifies four problems:
● Lack of an operating theatre reserved for emergencies;
● Inadequate intensive care facilities, leaving some operations for old and sick people little chance of success;
● Emergency operations at night on old and sick patients, by unsupervised doctors in training grades;
● Poor standards in the appointment of locum doctors.

Some 7,000 consultants were invited to take part in the investigation, but 24 per cent declined to do so, often because they could not find the case notes or other medical records.

Professor John Blandy, chairman of the inquiry, said: "There are roughly 3 million operations per annum in this country and about 18,000 deaths — a rate of 0.6 per cent — almost entirely restricted to the very old and the very sick."

The death rate has remained unchanged since a previous survey. "The vast majority of operations for the vast majority of patients are safe," Prof Blandy said. "However, this report is an effort by anaesthetists, gynaecologists and surgeons to see if they can't do better."

Prof Blandy said some of the large-scale desperate operations on very sick patients were carried out to reassure relatives that everything possible was being tried, but it some cases it was difficult to understand why they had been done.

He said patients, as well as health districts placing contracts, should ask questions about the surgical facilities available in hospitals.

The report says it "is no longer acceptable" for trainees to work alone without suitable supervision and direction by consultants.

Some patients are being given far too much fluid while they are unconscious and unable to pass urine. This can build up until it damages the heart and lungs, says the report.

Some examples of "hopeless" operations given in the report included that of a 74-year-old woman with a head injury who was operated on although she appeared lifeless. She later died from broncho-pneumonia.

A 68-year-old man with inoperable spread of cancer in the brain was recommended for surgery, and later received a second operation the same day to relieve fluid pressure in the brain. He died soon afterwards.

A senior registrar operating on an 80-year-old woman with a perforated duodenal ulcer also discovered she had womb problems. He carried out a hysterectomy, but the patient died from a heart attack. "There was no justification for this hysterectomy," the report said.

The report of the National Confidential Enquiry into Perioperative Deaths 1991/1992; 34-35 Lincoln's Inn Fields, London WC2A 3PN; £9.00.

Source: *The Guardian*, 8 September 1993

Case study

Care in the community: Alice's tale – the long bereavement

Alice had been a professional with 15 people working under her. She had responsibility for care of several hundred children. She and her husband moved to a large house in the country before they both retired with the aim of following their joint interests in gardening.

About two years after she retired, friends and family began to notice small changes. Alice was constantly talking about her old job as if she were still there. She still remembered the grand-children's birthdays, but the presents didn't reflect the fact that they were growing up. She started to forget what she had said and so often repeated herself. Everybody put it down to the delayed reaction following her retirement from a job she had enjoyed and done well.

Her GP gave her a check up and initiated treatment for high blood pressure. He continued for the next two years to repeat prescriptions and have infrequent check-ups. People close to Alice didn't notice much change other than she was starting to slow down and needed more time to think.

Four years after her retirement, her forgetfulness started to show more clearly. She needed prompting to recognise her daughter, visiting her after a long absence. She called her son by her brother's name. Alice's husband started to become concerned when what he had not noticed as major changes were pointed out to him. The GP arranged for an appointment with geriatrician.

The next six months showed a sharp decline in Alice's health. She became very forgetful and also very angry towards her husband. She became incontinent, especially at night, and so her husband's work load increased with all the extra washing.

Eventually a care plan was agreed, with Alice attending a day centre three days a week and going into residential care one week in four. Also domiciliary support would be provided to help wash and dress Alice on two days a week.

Over the period of time before the next six monthly review Alice deteriorated. It became more difficult to get her into the car and take her to the day centre. She became incontinent during the day, putting an even greater work load on her husband. Also, for financial reasons, it was decided to reduce the residential weeks to one in five. Alice's husband is awaiting the review of her case under the Care in the Community legislation.

Clearly he is coping, and making a limited use of the social services resources. The care plan originally agreed needs urgent review, but because he can cope and Alice's needs are being met there is likely to be little change – possibly more domiciliary support and collection from home by ambulance as she will soon find it impossible to travel by car. It is unlikely that full-time residential care will be available because Alice's needs are being met by care in the community.

Care in the community is working for Alice. But for her husband it is not. He retired with plans for his garden – it is a wilderness. He looks forward to the respite care time to get basic housework done. He is unable to go out as Alice cannot travel far by car and when he goes anywhere with her, it has to be somewhere that can cope with Alice's needs. Like many people in his situation he will be alone for Christmas. His only conversation will be with relatives and friends over the telephone. He could be with family but refuses to allow them to 'ruin' the young grand-children's Christmas by taking them away from home.

Alice has Alzheimer's disease. She cannot talk, feed herself or in any way care for herself. The personality her husband married is no longer there, it has died and only the living body remains. He and his family know the meaning of the other name for the disease – 'the long bereavement'.

Activity

Read the case study above and, referring to Chapters 5, 6, 13 and 14, answer the following questions:

a What are Alice's needs? How are they being met?

outcomes, in recognition of the changing needs and preferences of clients. The principles and process outlined above implies a shift towards a problem-solving approach, which for many workers involves a significant change from traditional practice.

The assessment process itself can be a powerful form of intervention. The assessor may stimulate a dialogue that might not otherwise have taken place. The fact that a worker asks questions about the way in which a client or carer functions may prompt those involved to a new realisation of the extent of the problem or of ways of alleviating it.

Assessment

Principles of assessment

Before examining the process of assessment in detail, it is necessary to consider the basic principles that surround the subject. An assessment carried out by a social worker, nurse or care worker is primarily an assessment of a person, their abilities, expectations and aspirations.

- Any assessment must be with the explicit consent of the client and, if appropriate, carers.
- The client should understand the process and agree to the assessment unless there is a clear statutory mandate for intervention, for example under the Mental Health Act or Children Act.
- Care should be taken to clarify with clients when the partnership is based on consent and when it is based on legal authority.
- Any subsequent intervention should be based on the views of all relevant carers and or family.
- Any services offered should be based on negotiated agreement with all concerned. This includes statutory, voluntary and private sector services
- Clients should have the greatest possible degree of choice in the services they are offered.

Identifying needs

It is most important that the client's own interpretation of his or her problems and needs is identified and considered. However, perceived need may bear little relation to the level of impaired functioning itself. Perception of need can be crucially affected by the attitude and motivation of the client and the degree of support they have from their friends or relatives. Assessment should reflect the following areas of client need:

- physical need
- emotional need
- social need
- psychological need
- cultural need
- identity needs.

There are two models of care assessment that you may encounter:

- Maslow's hierarchy of needs
- activities of daily living.

Maslow's hierarchy of needs

This is a useful starting point, first put forward in 1943. Maslow suggests that human needs are arranged in a series of levels, a hierarchy of importance.

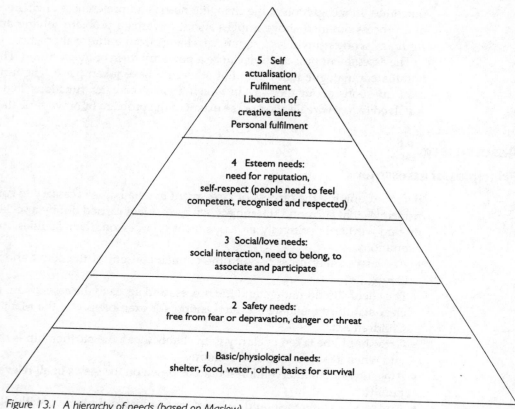

Figure 13.1 A hierarchy of needs (based on Maslow)

The hierarchy ranges through five levels from the lowest level, physiological needs, through safety needs, love needs, esteem needs, to the need for self-actualisation or fulfilment at the highest level (Figure 13.1)

The needs shown at the bottom of the pyramid are the basic, essential requirements for any individual. The more complex needs shown in the middle of the pyramid only come into play when the basic needs have been taken care of. The theory also impliess a thinning out of needs as people progress up the hierarchy. Maslow assumes that for an individual to be functioning at his or her highest potential, all the needs shown should be considered and provided for.

Basic/physiological needs These include homoeostasis (the body's automatic efforts to retain normal functioning, see page 89) such as satisfaction of hunger, thirst, the need for oxygen and to regulate body temperature. It also includes the need for sleep, sensory pleasures, maternal behaviour and sexual desire. If people are denied any of these needs, they may spend periods of time looking for them. For example, if water is not readily available or food then a person's energies will be directed to obtaining a supply.

Activity

Read a selection of daily newspapers and note any situations in which you think that people might spend a lot of time and energy looking for food and water.

Safety needs If physical needs are met, our next concern is usually safety and security, freedom from pain, threat of physical attack, protection from danger or deprivation and the need for predictability and orderliness.

Love/social needs These include affection, sense of belonging, social activities, friendships, and the giving and receiving of love.

Activity

Read the sections in Chapters 1, 7 and 8 on socialisation. Discuss with your class colleagues what it means to not have any or some of your social needs met.

Self-esteem needs These include self-respect and the esteem of others. Self-respect involves the desire for confidence, strength, independence and freedom and achievement. Esteem of others involves reputation, prestige, status, recognition, attention and appreciation.

Activity

a List as many situations as you can in a residential care setting where self-esteem needs might not be recognised. For example, not allowing residents to chose when to retire for the night.

b Discuss how self-esteem needs may be met in a residential establishment.

Self-actualisation/self-fulfilment needs This is the development and realisation of one's full potential. To function at this level then all the needs identified in the model should be considered and provided for.

Activity

List some examples of need under the following headings and discuss with your class colleagues at which of the five levels of Maslow's hierarchy these needs could be met:

a religion needs

b sexuality needs

c nutritional needs

d learning needs.

Maslow's model has been used as a basis for assessing individual need in social care and health settings. The assessment of the individual is the key element in any process. The approach and skills are essentially the same for the assessment of any health or social care need.

Activities of daily living

Using this model the assessor starts with an examination of the everyday activities that people (need to) carry out every day. The list of activities to discuss with the client could be as follows:

- **safe environment** – Are you free from pain? Are you comfortable?
- **body functions** – Are you breathing comfortably? Passing urine and faeces regularly? Maintaining body temperature, etc.
- **nutrition** – healthy diet, ability to eat, adequate and suitable fluids

- **personal cleaning and dressing** – mouth, teeth, eyes, ears, skin, clothing, ability to dress or undress
- **mobility** – Are you able to get out of bed or exercise?
- **sleep** – sleep pattern, Do you wake during the night?
- **leisure and work** – recreation, rehabilitation
- **sexuality** – ability to express feelings, ability to enter into meaningful sexual relationships
- **religion** – cultural needs of client, freedom to worship
- **communication** – ability to communicate verbally, express emotions, using smell. touch , task, hearing, etc.

Activity

Identify a client that you have been supporting in your work placement. Observe their behaviour over a period of time.

a Using Maslow's model, list the needs that you think are been met and those not met. Explain your observations.

b Repeat your observation using the activities of daily living model.

The scope of assessment

Most clients or carers face the prospect of an assessment interview with anxiety. The interview may signify their sense of failure to manage their own affairs. People who have been active and independent may resent their move towards dependence. In such cases it is not unusual for clients or carers to give vent to their anger and frustration on the assessor. The worker must be prepared for such eventualities and to spend time discussing with the client their feelings about asking for help. The ideal place in which to make an assessment of a client is in their own home. Usually the health and social care worker has the advantage of being able to do this, although assessment is also carried out in many other situations such as hospitals, residential establishments, schools, clinics or day centres.

The advantage for the client of being assessed in their own home is that they can operate in a situation in which they are most confident and competent. Their capabilities and limitations in their everyday setting can also be observed at first hand. Their interaction with other members of the family, with carers and friends can be noted.

The expectations and understanding of those around the client also represent important facts to be borne in mind. Need is not usually perceived and defined in the same way by all those involved, the client, carer and various agencies. The assessor must therefore aim for some degree of consensus. However, the client's views must carry the most weight. If it is impossible to reconcile the different perceptions, this should be acknowledged and recorded.

When recording the definition of the client's needs, the assessor must clearly distinguish between facts and the assessor's interpretation of those facts. By asking questions and guiding discussion, the assessor can help the client and carer to appreciate more fully the nature of the problem. The assessor can disentangle complex issues that have led to misunderstandings and inappropriate responses previously. To obtain a full objective picture of the situation a structured discussion is a necessity.

Activity

A GP has referred 6-month-old Mary to the hospital as she has a dislocated shoulder. The GP believes she may have received this injury as a result of physical abuse from her parents. The health visitor states that she feels Mary's mother may be aggressive to the child. Mary's father has left home.

List the factual information and the information that is based on personal opinions (i.e. not based on fact or observed fact) in this case.

What information is necessary?

When gathering the facts or taking a history of the client, it is most important that the assessor explains the reason for the interview so that the client is aware that the information they give will be purposefully utilised in planning their care. In gathering information, the worker is primarily concerned with establishing facts. What is the client's and carer's condition? What prevents them from functioning effectively? What aspects in their everyday life cause them most difficulty? How do they cope with dressing, cooking, cleaning, meals, walking and general household tasks?

To aid assessment, a certain amount of personal information from the client is necessary. However there must be a rationale for asking a particular question, and a individual judgement should decide on the relevance of particular questions in each situation. Simple needs, such as a request for meals-on-wheels will require less investigation than more complex one such as a request for support after discharge from hospital after a serious accident. The assessment process should be kept as simple, speedy and informal as possible. Exploration of areas other than those about which information has been volunteered, should only be undertaken with the consent of the client.

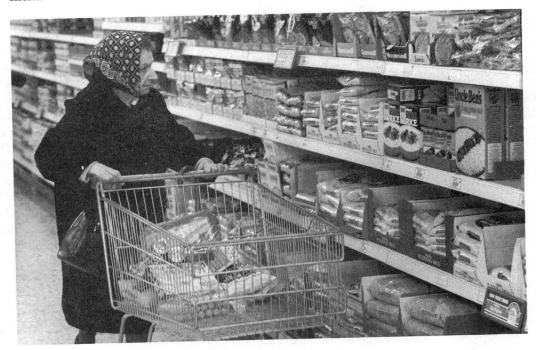

How motivated and able is the client for self care?

The broad areas that should be covered in a comprehensive assessment include:

- **basic biographic details of the client** These include date of birth, gender, marital status, ethnic origin, physical or sensory disability, address, telephone number, household composition, next of kin and GP
- **how motivated and able the client is for self care** This includes basic activities such as eating, dressing, bathing mobility and the ability to carry out tasks such as shopping or cooking
- **abilities, attitudes and lifestyle** Perceived needs derive from aspirations and expectations of life as from any disability itself. A client's ability to cope depends as much on their personal resources and motivation as on the extent of the disability. Two people with similar problems will manage differently and need different levels of support.
- **personal history (if relevant)** Information relevant to personal resources and how clients have coped with similar situations is very useful in determining how the client may handle the present problem
- **race and culture** It is important that the assessor takes account, and has an appreciation, of racial and cultural differences, their differing perspectives and the impact of racism
- **physical health or mental health** It is not usually the task of a social care professional to assess a client's physical or mental health. However, the assessor must be able to decide whether the client may need to be seen by a health specialist
- **contribution of relatives, friends and neighbours** Where a client is supported or is dependent upon relatives or friends, the assessor should be in a position to gauge their contribution to any care package. To achieve this the assessor will need to take account of the status of the carer and their relationship to the client, the care they provide, their physical or mental health, their other commitments, the emotional or physical stress they may be experiencing, their future capacity or willingness to care and their wishes and preferences
- **need for care services, housing, finance, transport**
- **risks arising from any health, behavioural, family, social or environmental hazard** The assessor must remember that social service departments have a duty in law to **protect** as well as **support** individuals. The right to intervene by social care staff is confined to childcare and mental health legislation and the National Assistance Act, where the client may be deemed a danger to themselves or others. However, the assessor must be alert to other risks occasioned either by environmental hazards (gas fires which may be left on by confused elderly people) or behaviour (psychotic episodes). The assessor has to weigh risks to the client against those faced by carers or the wider community in arriving at a balanced judgement
- **other needs such as leisure, employment or education** Under the NHS and Community Care Act all the community needs of the client must be considered. These considerations extend beyond health or housing needs to such areas as education, employment and leisure.

Activity

Mr Jones has been referred to the social services by a neighbour because she thinks that he needs meals-on-wheels. Mr Jones agrees with his neighbour but he doesn't think he needs any other help. When the assessor arrives to see Mr Jones it is obvious that he could also be helped by the support of a home help.

What course of action would you take?

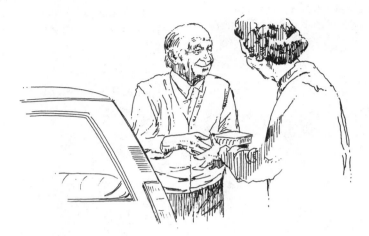

Facts about people are never straightforward, a client may say that they cannot bath themselves, but there may be no physical reason for not doing so. It may be that they are depressed or afraid they might fall when getting into or out of the bath. It is very important therefore to understand the client's perception of their problem, if indeed they see it as a problem. How they feel about a situation is just as much a fact as whether they can or cannot carry out a task. Each fact is a meaningless piece of information until it is compared with others to build up a picture of the client and their needs.

The assessor needs to ask themselves:

• What do these facts mean?
• What is it like to be this client?
• What can the client do for themselves?
• What support can family, friends, neighbours or carers give?
• What aspects of the client's needs or functioning are outside the assessor's competence and who else should be involved in the assessment process?

Ultimately, the assessor is responsible for defining the client's needs. They have to define, as precisely as possible, the cause of the client's difficulty, remembering that the same apparent need may have a number of different causes. For example, a child refusing to go to school may be suffering from fear of bullying, loss of confidence, depression or it may be as a consequence of some breakdown of relationships within the family. The proper identification of the cause of the problem is the basis for selecting the appropriate service to support the client.

Accepting what clients say is the first step. Any probing for underlying problem information only be done with the client's consent. If the client requests a home help this should be accepted on face value as a simple request for that type of support. It may be important to enquire what incident has made it necessary for help to be sought at this point in time. Sometimes the reason is easily understood. The client may have had a fall, or just been discharged from hospital. On the other hand, the service may be required because the carer cannot cope any longer or perhaps a neighbour is anxious about the risks the client has chosen to take.

277

The assessor cannot discard their own personality, prejudices and assumptions. The assessor should try not to do this and should display judgement and integrity by being aware of their own reaction to disability and human needs. However, the assessor is a product of society and will inevitably make judgements based on his or her own life experience unless they receive the appropriate training to help them not to do this.

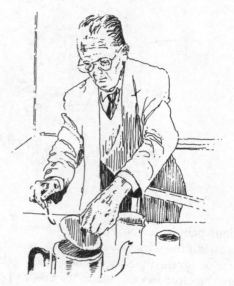

What can the client do for himself?

Types of assessment

There are two main types of assessment:
- self-assessment
- observation.

Self-assessment

Self-assessment reinforces the importance of the client's own views. It actively promotes the participation of the client and carer and their assumption of responsibility within the process. This method also enables professional staff to have an understanding of the client's perspective. One example of self assessment is when a client fills in a form, from which they can see if they are eligible for the service. Some welfare benefits fall into this category. This method of assessment has some disadvantages:
- it favours the more able and articulate
- it allows difficulties to be concealed
- the reliability of the assessment will vary with the self-knowledge of the client.

Observation

Observation methods of assessment tend to be associated with health care rather than the social care field. The findings of observation assessments should be treated with caution as they may not be typical of every situation in which the client may function. Clients behave in different ways in hospital than in their own home. The place where an assessment is conducted may have a material effect on the outcome. As a normal rule,

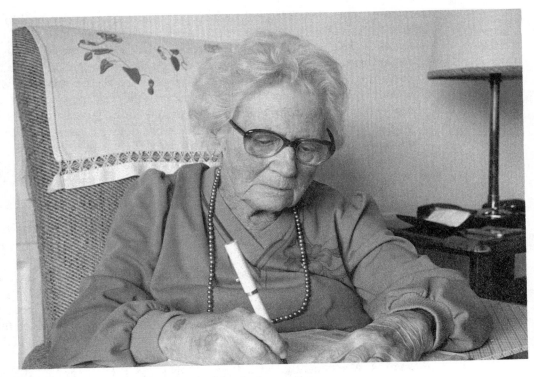

Self-assessment reinforces the importance of the client's own views

assessment is best undertaken in the normal environment of the individual. However, contrast between behaviour in different settings can be illuminating of the client's needs. Care should be taken not to expose the client to any unnecessary disruption.

Individuals do not exist in isolation from their social situation, so it is rarely possible to isolate needs from their social context. One of the tasks of assessment is to define the scope of the social network that it is necessary to explore in order to have an understanding of the client's needs and, as a consequence, where any services are best targeted. Obviously in the interests of time, the assessor has to set a limit on the number of people, places and activities that are deemed to be significant to the assessment of the client's needs.

Activity

a Obtain as many DSS pamphlets as possible and discuss with your class colleagues how many of them call for a claimant to self-assess themselves.

b Arrange an interview with a representative of your local social services department and find out how many referral situations fall into the self-assessment category.

Levels of assessment

A number of 'levels' of assessment have been developed which enable specialist and complex assessments to be targeted to those clients and their families with most need. Specialist assessment staff will usually see all referrals to the social service department in the first instance. Following an initial assessment, where there is a need for a continued service or where specialist help is needed (childcare or mental health), the referral is passed on to staff with experience and qualifications in those fields.

- **Level 1** This is usually the initial contact that a client has with the social services department. At this stage the assessor collects basic information from the client, on the basis of which a decision is made as to whether the client's needs fall within the remit of the department or another agency, such as the health services. At this stage, such requests as bus renewals or car badges (orange car badge scheme for the disabled) can be met immediately. Other requests for more detailed assessment are passed on to specialist staff (childcare, mental health, domiciliary care or occupational therapy, for example).

- **Level 2** This is for the client whose needs cannot be met at the level 1. The outcome of action at this level might be:
  - giving advice or immediate counselling
  - redirecting the client to another agency more appropriate to their needs
  - the collection of information so that a more complex assessment may be made in the client's home, if they wish.

- **Level 3** Assessment at this stage results from the client's need for a more detailed assessment of their health and social care needs which will involve personnel from other agencies. Assessment at this level attempts to change the focus of assessment from assessing for one specific service to building up a profile of the client, their environment and support networks. After consultation with all involved, a care plan is drawn up and resources made available to meet such a plan.

- **Level 4** Assessment is carried out at this stage if it is clear that the client has very complex needs, has been assessed for residential care or is to be rehabilitated from hospital to community.

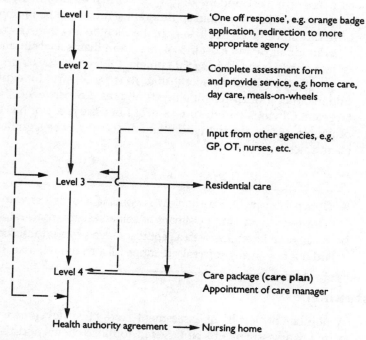

Figure 13.2   The assessment process for a client living in the community

Assessment check-list

- Has the assessment been negotiated with the potential client? Is the client aware that they are been assessed or do they think the discussion is an informal one? Has the assessor explained their role and why they are there?
- Has the appropriate setting for the assessment been chosen – The client's home, day centre, home for elderly persons, school, etc? It is important that both the assessor and client are comfortable and at ease.
- Have the client and carer been empowered to take part in the process, taking into account their ethnic, cultural or communication needs?
- Has the client access to someone who can speak on their behalf if appropriate?
- Have any differing perceptions of need been clarified and, if so, have they been recorded?
- Does the client know if they are eligible for the service they have requested?
- Have the client's needs been prioritised and have objectives been set for each of those needs?
- Has the client seen and agreed the written record of the assessment?
- Does the client know when they may request reassessment?
- Does the client understand the means of complaining if they are dissatisfied?
- Does the client know that they may decline assistance if they wish unless there is statutory intervention?

Case study

George is a very elderly confused gentleman. He has lived alone for many years in a very large house and has managed to cope on his own until his recent bout of flu three months ago. Since his illness he has become more and more confused.

He has no relatives or close friends living near (he has a daughter living 20 miles away) and has difficulty getting out to get his pension every week or to get to the local pub, as he used to three or four times a week. He is now so frail that he can no longer cook his meals or clean the house. Recently, he has developed leg ulcers. George is a very educated man, but because his eyesight is poor he can no longer can read his books.

Review questions

Read the case study above and then answer these questions:

1 At a care planning meeting how could you make sure that George's views are represented.
2 George has asked you to explain what the role of a care manager is in the new assessment process. What is the principal aim of the role of a care manager?
3 Which of the statutory health and social care agencies (since April 1993) has the primary responsibility for co-ordinating the care planning process with George?
4 Explain the process involved in the monitoring of any services which might be offered to George.
5 As George's social worker, it is your responsibility to interview him to assess his individual needs. Which interviewing technique should you use?
6 When you are reviewing the care plan with George and other agencies, you should use secondary and primary sources of information. Give one example, from the case study,

of each source of information.

7   Many people may be involved in formulating a care plan with George. One of these will be the key worker. Explain to George what the role of the key worker will be?

8   From the details in the case study, identify one social need that George may have.

9   There are four principal objectives of a care plan for promoting independence. Give two examples.

10 What broad issues would you want information on in order to be in a position to make a comprehensive assessment with George of his situation?

Assignment 13
Assessment and review of individual needs

This assignment develops knowledge and understanding of the following elements:

7.1 Describe the development of care plans

7.2 Describe methods of assessing client need

7.3 Identify the purpose of monitoring and evaluation approaches within care plans

It supports development of the following core skills:
Communication 3.1, 3.2

In this assignment you are required to assess and review the needs of George, the subject of the case study on page 281.

Your tasks

Planning

In implementing any care plan for George remember that the following principals of assessment should be adhered to:

- Assessment should be with the explicit consent of George.
- George must understand the assessment process. If there is a statutory mandate for intervention this should be explained.
- The client should always understand when the assessment partnership is based on consent or on legal authority.
- Any intervention must be based on the views of all relevant carers and or the family.
- Any services offered to George should be based on negotiated agreement with all agencies.
- George should have the greatest possible degree of choice in the services that are offered.

Assessment

1   Using a copy of the following grid, identify how you would attempt to meet George's needs.

	Need	Possible support
Physical needs		
Social needs		
Cultural needs		
Emotional needs		
Cognitive needs		
Behavioural needs		
Identity needs		

2 Using a copy of the following grid, set objectives for George's care plan that can be monitored and reviewed by all the supporting agencies. Identify:
- the agencies or individuals that George might obtain support from
- the objective of such support
- the likely time-scale of any support offered.

	Support from	Objective	Time scale
Domestic abilities			
Self-care			
Social needs			
Intellectual needs			

- **as an aid to monitoring and evaluation** Monitoring and evaluation are integral to the care planning process. Without adequate records it would be impossible to judge progress and without evaluation it would be impossible to move on to the next stage. An appropriate distribution of resources will depend on adequate information.

The effectiveness of written records will be affected considerably by the structure and efficiency of the notes kept. Information derived from assessment interviews must be recorded on some kind of proforma. These documents should be a help and not a hindrance to the process of understanding the needs of the client or carer. Unnecessary data should not be collected and the assessor must remember that, in the course of recording, the individuality of the client and any needs identified must not be lost. Clients should know how this recorded information is going to be used. The assessor is not free to use it for other purposes and the client is entitled to believe that any information is used only for assessment purposes.

A recording system will reduce the professional's dependence on memory for individual pieces of information. Recording also provides a logical approach to systematically planning care and will also help co-ordinate team effort.

The components of a good record are:

- an initial assessment and data collection record
- generation of a needs list (prioritised)
- an initial plan agreed by all
- progress notes of how the agreed plan is working
- end summary.

When recording and completing a care plan, the assessor must be aware of the difference between subjective data and objective data.

Activity

List of six types of subjective data and six types of objective data which could be used in the assessment recording process.

Implementation of the care plan

The aim of implementing the care plan is to achieve the objectives set by the assessor and the client or carer. Only one person should be responsible for implementing the care plan and this person will be accountable to both the client and agencies involved. If possible the person who drew up the care plan should also implement the objectives. The assessor will have the benefit of having established a relationship with the parties concerned.

The role of the person responsible for implementation can be summarised as follows:

- **Agreeing the scope of the client or carer participation** All recommendations and inputs should be geared to support the client's or carer's contribution to the care plan. A successful care plan is one that enhances rather then undermines any arrangement that may have operated before the assessor's intervention. Clients should play as active a part in meeting the care objectives as their abilities will allow. The client may require a considerable amount of reassurance and persuasion to accept support. If a client is unable to participate or represent themselves, someone should be appointed to speak on their behalf.
- **Agreeing on the speed of the implementation of various objectives** Once the care

plan has been finalised, how it is implemented and the pace of implementation should be negotiated with the client and carers. How this is carried out may be a determining factor in the acceptance of the plan by the client.

- **Checking the availability of services** The assessor's role is to confirm the availability of the agreed services. If any negotiated service becomes unavailable or subject to charging arrangements it should be re-negotiated with the client.
- **Revising the care plan** The care plan should be revised in the light of any changes that have been made during implementation. The reason for any such changes should be recorded. For example, if an agreed service becomes unavailable, the fact should be recorded and brought to the attention of the assessor's senior manager. All parties to the care plan (client, carers and other agencies) should be told of any change in the plan.

Case study

Robert was a 7-year-old boy with learning difficulties. He had been soiling since he was 3, the onset coinciding with his start at nursery school. Prior to this, he had been toilet-trained. He was prone to constipation. He had been seen several times at the local hospital and been admitted for an in-patient stay to clear his bowel. Robert's parents accepted his soiling as a permanent problem.

Robert was being made fun of by his peers at school because of his soiling and constipation. He complained of 'tummy ache'.

Solutions to help Robert:
- Community nurse to help with bowel-training programme. The nurse agreed the following with Robert's mother:
  - Three enemas to be given regularly during fortnightly periods for a three-month span. This was to ensure that Robert's bowel was cleared at frequent intervals.
  - Introduction of more bran into Robert's diet to build up over a period of weeks.
- A behaviour programme. Robert's mother was asked to check his pants on an hourly basis during the day so see if he was clean. When he was clean he was praised and given a cuddle by his mother.

Over a period of time the programme became more successful. The soiling reduced and Robert gained more self-confidence.

Monitoring, evaluation and review

Monitoring the care plan

Monitoring is a proactive form of surveillance which supports the achievement of the objectives set in the care plan. As a result of the monitoring process the objectives may be adapted to the changing needs of the client. How the monitoring is carried out will depend on the scale of intervention.

The purpose of any monitoring should be discussed and explained to the client and any others involved in the delivery of the care plan. Monitoring will be undertaken by a number of individuals:

- the client
- the carer

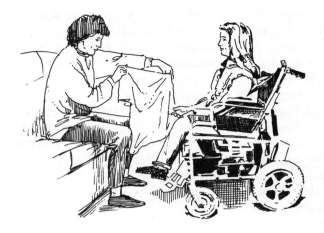

- neighbours, friends relatives
- key worker
- service providers
- quality assurance and inspection units.

Monitoring involves a number of tasks:

- **Monitoring the objectives of the care plan** The aim of this function is to see that the objectives of the care plan are achieved. Each member of the team delivering services is observed to see if they are keeping to the agreed objectives. Progress is measured against the criteria or performance indicators defined and agreed in the care plan.
- **Co-ordination of the inputs to the care plan** The more agencies and individuals involved in the delivery of care, the more important the role of the monitor becomes. Any changes in the pattern of care must be co-ordinated in such a manner that the continuity of care is not interrupted.
- **Ensuring that agencies and individuals are carrying out their inputs according to agreed specifications** Make sure that the care given to the client is of an adequate quality.
- **Fine tune the care plan** The monitor should be alert to any changes in the needs and preferences of the clients or carers. Any new needs should be identified and minor adjustments made to the care plan. Any major changes identified should only be sanctioned by a full review of the case involving client, carer and all agencies involved.
- **Contribution to the review process** Monitoring provides the evidence on which care plans are re-evaluated and which should be recorded in a systematic way. Any review should record progress, or lack of progress, in achieving the agreed objectives. A monitoring programme will also provide evidence of any difficulties that might point to the need for a early review.

Reviewing the care plan

Care plan reviewing is the process by which changing needs are identified and service delivery adapted accordingly. The review process will help determine whether the objectives that were set have been achieved. Reviewing is needs-based, focusing on the need of the client or carer, and not on the services available to meet any identified need. The views and preferences of the client must be the focus of the review which should be held at regular intervals as appropriate.

The scope of the regular review will depend upon a number of factors, the complexity of need and the level and complexity of services delivered.

The review should be held at an appropriate venue suitable to the client. The client's home should be considered if the client so wishes.

Normally the review will be undertaken through a meeting of all concerned parties, but in some cases consultations by telephone or letter may be appropriate. Large-scale review meetings may be intimidating to clients or carers. However, if they are necessary their purpose should be clearly defined. They should be chaired and a full record of the proceedings should be made. Client or carers should be clearly informed that they may be represented or accompanied by a third party. Large-scale reviews should only be contemplated if:

- needs have changed
- new arrangements have to be agreed
- there has been a lack of co-ordination between agencies or individuals involved in the delivery of care.

Purposes of the review

- **Review the achievement of the care plan objectives** The perception of the client should be the starting point for any review. Their view of what progress has been made in achieving the objectives of the care plan is most important. The views of the client or carer can then be measured against the views of the agencies or the individuals delivery the services that were agreed.
- **Examine the reasons for success or failure** The reasons why the objectives have been met or not should be discussed and analysed so that lessons can be learned and objectives reviewed. Was the objective partly achieved? Was the objective understood by all involved, the client and workers? Was the appropriate support offered to allow the objective to be achieved?
- **Evaluate the quality of care provided** The review situation gives an opportunity for the formal evaluation of the quality of services delivered. The reasons for any shortcomings or failure can be discussed and explored.
- **Re-assess current needs** The review also allows the opportunity to consider whether any new needs have arisen since the original assessment. A client's needs will constantly change and the assumption should be that the care plan will change to meet those new needs.
- **Reappraise eligibility for services** The review will give the multi-disciplinary team the opportunity to decide whether the client's eligibility for services has changed. The level of service delivery may need to be adjusted and this should be explained to the client and reasons given.
- **Revise the care plan objectives** The review gives the opportunity to re-evaluate the objectives set at the original assessment. The short- and long-term objectives can be examined and any changes made. The client should be as fully involved in this process as they were in the original assessment
- **Redefine the service delivery requirements** Any changes in the care plan may require the client to agree to a new care plan contract and, if appropriate, new levels of charges.

- **Set date for next review** The dates of the next review should be set taking into account the complexity of the care plan and the client's wishes.
- **Record the findings of the review and circulate to all parties** The findings of the review should be recorded and a copy given to all parties, including the client or carers The focus of the review should not be on the services provided, but on the needs, views and preferences of the client and their carers. The outcome of the review should be an enhanced understanding of the needs of the client and their perceptions of the services provided. This should lead to a re-definition of the objectives of future intervention and an allocation of responsibility for their achievement.

Review questions

1 How would you assess a client's cultural needs?

2 What is the function of the initial assessment process?

3 Why is the monitoring process such an important aspect of the care plan?

4 In drawing up a care plan, how would you ensure the independence of the client?

5 What is the purpose of the review process?

6 Give two examples of how you would assess the cognitive needs of a 5-year-old child.

7 Give an example of how in the assessment process you would display respect andvalue for the client's identity.

8 What is meant by the term 'cultural needs'?

9 How could you monitor freedom from discrimination in the care planning process?

10 How would you ensure that a client's religious needs were met?

Assignment 14
Assessment and review of the needs of a disabled child

This assignment develops knowledge and understanding of the following elements:

7.1 Describe the development of care plans

7.2 Describe methods of assessing client need

7.3 Identify the purpose of monitoring and evaluation approaches within care plans

It supports development of the following core skills:

Communication 3.1, 3.2

Mary is a very physically disabled, wheel-chair bound, 7-year-old girl, living with her father who has moved to this part of the country due to a change of job. Mary's mother lives many miles away. She still loves Mary and wishes to continue to have as say in her future. Mary's present accommodation is a large victorian house in a suburb of a large city with good health and social care support services. The local education authority's policy is to integrate all children with a disability into main stream education.

Table 15.2 The advantages and disadvantages of the survey

Advantages	Disadvantages
When the research is concerned primarily with social characteristics and with information that lends itself to numerical presentation, survey research is the best way to operate Results are valid, a concept that will be discussed later, validity is not a question of 'more' or 'less', something is simply valid or not. Can measure attitudes, values and beliefs Relatively inexpensive	Emphasis on scope rather than depth Interviewers may reveal biases and influence respondents answers. Even trained interviewers are not necessarily going to get over this problem as personality factors intervene, for example 'trust', an intuitive judgement made by interviewee, can be 'taught' to interviewers

Questionnaires

Methods such as observation are adequate for certain survey situations, but if the researcher wants to find out what a person thinks, or what he or she did last week or why they read a certain newspaper, one must ask questions and rely on the answers. The main distinction between the personal interview, discussed below, and the questionnaire is that in the questionnaire the respondent records the answer themselves. The postal questionnaire is regarded as an impersonal survey method, however under certain conditions this might be useful. Questionnaires have to be carefully designed so that the respondent has no difficulty in understanding the questions and in knowing exactly how to record the answers (see Chapter 16).

Table 15.3 The advantages and disadvantages of questionnaires

Advantages	Disadvantages
Cheaper than other methods Generally quicker than other methods Avoid the problems associated with the use of interviewers (interviewer bias, attitudes of interviewer, sex of interviewer, etc.) People tend to be more honest and less embarrassed at answering personal questions (in self-administered questionnaires) People can take their time and consult documents to clarify answers	Non-response (people may not respond) – a response rate of about 30–40 per cent is not uncommon for postal questionnaires Questions must be simple and easily understood with the help of printed instructions Answers have to be accepted as final. No opportunity arises to probe beyond the answer given Mail questionnaires are inappropriate where spontaneous answers are required There is no opportunity to supplement the respondents answer by observational data

Activity

In small groups, each select one of the disadvantages of the postal questionnaire. Discuss why it might be important to be aware of the problems caused by the disadvantages. For example, why might it be important to probe beyond the answers give in some situations?

Interviews

The personal interview is the method most used in social surveys to collect data. It is the most appropriate method in most cases even, though it introduces various sources of error and bias, discussed on page 321.

A personal interview is a face-to-face interpersonal role situation in which the interviewer asks respondents questions designed to obtain answers pertinent to the research they are carrying out. The interviewer may use an interviewing schedule which lists the questions to be asked and makes provision for recording the answers. Interviewing conducted by researchers has the same pattern as that used by curious non-researchers. The major difference is that the answers the researcher receives are usually carefully recorded and reviewed in terms of concepts and theories relating to the research. The interview allows the researcher to probe the intensity of an individual's feelings about a given social phenomenon, their definition of it and how it relates to other area of their life.

The schedule-structured interview The most structured form of personal interview is the schedule-structured or highly structured interview, in which the questions, their wording and their sequence are fixed and are identical for every respondent. The respondents in this situation do not have the opportunity to enlarge on any of their answers. This type of interview is based on three crucial assumptions:

- that the respondents have a sufficiently common vocabulary so that the interviewer and respondent have the same understanding of the words used in the question
- that all the questions are phrased in a form that is equally understood by all the respondents
- that the sequence of the questions must be the same for all the respondents.

The semi-structured interview In the semi-structured interview the respondent will have opportunities to answer outside the structure of the interview schedule. With little or no direction from the interviewer, respondents are encouraged to relate their experiences, to describe whatever events seem significant to them and to reveal their opinions and attitudes as they see fit. The interviewer has therefore a great deal of freedom to probe various areas and to raise specific queries during the course of the interview.

Example

'Do you think that people who kill policemen should be hanged?'

In a semi-structured interview, both those people who answer 'yes' and those who answer 'no' may be asked why they gave that answer. In a structured interview they cannot do this.

Interviews may however consist of structured and non-structured elements. This will usually depend upon the purpose of the study.

Experimental research

The classic experimental design is usually associated with research in the biological and physical sciences. The main difference compared with most other methods is that the research situation is manipulated by the researcher. Classical experiments are usually associated with studies in a laboratory rather than with the study of group behaviour or, say, the attitudes of residents in a hostel or voters before an election. Most classic experiments are based on the principle of an **experimental group** and a **control group**. The groups are as similar as possible in all respects except that the experimental group receives the input of the factor whose effect is to be studied. This factor is referred to as the 'independent variable'.

Examples

1 A study of the effect of a particular drug on a group of individuals would need at least two groups selected for their similarities, i.e. age, sex, weight, illness. One group would be given a placebo, that is, for example, a tablet or pill made of chalk which would not affect the individual in any way, while the other group would be given the drug to be tested, the 'independent variable'. The two groups are observed for any for changes as a result of taking the drug. Differences in the groups could then be attributed to the drug taken, the 'experimental factor'.
2 An ideal test to determine whether smoking causes lung cancer would be an experiment in which one group of people (subjects) were made to smoke, say, 40 cigarettes a day for ten years, and a second group of subjects, matched in all respects to the first, were prohibited from smoking. If the first group subsequently developed cancer, one could conclude with reasonable confidence that smoking (the independent variable) was a direct effect on the incidence of lung cancer (the dependent variable).

Activities

1 How would you design a research test to find out if drinking was a factor in causing accidents?
2 Working in small groups, discuss and list as many situations as you can think of in the health and social care field where research may intrude on the rights of the individual.

It is clear that experimental methods have only limited applications in social research because they are impractical and may involve too great a restriction on human rights. Why then do we need to discuss this type of research? The classic experimental design helps us to understand the logic of all research designs. The experiment is treated as a model against which other designs can be evaluated. It also allows the researcher to draw causal inferences and observe, with little difficulty, whether or not the independent variable caused the changes, i.e. did the smoking cause the cancer?

Table 15.4 The advantages and disadvantages of experimentation

Advantages	Disadvantages
Can usually be repeated again and can contribute to build up a body of data Theoretically the most objective method likely to counteract experimenter bias	In the social science field there is the difficulty of selecting and keeping two similar groups constant

Activity

A researcher comparing the activities of children in two separate playgroups may have difficulty in duplicating the research with the same groups. List as many reasons as you can why this may be so.

Sources of information

Primary sources

Primary sources are usually the first publication of a work, article or paper. Primary sources contain the original data collected in carrying out research such as measurements from laboratory experiments, data from field observation, archive data, information gathered by questionnaires and interviews.

Secondary sources

Secondary sources are generally in the form of indexes and classifications of primary sources, such as text books, subject abstracts and monographs. This type of data varies from the highly quantitative statistics to the more qualitative documents such as autobiographies, log books or diaries. These sources will suffer from the problem that they were collected for purposes other than the researcher's present work and will suffer also from the biases and inaccuracies of the author.

Major sources of secondary data are technical publications, books and journals, official publications, trade association data and computer databases.

However, secondary data has considerable attractions for the research student particularly in the social sciences and especially if they are engaged in short research projects. They are more quickly available than primary sources and they exist in considerable quantities.

Activity

Choose an area of study such as residential care, day care, out-patient departments. Using the resources in your school or college library make a list of primary and secondary sources of information or data for your chosen subject.

Tertiary sources

This category of data includes sources which facilitate the location of primary and secondary sources such as handbooks, bibliographies and encyclopaedias.

Sampling methods

Selecting a sample

At first glance, it sounds a very simple exercise to select a sample. We sample things every day, for example people sample wine or food in a supermarket. In practice , good sampling is a far from easy matter. For example, to be fully comprehensive and accurate a survey should be filled in by everyone to whom it applies. If you wish to find out about

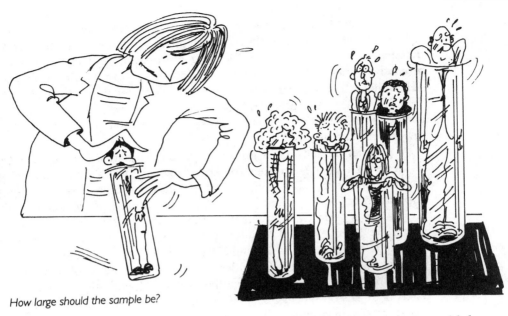

How large should the sample be?

how users of a cinema feel about it, you should ask every user. This would, however, take too long and would be very expensive. You must therefore question a sample of the users.

Activity

Asking your friends in a pub about drinking would be likely to give you a biased set of answers. Discuss with your class colleagues why this would be so?

The size of the sample will depend on what you want to do with the results. If you want to generalise, then you must interview as large a sample as possible. If you only interview six mothers who use a day nursery on a Friday, you cannot state that their views represent those of the users on the other days of the week. If you want to generalise about users of the day nursery, you must interview all users or a sample of those who use it every day.

Activity

a If you wanted to find out how people in your locality feel about their local councillors and it was only possible to interview people in the high street one morning at 11 a.m., which groups of people might be missed out on any day?

b How would you go about getting a fully representative sample?

The size of the sample is important but to believe you have a good sample is not just a matter of knowing how large the sample is. It also depends on how well you have chosen the sample. The principles underlying all sample design are:
• to avoid bias in the selection procedure
• to achieve the maximum precision for the resources available.
The goal of science is to find uniformities or 'patterns' in nature. The scientist obviously

cannot examine all instances of the data they are studying. For example, the botanist cannot look at all plants, or the social scientist all juvenile car theft. A poor sample can be disastrous – it can provide misleading information and result in errors. Even if the researcher cannot observe all of the population, for example all people with an experience of hospital admission, they will wish to be able to generalise to all similar cases from the data they collect. The problem is how can the researcher be sure that the sample studied will be representative or similar to the rest of the people (population) who were admitted to hospital at some time?

A **population** may be a group of people, students, people over 65 years of age, residents of a home, shoppers or home owners. The specific nature of a population depends on the purpose of the investigation or research. The first step is to define the population to be sampled. This task is not as easy as it sounds. No sample of a population is perfectly representative, the smaller the sample, the more unrepresentative it will be. If you wished to interview students in your college or school about their attitude to a particular issue, could you interview every student. Would you chose five from every class or form? If you decided to do this, how would you select them? Would they be representative of the rest of the students? If you wished to interview people who used a meals-on-wheels service, would those who used them on Monday be representative of people who received them at weekends?

If you are going to generalise from your results to the general population then you must chose your sample according to the rules of statistical theory. It may be wrong to select say volunteers, friends or people who happen to be at hand. The idea of sampling is not new and it is economical. It is obviously cheaper to collect information form 100 students than from 1,000. Sampling also saves labour and time.

Random sampling

Random does not mean 'haphazard'. In fact it means the very opposite. It implies a very careful pre-selection plan. A random method of selection is one which gives each of the **units** (people) in the population to be studied a calculable probability of being selected. Each member of the population to be studied has an equal chance of being selected for the sample. How might we draw a random sample? First as already mentioned, you need to define the population which you wish your sample to represent.

Example

If you wish to study students at your particular college, you first need to define what you mean by a student.

- Who is included in the population?
- Do you want to include full-time and part-time students?
- Do you wish to include Youth Training trainees?
- Do you wish to include students over 65 years of age?

When you have clarified the target population, you need to locate or complete a list of all of its members, say every full-time student under 65 years of age. If you do not have such a list then random sampling cannot be used and other methods will be more suitable. Many lists are suspect and do not list all the population. A telephone directory is not an adequate listing of people in a town because it will not include people who cannot afford a telephone or those who wish their telephone number to be unlisted.

Assuming that you have a list of all the members of the population you wish to study, how do you select your sample? There are a number of methods of probability sampling.

Simple random sampling

Simple random sampling is the basic probability sampling design. It gives each of the N (known) sampling units of a population an equal and known probability of being selected. To ensure that this happens one of the following methods may be used:

- **The lottery method** Each member of the population is represented by a disk or a piece of paper with their name or a number corresponding to their name on the list. The pieces of paper or disks are placed in a box, mixed well and a sample of the desired size is drawn. Every member of the population has an equal chance of being selected.
- **Table of random digits** The random number tables were devised to meet the two criteria of random selection:
  - each number has the same chance of being selected
  - each number is independent of the others.

The procedure is simple. Each member of the population is listed and numbered. A number is selected from a table of random digits. Each digit that appears in the table of random digits corresponds to the numbering of a sample unit in the list, that sampling unit is selected for the sample. The process is continued until the desired sample size is reached. Random numbers can also be generated by computer.

Table 15.5 1,000 random digits

	1–4	5–8	9–12	13–16	17–20	21–24	25–28	29–32	33–36	37–40
1	36 45	88 31	28 73	59 43	46 32	00 32	67 15	32 49	54 55	76 17
2	90 51	40 66	18 46	95 54	65 89	16 80	95 33	15 88	18 60	56 46
3	98 41	90 22	48 37	80 31	91 39	33 80	40 82	38 26	20 39	71 82
4	55 25	71 27	14 68	64 04	99 24	82 30	73 43	92 68	18 99	47 54
5	02 99	10 75	77 21	88 55	79 97	70 32	59 87	75 35	18 34	62 53
6	79 85	55 66	63 84	08 63	04 00	18 34	53 94	58 01	55 05	90 99
7	33 53	95 28	06 81	34 95	13 93	37 16	95 06	15 91	89 99	37 16
8	74 75	13 13	22 16	37 76	15 57	42 38	96 23	90 24	58 26	71 46
9	06 66	30 43	00 66	32 60	36 60	46 05	17 31	66 80	91 01	62 35
10	92 83	31 60	87 30	76 83	17 85	31 48	13 23	17 32	68 14	84 96
11	61 21	31 49	98 29	77 70	72 11	35 23	69 47	14 27	14 74	52 35
12	27 82	01 01	74 41	38 77	53 68	53 26	55 16	35 66	31 87	82 09
13	61 05	50 10	94 85	86 32	10 72	95 67	88 21	72 09	48 73	03 97
14	11 57	85 67	94 91	49 48	35 49	39 41	80 17	54 45	23 66	83 60
15	15 16	08 90	92 86	13 32	26 01	20 02	72 45	94 74	97 19	99 46
16	22 09	29 66	15 44	76 74	94 92	48 13	75 85	81 28	95 41	36 30
17	69 13	53 55	35 87	43 23	83 32	79 40	92 20	83 76	82 61	24 20
18	08 29	79 37	00 33	35 34	86 55	10 91	18 86	43 50	67 79	33 58
19	37 29	99 85	55 63	32 66	71 98	85 20	31 93	63 91	77 21	99 62
20	65 11	14 04	88 86	28 92	04 03	42 99	87 08	20 55	30 53	82 24
21	66 22	81 58	30 80	21 10	15 53	26 90	33 77	51 19	17 49	27 14
22	37 21	77 13	69 31	20 22	67 13	46 29	75 32	69 79	37 23	32 43
23	51 43	09 72	68 38	05 77	14 62	89 07	37 89	25 30	92 09	06 92
24	31 59	37 83	92 55	15 31	21 24	03 93	35 97	84 61	96 85	45 51
25	79 05	43 69	52 93	00 77	44 82	91 65	11 71	25 37	89 13	63 87

- **Systematic samples** Using this method, each member of the population under study is given a number, and then a subgroup is taken for study. For example if we wished to study a subgroup of your school or college. every student would be given a number, and then the sub group, say a particular class or students of a particular age or hair colour, would be taken for study. Systematic sampling consists of selecting every Kth (10th, 20th or 30th) sampling unit of the population after the first sampling unit is selected at random from the first K sampling units. So if you wished to select a sample of one hundred students from a population of 1,000 at a college, you take every 10th student ($K = N \div n$, where K is the interval of selection, N is the total population and n is the sample, so $1,000 \div 100 = 10$). The first selection must be chosen by the random process. Suppose the fourth person was selected, the sample would then consist of students numbered 4, 14, 24, 34, 44, 54 and so on.
- **Stratified sampling** This method can only be used when there is detailed knowledge of the population under study. Stratified sampling is used primarily to ensure that different groups of a population are adequately represented in the sample. For example, if you knew that the student population was made up of 20 per cent female students and 80 per cent male, a simple random sample might not give you a representative sample of these groups. The answer to this problem is to draw from each group a random sample proportionate to the size of the group, you will then be sure of having both male and females in your sample.

Non-probability sampling

If a list of a population is not available this type of sampling may be used. In non probability sampling, there is no way of specifying the probability that each unit has been included in the sample, there is no assurance that every unit has some chance of being included. The major advantage of this type of sampling are convenience and economy.

Convenience sampling

A convenience sample is obtained when the researcher selects whatever sampling units are conveniently available. Thus you may select only students in your class or the first 100 people you meet in the street who are willing to be interviewed.

Purposive sampling

Sometimes this method is referred to as judgement sampling. The researcher attempts to obtain a sample that appears to them to be representative of the population they wish to research. The chance that a particular person will be selected depends on the subjective judgement of the researcher.

Quota sampling

The aim of this method is to try and select a sample that is as closely as possible a replica of the population to be researched. For example, if it is known that the group to be researched has equal numbers of male and female, the researcher selects an equal number of both. If it is known that the group or population has only 20 males then the researcher would select an appropriate percentage.

Review questions

1 List the most common purposes of research.
2 Carrying out a research project raises a number of ethical issues. What questions

should you ask yourself before you embark on any research project? Explain your answers.

3 Explain what is meant by qualitative research.

4 Explain what is meant by action research and discuss its advantages and disadvantages.

5 Outline the differences between experimental and observational research. Give an example of each.

6 Explain what is meant by primary and secondary data. Give an example of each.

7 a Identify appropriate examples of the main advantages of using the following data collection techniques:
   - structured questionnaire
   - observation.

   b In which situations would you use these methods?

8 Define what is meant by the following sampling methods:
   a random?
   b stratified?
   c quota?

Assignment 15
The in-depth interview

This assignment develops knowledge and understanding of the following elements:

8.1 Investigate types of research used in health and social care
8.2 Construct a structured research instrument to survey opinion
8.3 Investigate methods of interpreting information

It supports development of the following core skills:
Communication 3.1, 3.2
Information Technology 3.1

One of the major tools of the social scientist – the indepth interview – is also a favourite of the average person in the street. Everyone at some time or other has used this technique to learn about a subject of interest. The researcher starts by asking a general question and following up the answers with increasingly specific questions until they have acquired 'an understanding' of the top.

Ordinarily an indepth interview will last about 1–1½ hours. You must carry out about five to ten such interviews to give the investigation some notion of the kinds of information that may be pertinent to the research problem. However because your time is limited, your assignment is to carry out four 30–45 minute interviews.

You will be required to word process this assignment and present it in that form for assessment.

Your tasks

Planning

1 Choose a subject for the interview – one that people usually have strong feelings about, such as child abuse, abortion, euthanasia, hanging or the government. Read as widely on the subject as you can before you begin to design any questions.

2 Think of a few neutral questions, say six, that will put the person you are interviewing at ease and that will lead them into your chosen subject.

3 Think of some more specific questions to follow that will give you a greater insight into their feelings on the subject.

4 Decide whom you will need as respondents. For example, if your chosen subject was abortion, you might consider interviewing:
   • rank and file respondents – people in the street
   • participants in positions of authority – ministers of religion, MPs, councillors, teachers
   • so-called 'well-informed people' – members of organisations for and against abortion, politicians, radio personalities, etc.

The interview

5 Depending on whom your are interviewing, talk to respondents about their feelings on the subject matter. Write down their answers as nearly verbatim as possible. This means in their own words, not in a summary by you.

6 Read over each interview before embarking on the next. Watch for points that you will want to follow up in this and subsequent interviews.

Presentation

7 By the time you have finished your interviews, you should have some interesting information concerning the topic you have chosen to investigate. Read your interviews and make notes concerning points you wish to make and the questions you wish to use in your report.

8 Write a report including the following:
   • a brief statement stating the topic of study and explaining what aspect of that topic you intend to study
   • a brief list of questions you asked in the order in which they developed, from the introductory ones to those that are more focused
   • an explanation of why and how you selected participants, your sampling technique
   • an explanation of why at least two other sampling techniques were not thought more suitable to use
   • a discussion of your findings and the supporting evidence, taken from interviews, to back them up
   • a discussion of the pertinent areas or hypotheses for further study
   • a discussion of the problems you encountered in carrying out the interviews and any suggestions you have for surmounting them in the future
   • a list sources of information and a bibliography.

16 Constructing a research project

What is covered in this chapter

- Defining a research problem
- Designing questionnaires and interviews
- Forms of response
- Analysis and interpretation of data
- Presentation of data
- Basic statistics

These are the resources you will need for your Research in Health and Social Care portfolio:
- examples of how data is presented in the media (newspapers, journals, etc.)
- examples from journals of research reports
- your written answers to each of the activities in Chapter 16
- your written answers to the review questions in Chapter 16
- your report for Assignment 16.

Defining a research problem

Considerable benefit can be gained by systematic planning A good definition of a research problem aims to develop a realistic plan of action with clear objectives which take account of resources, constraints, and has a high probability of being achieved. To achieve this it is helpful to complete a **topic analysis**. A topic analysis is a convenient way of summarising various aspects of potential topics for research (see Figure 16.1).

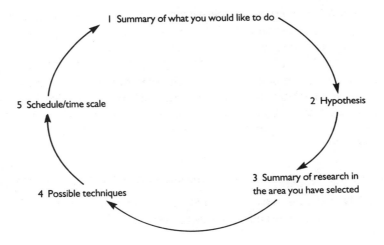

Figure 16.1 A typical topic analysis

Hypothesis

The first stage in research is to formulate a **hypothesis** – a proposition that can be tested, or the naming of the phenomenon which is to be tested. Any idea or theory which makes provisional predications is called a hypotheses. For example:

- All social care students are female.
- All engineering students are male
- Sports enthusiasts are less likely to smoke than people who take no part in sports.

The view of the issue that the researcher holds has an impact on the formulation of the hypothesis. The researcher sets out to support or contradict their hypothesis.

The difference between problems and hypotheses

A few examples will help clarify the distinction between problems and hypotheses, and how hypotheses are constructed and expressed.

Problems are general questions. For example:

- What causes inflation?
- Who uses a playgroup?
- What types of student pass examinations?
- What causes football violence?
- Who becomes a leader in a group?
- What causes child abuse?

The researcher can then generate a hypotheses based on a general question.

Examples

1 From the general question, 'Who becomes a leader in a group?', a hypothesis about how leaders develop in a group could be expressed as follows:

'As intergroup conflict increases, those people who are more aggressive and who are able or articulate are given power by the group.'

The researcher will then devise a strategy to observe behaviour in one or more groups to support or contradict the hypotheses.

2 'What causes child abuse?' The researcher may feel that those who have suffered abuse as a child are likely to abuse their own children. The hypothesis could be formulated as follows:

'Individuals who have experienced violent and abusive households are more likely to grow up to become child abusers than individuals who experience little or no violence in their childhood.'

Hypotheses can be derived from theories, observation, intuition or a combination of all. Ideas and background to any potential idea can be obtained by consulting bibliographies, indexes, abstracts, professional journals, and statistical sources. It does not matter if your research findings don't support your hypotheses. Unexpected findings often are the most interesting.

> **Research problems** are intellectual stimuli calling for an answer.
>
> **Hypotheses** are tentative answers to research problems. Hypotheses should be clear, value-free and amenable to testing.

Activity

Generate a hypothesis based on the following general question:
Does having a certain number of GCSEs indicate whether students can obtain a
qualification at GNVQ Advanced level?

Designing questionnaires and interviews

When the researcher has formulated a hypothesis he or she has to decide how to gather
or collect data. In the social sciences the most widely used methods are   the
questionnaire and the **personal interview**.

The foundation of all questionnaires is, of course, the question. Instead of observing
what people do, would you get more relevant information if you asked people what they
are doing or asked them their views on what they are doing? A questionnaire is simply a
list of questions which provides a relatively fast, effective and cheap method of obtaining
information.

The personal interview is a face-to-face, interpersonal situation in which the
interviewer's questions are designed to obtain answers which are relevant to the research
hypotheses. The interview can be tightly structured, with the interviewer asking
questions from a prepared questionnaire or it can be open with scope to ask further
questions in order to probe the respondent's feelings more deeply (see Types of
interview, below).

Sometimes the researcher may make use of the **self-administered questionnaire** (see
page 326).

A good questionnaire requires a lot of thought and planning You must ask yourself:

- What questions am I going to ask?
- Who am I going to ask?
- How am I going to record the answers?
- What am I going to do with the results?

Summary of research

Before you construct a questionnaire or an interview you must carry out some
background reading and research into the subject of your research. This will give you
some ideas of the questions that should be asked. You should read books, journals and
leaflets to gain some general ideas about your project. It might also be useful to read
other research projects which involved questionnaires and other publications and
statistics relevant to your area of study.

If you want to draw up tables and graphs from your data you will need to ask
questions which allow for only a limited number of answers. This will allow easier
analysis of the results.

Types of interview

There are two main types of interview:
- the structured interview
- the unstructured interview.

Structured interviews

The structured form of interview is one in which the questions, the wording and their sequence are fixed and identical for each respondent. Any variations which appear in the responses can be attributed to the actual differences between the respondents and not to variation in the interview.

Structured interviews provide an objective exercise and the tendencies toward bias are less than with observation or unstructured interviews. A major advantage is that the information can be easily coded and analysed by computer.

It is important to give a lot of thought to the design of the questionnaire, as structured interviews are only as good as the questions asked. It is also important to frame the questions in a language that the respondents will understand:

- avoid woolly generalisations
- avoid bias that might encourage the respondents to give an answer that you want them to give.

Example

```
How often do you watch soaps on television?
Never                        ☐
Every week                   ☐
Two or three times a month ☐
Once a month or less         ☐

How much money do you spend on cigarettes each month?
Less than £50        ☐
£51-80               ☐
£81 or more          ☐

Do you go to the cinema?    Yes/No
If your answer is no, is it because:
You don't like what's showing?              ☐
You prefer to watch it on video?            ☐
It costs too much money?                     ☐
You are worried about the cigarette smoke?  ☐
Other reasons please state:

_____

_____
```

There are many problems with framing questions for structured questionnaires. Some questions may be unclear, or use words that the respondent may not understand:

- **Leading questions** These questions encourage the respondent to say 'Yes' Therefore, the following two questions are biased:
  - Do you think that women should not work until their children are old enough?
  - Don't you agree that there is too much violence on television?
- **Questions which presume** These questions presume that the respondent has done the actions defined in the question:
  - When did you last go to a pop concert?
  - How many cups of coffee have you had?

- **Double questions** These are questions with more than one part:
  - Do you think that the college should spend less money on books and more on sports facilities?
  - Do you think that there is too much violence at football matches and that this is responsible for the lowering of standards in society?

Activity

Compare the following two questions. Which question expects the answer 'yes' and which the answer 'no'?

a Do you think people should be free to provide the best medical care possible for themselves and their families, free of interference from the state?

b Should the wealthy be able to buy a place at the head of the queue for medical treatment, pushing aside those with greater need, or should medical care be allocated only on the basis of need?

Unstructured interviews

The least structured form of interviewing is the unstructured, or non-directive, interview in which respondents are given no direction from the interviewer. They are encouraged to relate their experience and to reveal their opinions and attitudes as they see fit. It allows the respondents to express their opinions as well as answer the questions. The respondents can let you know their real feelings about the subject of the question and, therefore, tend to answer more freely and fully.

Example

Your task is to discover as many specific kinds of conflicts and tensions between children and parents as possible. The four areas of possible conflict we want to explore are listed in question 3. The first two are to allow you to build up a rapport with the respondent.

> 1 What sort of problems do teenagers have in getting along with their parents?
> 2 What sort of disagreements do you have with your parents?
> 3 Have you ever had any disagreement with either parent over:
>   staying out later? ☐
>   friends of the opposite sex? ☐
>   dating? ☐
>   smoking? ☐
>   drinking? ☐

Activities

1 When interviewing, do you think that there are situations when the respondent might feel inhibited?

2 Discuss with you class colleagues the effect on outcome of an interview that the following scenarios might have:
   a a white interviewer and a black respondent
   b a male interviewer and a female respondent.

The principles of interviewing

The aim in interviewing is to get the desired information. This can be done by following a few simple guide-lines:
- The person you are interviewing needs to feel that the interview will be pleasant and satisfying.
- Interviewers should present themselves as being understanding and easy to talk to.
- The people being interviewed need to feel that the study is worthwhile.
- The interviewer also needs to overcome the respondent's suspicions.
- The interviewer should explain in a friendly manner the purpose of the study and the confidential nature of the interview.

How can you put people at ease?
- Tell the respondent who you are and who you represent and explain to them what you are doing in a way that will make them interested in your research.
- Tell the respondent how and why they were chosen to be interviewed. Any instructions should be brief.
- Create a relationship of confidence between yourself and the person you are interviewing.

Types of question

There are basically two types of questions:
- factual questions
- opinion or attitude questions.

Factual questions
Factual questions elicit objective information. The most common type of factual questions obtain information such as sex, age, marital status, education or income of respondents.

Example

At what age did you get married?

```
16 years      □
17 years      □
18 years      □
19 years      □
20 years      □
21 years      □
Over 21 years □

Please tick the appropriate box.
```

Other factual questions could elicit information about a respondent's social environment, for example 'How may people are living in your household?' or their leisure activities, 'How often do you go to the pub?'

Opinion or attitude questions

Opinion or attitude questions are more difficult to construct. Before we examine how to develop an opinion or attitude question, we must first examine the difference between an 'attitude' and an 'opinion'.

> An **attitude** is the sum total of a person's prejudices, ideas, fears and convictions about any specific topic. **Opinions** are the verbal expression of attitudes.

Activity

Which of the following are opinions and which are attitudes?
a John says he likes Liverpool Football Club.
b Mary refuses to allow her son to marry an Irish girl.
c Jim is convinced that anyone over 65 years of age should not work.
d Peter says that a woman's place is in the home looking after children.
e Jim refuses to allow his wife to go out to work after the birth of their first child.

To obtain data about factual matters or attitudes, you can ask two types of question:
- closed questions
- open questions.

Closed questions In closed questions respondents are given a set of answers from which they are asked to choose one that closely represents their views (Example 1).

Closed questions are easy to ask, quick to be answered and their analysis is straightforward. Answers can be more elaborate than open questions (Example 2).

Examples

1
```
Managing is a man's job.

Strongly agree        ☐
Agree                 ☐
Disagree              ☐
Strongly disagree     ☐
```

2
```
Do you feel that you are really part of your class group?

Really a part of my class                    ☐
Included in most ways                         ☐
Included in some ways, but not in others      ☐
Don't feel that I really belong               ☐
Don't fit in with any class                   ☐

Please tick the appropriate box.
```

Open questions Open questions are not followed by any kind of specified choice – the respondents' answers are recorded in full. For example, the question 'What do you personally feel are the most important problems the government should try to tackle?' is an open question. The virtue of this type of question is that the respondent can express their thoughts freely, spontaneously and in their own way.

What type of questions should you use?

In which situations should you use the different type of questions? The following points should be considered:

- **The objectives of the questionnaire** Closed questions are suitable when you want to find out if the respondent agrees or disagrees with a point of view. If you want to find out how the respondent arrived at this view, an open question is more appropriate.
- **How much does the respondent know about the topic in question?** Open questions give you the opportunity to find out how much the respondents know about the topic. Obviously, it is futile to ask any questions that are beyond the experience of the respondent.
- **Communication** How easily can the contents of the answers be communicated by the respondent?
- **Motivation** What is the extent of the respondent's motivation to answer the questions?

How to encourage people to complete and return questionnaires

With all surveys there is the problem of people who may refuse to fill in your questionnaire or simply forget to do so. This makes your results less accurate. If your response rate is low, what can you do to improve it?

There are various methodsthat you can use to improve the response rate, including:

- **Follow-up** Write or telephone the people who have not responded.
- **Length of questionnaire** The shorter the better, as longer questionnaires tend not to be answered.
- **Who gave out the questionnaire** If the respondents know you or the college, then they are likely to reply. However, where questions are of a confidential nature this may not be the case and in these instances you must stress confidentiality in your introductory letter.
- **Introductory letter** An appeal to the respondents to emphasise that they would be helping the interests of everyone seems to produce the best results.
- **Method of return** A stamped addressed envelope produces best results.
- **Format of the questionnaire** A title that will arouse interest helps, as does an attractive and clear layout with plenty of room for hand-written answers.

The self-administered questionnaire

The self-administered questionnaire, as a method, is cheaper than others and avoids the problems, such as bias, associated with the use of interviewers. It may handed out to people or sent through the post, to be completed in their own time.

The self-administered questionnaire has some positive advantages. People are more likely to express less socially-acceptable attitudes and feelings when answering a questionnaire alone than when confronted by an interviewer. The greater the anonymity the more honest the response. Aside from the greater honesty that they may produce, self-administered questionnaires also have the advantage of giving a respondent more time to think.

This type of survey gives no opportunity for the respondent to probe beyond the answer given. The questions should be simple and straight forward, and be understood with the help of minimal, printed instructions.

Forms of response

Rating

One of the most common formats for questions in social science surveys is the rating scale. Here, respondents are asked to make a judgement in terms of strength of feeling.

Example

```
Old people should not be allowed to live on their own if they are
very dependent.

1 Strongly agree        ☐
2 Agree                 ☐
3 Disagree              ☐
4 Strongly disagree     ☐
5 Don't know            ☐

Please tick the appropriate box.
```

These responses reflect the intensity of the respondent's judgement.

Ranking

Ranking is used in questionnaires whenever the researcher wants to gather data regarding the degree of importance that people give to a set of attitudes or objects. For instance in a survey on the quality of life of students, respondents could be asked to rank order various dimensions they considered important to student life.

Example

```
I would like you to tell me what you have found important in
student life. Would you please look at this card and tell me which
of these is most important to you as a goal in your student life,
which comes next in importance, which is third and so forth?
```

```
Meeting other students
1st rank
2nd rank
3rd rank
4th rank

Academic life
1st rank
2nd rank
3rd rank
4th rank

Sport activities
1st rank
2nd rank
```

```
3rd rank
4th rank

Student's Union
1st rank
2nd rank
3rd rank
4th rank
```

Ranking is a useful device in providing some sense of relative order among judgements. It is important particularly in the social sciences where a 'numerical value' cannot be applied.

The rank order method is an extremely easy method to use. One of the most basic assumptions is that attitudes towards various objects may be expressed along a continuum from least to most favourable.

Semantic differential measuring instrument

The semantic differential measuring method is one of the most adaptable yet, ironically, under-utilised scaling methods in the social sciences. This scale with minor variations, is adaptable to any attitude measurement. The semantic differential measures a subject's responses to stimulus words, concepts or phrases in terms of bipolar adjective ratings. An example is shown in Figure 16.2.

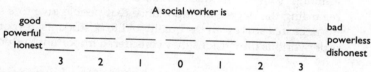

Figure 16.2 A bipolar adjective rating scale

With a list of such bipolar adjective scales, it is possible to measure the affect experienced by any person towards any object.

Activity

Design a bipolar adjective scale to measure peoples' attitudes to the role of the police.

Analysis and interpretation of data

Validity

Validity is defined as the degree to which the researcher has measured what he or she set out to measure. Validity also provides a direct check on how well the questions fulfil their function, the determination of which usually requires independent, external criteria of whatever the questionnaire is designed to measure. Validity refers to whether the researcher is really measuring what he or she says is being measured.

Do the questions asked in a survey actually measure the concepts the researcher intended them to measure? For instance, from the wording of a question, the researcher assumes that the respondent who agrees that 'all policemen are hostile' is indicating a distrust of the police. Undoubtedly one of the most important questions that needs to be raised regarding any questionnaire relates to the validity of the questions, i.e. do the questions actually measure what they purport to measure?

Example

A measuring tape may measure in feet or metres, not in pounds or grams. You do not measure height by standing on a weighing scale.

Tests for validity

One of the common tests for validity is **face validity**. For example, if the concept the researcher wishes to measure is 'How satisfied is a person with their car?', the question 'Do you like your car?' has face validity because it is relevant to the concept in question and it is unambiguous. Face validity can be checked by discussing the questions in a questionnaire with respondents, who can give their opinion as to their validity.

The question the researcher should, therefore, ask themselves is, 'Will the question-naire look valid to the subjects who respond to it and to the personnnel who make use of it?'

Reliability

Reliability should be distinguished from validity. It refers to **consistency** – to obtaining the same results again and again under similar circumstances. Will the same methods used by other researchers produce the same results? Reliability refers to consistency between independent measurements of the same phenomenon.

Many argue that in the social sciences 'true' answers do not exist. True answers may exist, but they may change over time. However, some sort of criterion is available which can be applied to the realm of 'factual questions' such as, 'Is bathing residents part of your job?' or 'Do you think that shaving residents is part of your job, or someone else's?' Such questions would produce a true answer, if the researcher could find time to observe the member of staff in their work. If another researcher asked the same staff the same questions the answers ought to be the same, i.e. show high reliability. If questions are poorly phrased and obscure, the respondent may answer differently to the same question on different occasions. The answers may reflect the respondent's current mood. It is rare for researchers to obtain perfect reliability between independent measurements.

Inferential statistics

Using statistics to help simplify and describe data is only the first step in analysing the results of a research study. The rest of the analysis is concerned not so much with the specific subjects that the researcher has tested (the sample), but with what those subjects can tell the researcher about a larger group (the population). The researcher uses statistical analysis of the data from the sample to draw inferences about a larger group. These statistics are called **inferential statistics**.

Presentation of data

Information or data can be presented in the form of:

- diagrams
- graphs

- pie charts
- tables.

Each of the four different methods helps you to present information in an understandable and logical way.

Diagrams

Diagrams are a way of presenting a lot of information in picture form. A good diagram will help you cut down on the amount of writing you would otherwise have to do to describe the information presented in the diagram.

Graphs

A bar chart or graph shows the relationship between two variables, usually one being quantitative and the other qualitative. Information can be presented in a variety of graphical forms. Graphs can be used to show changes in a particular variable over a given period of time. The graph can be used to reinforce points made in writing.

Bar graphs

Examples of bar graphs are shown in Figures 16.3, 16.4 and 16.5.

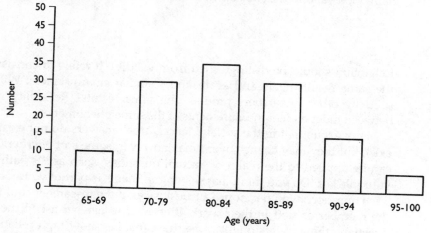

Figure 16.3 Bar graph to show the number of elderly people admitted to day care in Uptown Local Authority, by age, 1993

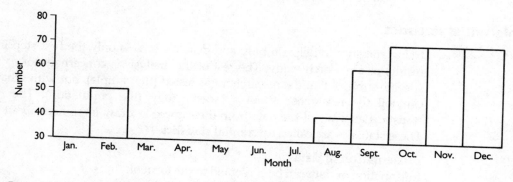

Figure 16.4 Bar graph to show the number of elderly people in residential care in Uptown Local Authortiy, by month, 1993

330

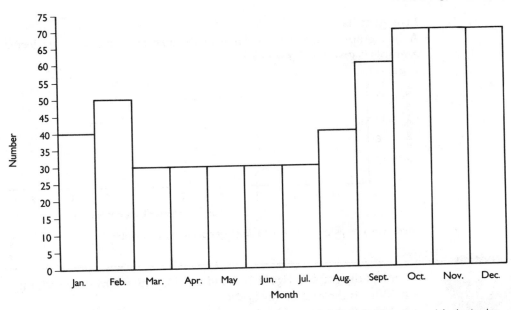

Figure 16.5 *Bar graph to show the number of elderly people in residential care in Uptown Local Authority, by month, 1993*

Activities

1 Construct a bar graph from the data in Table 16.1.

Table 16.1 Children on child protection register at 31 March 1993, by age

Age	Number
1–4	200
5–8	67
9–12	100
13–15	75
16+	8

2 Look at the graphs in Figures 16.4 and 16.5 Although they give the same information, do they look different. Do they seem to be conveying the same message? Discuss the reason why they look as if they are giving different messages based upon the same data.

3 From the data in Table 16.2 construct a bar graph.

Table 16.2 Referrals for home care support to Downside Social Services Department, 1993

Month	Number	Month	Number
January	100	July	55
February	81	August	50
March	84	September	60
April	81	October	70
May	73	November	75
June	60	December	85

Line graphs

A line graph is another useful way to illustrate increasing or decreasing values. An example is given in Figure 16.6.

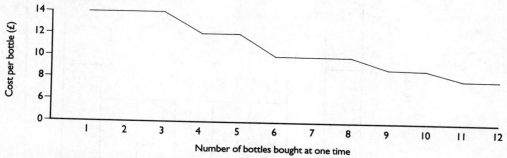

Figure 16.6 Line graph to show the advantages of buying wine in bulk

Activities

1 Look at the graph in Figure 16.6 and consider the following questions:
   a What is the cost of one bottle?
   b What is the cost of five bottles?
   c What is the cost of seven bottles?
   d What is the cost of ten bottles?
2 Compare Figures 16.6 and 16.7. Why does it look as if a bottle of wine is more expensive in Figure 16.7?

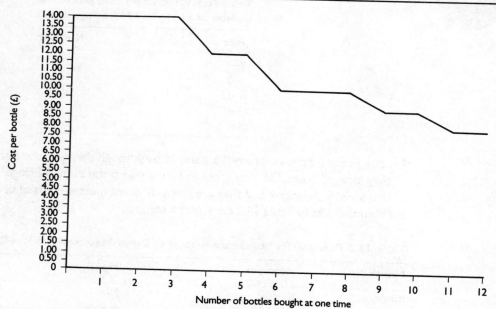

Figure 16.7 Line graph to show the advantages of buying wine in bulk

How do you arrive at a percentage?

Look at Table 16.1 which shows the number of home care referrals. We can work out the percentage of referrals for the month of April as follows:

Divide the number of referrals for April by the total number of referrals for the year:
Total referrals for the year   = 525
Number of referrals in April = 81
                  81 ÷ 525   = 0.154
Then multiply by 100 to obtain the percentage:
          0.154 × 100   = 15.4
The percentage of referrals for the month of April is 15.4 per cent.

Activity

Look at the information in Table 16.3. Copy the graph axes and draw either a bar chart or a line graph using the data in the table.

Table 16.3 Health care assistants by age

Age	Number	Percentage
Under 20	19	1.5
20–29	163	9.0
30–39	433	24.0
40–49	643	36.0
50–59	418	23.5
60+	101	6.0
Total	1,777	100.0

Pie charts

A pie chart is a visual presentation which breaks down a total figure into different components. Look at the pie chart in Figure 16.8 which illustrates the percentages of patients attending out-patients at a hospital.

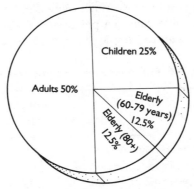

Figure 16.8 Pie chart to show the percentage of patients attending outpatients at St Jack's Hospital

The percentage figures were derived from Table 16.4

Table 16.4 Number of patients attending outpatients at St Jack's Hospital

Type of patient	Number of patients
Adults	400
Children	200
Elderly 60–79 years	100
Elderly 80+	100
Total	800

Activity

Construct a pie chart to illustrate the data in Table 16.5.

Table 16.5 Qualification held by Uptown Social Services Staff

Qualifications	Number	Percentage of staff
Cert. Social Service (CSS)	86	9.9
Diploma in Social Work	180	20.7
Management	20	2.3
GNVQ	26	2.6
Other	23	2.3
None	532	61.5
Total	867	100.0

Tables

Tables enable you to show much more data than, for instance, in a bar graph. Table 16.6 shows the response rate to a postal questionnaire which was sent to a sample of home helps (Group A) and a sample of auxiliary nurses (Group B) in a national survey.

Table 16.6 Response rates to a postal questionnaire

	Group A No.	%	Group B No.	%
Questionnaires distributed	1,302		100.0 1,961	100.0
Questionnaires returned	1,170		1,482	
Uncompleted questionnaires	133		144	
Total analysed	1,037		79.6 1,338	68.2

From the data in Table 16.6 we can see that although Group B were sent more questionnaires (1,961), the percentage response (68.2 per cent) was lower than in Group A (79.6 per cent)

Basic statistics

Frequency distribution

Finding a single figure that indicates the location of a distribution is not easy. The distribution may be spread out over a wide range of values and to chose one to represent its location is like trying to find a single person who can represent one student in a college or one patient in a hospital. When data is purely quantative, the simplest way to deal with then is to count the number of cases in each category.

Example

Analysis of the census of students in a large college, one of the variables of interest was the number of males and females in each faculty. To summarise the data, we count the number of students in each faculty by sex. The results are shown in Table 16.7.

Table 16.7 Number of students by faculty by sex

Faculty	Engineering	Social care	Science	Art
Male	300	20	400	250
Female	20	200	100	200
Total	320	220	500	450

The count of individuals having a particular quality is called the **frequency** of that quality. The frequency for male students in the science faculty is 400. The proportion of individuals having that quality is the **relative frequency** or **proportional frequency**. The relative frequency of male students in the science faculty (of all students) is $400 \div 1{,}490 = 0.26$ or 26 per cent. The set of frequencies is called the **frequency distribution** of the variables.

Shapes of frequency distribution

If we collect a large number of results we could split up the total range of values into a large number of small intervals and calculate the proportion of results falling into the intervals. If we mark in this proportion at the midpoint of each small interval and then join up the points we get a frequency distribution. For any given distribution researchers want some measure of the centre of the distribution. The most widely used is the **mean**.

Mean (or arithmetic mean) The mean is the measure to which we usually refer in everyday life when we use the word 'average'. It can be defined as the value each item in the distribution would have if all the values were shared out equally among all the items. It is a measure of central tendency. For a sample the mean is simply calculated by summing up all the values and dividing the result by the total number of values.

Table 16.8 Age of residents in Summervale Residential Home

Residential	Age
Joan	80
Mary	75
Jack	78
Peter	70
Jose	86
Ken	90
Alice	88
Mark	94
Total (8)	661

From the data in Table 16.8 the mean age for this sample is 82.6 years. This was calculated as follows:

List the numbers (ages) in a vertical column
Add the numbers (ages) together = 661 years
Count the number of items (residents) making up the list to get N
As the list comprises 8 residents therefore N = 8
Divide the total (661 years) by the value of N (8): 661 ÷ 8 = 82.6
so the mean, or average age, of residents is 82.6 years

Activities

1 Calculate the mean of the following, 36, 21, 6, 18, 78, 90,5, 67, 66.
2 Is the following set of data a suitable on which to use this formula (the mean)?
   30, 30, 30, 30, 30, 30, 56, 78, 30, 30, 30.

The median The median measure of the central or middle point of the distribution is the values. This is the value of the central result when the results are arranged in order of magnitude. If we have an odd number of results then the median is simply the value of the middle result. If we have an even number as in Table 16.9 then there is no single middle result, can we take the average of the two middle results. The two middle results are 80 years and 86 years 80 + 86 ÷ 2 = 83 years

Table 16.9 Age of residents (in order of magnitude) in Summervale Residential Home

Resident	Age
Peter	70
Mary	75
Jack	78
Joan	80
Jose	86
Alice	88
Ken	90
Mark	94
Total (80)	661

For a frequency distribution based on a whole population of values the median is the value that splits the area under the curve into two equal areas. Half the values would be above the median, and half below.

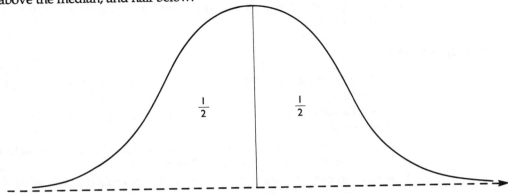

Figure 16.9 Frequency distribution curve showing the median

The median is sometimes a useful estimate of the middle of a distribution when the distribution is not symmetrical, i.e. when there is a long tail on one side and not on the other. An example of this would be salaries where most people have fairly moderate salaries, but a small number have very large ones. Most people would have salaries below the mean. This kind of distribution, which is not symmetrical, is called skewed. In this case, the median salary would be a sensible estimate of the middle of the frequency distribution of salaries. Half the individuals would have salaries below this and half above.

Activity

Calculate the median for the following values:

a 22, 33, 45, 46, 48, 89, 99

b 4, 6, 9, 23, 44, 44, 48, 78, 90

Mode Another measure of the middle of the distribution is the mode, which is the most popular value, or the value that occurs most often.

In the following set of figures the number 11 occurs most often so it is the mode: 2, 3, 6, 7, 11, 11, 11, 11, 13, 15, 17.

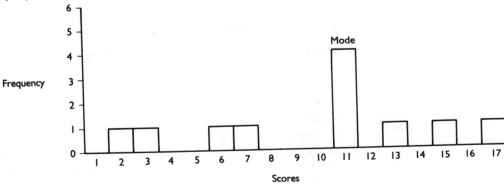

Figure 16.10 Frequency distribution showing the position of the mode for the above data

The mode is a useful measure of the middle of a distribution when the variable the researcher is interested in is discreet, that is, it is confined to certain restricted values. For example, it would be useful as a measure of the number of children in a family in this country. If the most frequent number of children in a family is, say, 2, then the modal value would be 2.

Review questions

1 Give an example of the main advantage of using observation as a data collection technique.
2 In what situation would an in-depth interview be the most appropriate way to collect information?
3 What are the main disadvantages of the observation method of collecting information?
4 Explain what is meant by the term 'random sample'
5 a Give an example of a rating scheme and why you would use it.
  b Devise a rating scale for a question of your choice.
6 Suggest two examples of how statistics may be misused.
7 Explain what is meant by the term 'measure of probability'?
8 Give two examples of a 'frequency count'?
9 What is meant by the term 'semantic differential'?
10 Give two examples of probes and prompts to support open questions.
11 Give an example of a situation in which you would use one of the following:
  a frequency count
  b mean
  c mode
  d median.

Assignment 16
The sociogram: A study of group behaviour

This assignment develops knowledge and understanding of the following elements:
8.1 Investigate types of research used in health and social care
8.2 Construct a structured research instrument to survey opinion
8.3 Investigate methods of interpreting information

It supports development of the following core skills:
Communication 3.1, 3.2
Information technology 3.1

Groups vary in their cohesiveness, every group has a 'preference structure' or a network of likes, dislikes and indifferences that links it members to one another. The **sociogram** (sociometry) was devised to enable relationships within groups to be more reliably detected than by direct observation. The essence of the technique is to ask individuals to indicate those other group members whom they most like or most dislike. A diagram called a sociogram is then constructed which summarises this information.

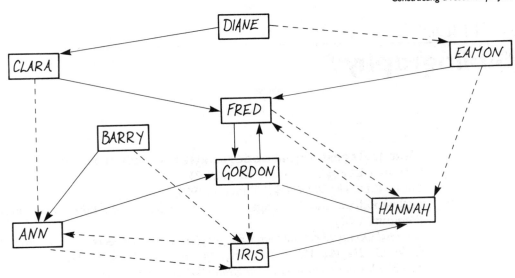

Figure 16.11 *Example of a completed sociogram*

Your tasks

1 Choose a small group for study, taking into account the following:
   - The person carrying out the experiment should be independent of the group. If you have relationships with the group members, they may be less likely to reveal their true feelings about the rest of the group. If it is not possible to find such a group, this difficulty must be recognised and taken into account.
   - It is best to carry out this experiment with a group which is to some degree compelled to remain in being, such as a class, tutorial group, sports team, people attending a day centre or residents in an old people's home.
   - The ideal size of a group should be between 6–10 members. If it is larger than this it becomes difficult to represent in diagrammatic form.
   The names of the group members should be listed and a copy of the list given to each group member.
2 Each group member should be asked to make, privately and without consultation, two choices:
   - one positive choice (Who would you like to sit next to? or Who are you most friendly with?)
   - one negative choice (Who would you least like to sit with? or Who are you least friendly with?).
   These choices should be marked with some appropriate symbol (for example, + or −) on the list of names of the group.
3 A chart should now be constructed which shows each member of the group. From the data you have collected, illustrate positive relationships with a unbroken line and negative relationships with a broken line (see Figure 16.11).
4 Explain in a report how useful a sociogram might be. In what kinds of social situations might it be particularly useful and revealing?

Bibliography

Unit 1: Access, equal opportunities and client rights

Goffman, E., *Asylums* (Doubleday, 1961)

Laing, R.D., *The Divided Self* (Penguin, 1960)

Littlewood, R. and Lipsedge, M. *Aliens and Alienists: Ethnic Minorities and Psychiatry* (Penguin, 1981)

National Occupational Standards for Care (Unit 0), Care Sector Consortium, 1992

Sacks, O., *The Man Who Mistook His Wife for a Hat* (Picador, 1985)

The Black Report, *Inequalities in Health* (DHSS, 1980)

Unit 2: Interpersonal interaction

Bateson, J. *Do we need service marketing?* Marketing Consumer Services: New Insights Report (Marketing Services Institute, November 1977)

Cowell, D.W., *The Marketing of Services* (Heinemann, 1984)

Gronross, C., *Strategic Management and Marketing in the Service Sector* (Swedish School of Economics and Business Administration, Helsinki, 1982)

O'Connor, J. and Seymour, J., *Introducing Neuro-Linguistic Programming* (Mandala, 1990)

Pease, A., *Body Language* (Sheldon Press, 1984)

Caring for Mary, a video-based learning programme that addresses many of the interpersonal aspects of health and social care, within the context of the care value base (available only from Educare, telephone or fax 0742 681075)

Unit 3: Physical aspects of health

A Manual of Nutrition (Ministry of Agriculture, Food and Fisheries)

Clare, A, *Psychiatry in Dissent* (Tavistock, 1980)

Clegg, A.G. and Clegg, P.C., *Man Against Disease* (Heineman) – unfortunately now out of print

Proposals for nutritional guide-lines for health education in Britain, prepared for the National Advisory Committee on Nutrition Education (NACNE, 1983)

Roberts, M.B.V., *Biology: A Functional Approach* (Nelson, 1986 [4th edition])

Simkins, J. and Williams, J.I., *Advanced Human Biology* (Unwin Hyman, 1987)

Unit 4: Psychological and social aspects of health and social care

Age Concern, *Abuse of Elderly People: Guidelines for Action* (Age Concern, 1992)

Bannister, A., Barrett, K. and Shearer, E. (eds), *Listening to Children* (Longman, 1990)

Bennett, O.J., 'Elder Abuse in Britain', *British Medical Journal* , 305: 998–999 (1992)

Committee on Medical Aspects of Food Policy, *Dietary Reference Values: A Guide* (HMSO, 1991)

Creighton, S ., *Child Abuse: Trends in England and Wales* (NSPCC, 1992)

Department of Health, *The Health of the Nation* (HMSO, 1992)

DHSS, *The Black Report: Inequalities in Health Report of a Research Working Group* (HMSO, 1980)

Eastman, M., 'Granny Abuse', *Community Outlook*, October 1988.

Holmes, T.H. and Rahe, R.H., 'The social readjustment rating scale', *Journal of Psychosomatic Research*, 11, 213–1218 (1967)

OPCS , *Occupational Mortality: Decennial Supplement 1970–1972* (HMSO, 1978)

OPCS, *General Household Survey* (HMSO,1982 and 1983)

OPCS, *Mortality Statistics 1989* (HMSO, 1992)

Parkes, M., *Bereavement: Studies in Grief in Adult Life* (Penguin, 1975)

Patrick, D.L. and Scrambler, G., *Sociology as Applied to Medicine* (Baillière Tindall, 1986)

Townsend, P. and Davidson, N., *Inequalities in Health* (Penguin, 1982)

Unit 5: Health promotion

Caplan, G., *Principles of Preventive Psychiatry* (Basic Books, New York, 1964)

I. Simmett, *et al.*, *Promoting Health: A Practical Guide to Health Education* (John Wiley, 1985)

Open University, *The Good Health Guide* (Pan Books, 1980)

Sarason, S.B., *Work, Aging and Social Change* (Free Press, 1977)

Most of the statistics in Chapter 9 were obtained from published government sources. An abstract of such information is published annually by HMSO in *Social Trends*.

Unit 6: Structure and practices in health and social care

Charities Digest (Family Welfare Association, 1993) – an annual publication

Guide to the Social Services (Family Welfare Association, 1993) – an annual publication

Hamm, C., *Health Policy in Britain* (Macmillan, 1992 [3rd edition])

Moore, S., *Social Welfare Alive* (Stanley Thornes, 1993)

Ottewill, R. and Wall, A., *The Growth and Development of the Community Health Services* (Business Education Publishers Ltd, 1990)

Stoyle, J., *Caring for Older People: A Multi-cultural Approach* (Stanley Thornes, 1991)

Tossell, D. and Webb, R., *Inside the Caring Services* (Edward Arnold, 1986)

Townsend, P. and Davidson, N., *Inequalities in Health* (Penguin, 1991)

Walker, A. (ed.), *Community Care: The Family, the State and Social Policy* (Basil Blackwell and Martin Robertson & Co. Ltd, 1982)

Unit 7: Care plans

Care Management and Assessment: The Practitioner's Guide (HMSO, 1991)

Caring for People: Information Pack for the Voluntary and Private Sectors (Department of Health, 1993)

Community Care in Lancashire: Care Assessment and Care Management, Paper 1, 1992

Hall, J., 'Assessing People and Patients' in Hall, J., *Psychology for Nurses and Health Visitors* (Macmillan, 1988)

Langan, M., and Day, S. (eds), *Women, Oppression and Social Work* (Routledge, 1992)

National Health Service and Community Care Act (HMSO, 1990)

Payne, M., *Modern Social Work Theory* (Macmillan, 1991)

Swain, J., Finkelstein, V., French, S. and Oliver, M. (eds), *Disabling Barriers – Enabling Environments* (The Open University/Sage, 1993)

Witz, A., *Professions and Patriachy* (Routledge, 1992)

Unit 8: Research in health and social care

Clegg, F., *Simple Statistics: A Course Book for the Social Sciences* (Cambridge University Press, 1982)

Everitt, W., Hardiker, P., Littlewood, J. and Mullender, A., *Applied Research for Better Practice* (Macmillian, 1992)

Moroney, M.J., *Facts from Figures* (Pelican, 1951)

Moser, C.A., *Survey Methods in Social Investigation* (Heinemann, 1969)

Oppenheim, A.N., *Questionnaire Design and Attitude Measurement* (Open University/ Heinemann, 1976)

Rowntree, D., *Statistics without Tears* (Penguin, 1983)

Townsend, P., *Poverty in the United Kingdom* (Allen Wall, 1979)

APPENDIX 2

Useful addresses

This list is by no means exhaustive, there are many small support groups throughout the UK. Many of the organisations listed below have regional offices, check in your telephone directory or *Thomson's Directory*.

Look at the beginning of your local *Yellow Pages*, where there is a section entitled 'Yellow Pages and Disabled People' which explains how organisations for the disabled have been classified.

You will find many useful local addresses in *Yellow Pages* under:

- Charitable Organisations
- Counselling and Advice
- Social Service and Welfare Organisations
- Youth and Community Groups.

Community Health Councils exist to help users of the National Health Service. Look in your telephone directory under the name of your local health authority. Local social services departments and Citizen's Advice Bureaux also supply information.

Pharmaceutical companies, food manufacturers and the large supermarket chains all produce their own health promotion literature, as do organisations such as the Milk Marketing Board.

Action for ME
PO Box 1302
Wells
Somerset
BA5 2WE
0749 670799

Action on Smoking and Health (ASH)
109 Gloucester Place
London
W1H 3PH
071 935 3519

Age Concern England
Astral House
1268 London Road
London
SW16 4ER
081 679 8000

Alcohol Concern
305 Gray's Inn Road
London
WC1X 8QS
071 833 3471

Alzheimer's Disease Society
158-160 Balham High Road
London
SW12 9BN
081 675 6557

Arthritis and Rheumatism Council
Copeman House
St Mary's Court
St Mary's Gate
Chesterfield
Derbyshire
S41 7TD
0246 558033

ASBAH
Association for Spina Bifida and
Hydrocephalus
42 Park Road
Peterborough
PE1 2UQ
0733 555988

Assocation for Residential Care
The Old Rectory
Old Whittlington
Chesterfield
Derbyshire
S41 7QY

Asthma Research Council
St Thomas's Hospital
Lambeth Palace Road
London SE1

Barnardos
Tanners Lane
Barkingside
Ilford
IG6 1QG
081 550 8822

British Diabetic Association
10 Queen Anne Street
London
W1M 0BD
071 323 1531

British Heart Foundation
14 Fitzhardinge Street
London
W1H 4DH

Carers National Association
29 Chilworth Mews
London
W2 3RG
071 724 7776

Centre for Policy on Ageing
25-31 Ironmonger Row
London
EC1V 3QP

Child Accident Prevention Trust
28 Portland Place
London
W1N 4DE
071 636 2545

Childline
Freepost 1111
London
N1 0BR
0800 1111

Child Poverty Action Group
4th Floor
1–5 Bath Street
London
EC1V 9PY
071 253 3406

Commission for Racial Equality
Elliot House
10–12 Allington Street
London
SW1E 5EH
071 828 7033

(Local community relations councils can
be found in your local telephone
directory.)

Contact-a-family
(links families of children with special
needs)
16 Strutton Ground
London
SW1P 2HP
071 222 2695

Cruse – Bereavement Care
126 Sheen Road
Richmond
TW9 1UR
081 940 4818

Cystic Fibrosis Trust
Alexandra house
5 Blyth Road
Bromley
Kent
BR1 3RS
081 464 7211

Department of Health
The Adelphi
1–11 John Adam Street
London
WC2N 6HT
071 962 8000

Disability Alliance
1st Floor East
Universal House
88–94 Wentworth Street
London
E1 7SA
071 243 8776

Disabled Living Foundation
380–384 Harrow Road
London
W9 2HU
071 289 6111

Down's Syndrome Association
155 Mitcham Road
Tooting
London
SW17 9PG
081 682 4001

Equal Opportunities Commission
Overseas House
Quay Street
Manchester
M33HN
061 833 9244

Family Welfare Association
501–505 Kingsland Road
Dalston
London
E8 4AU
071 254 6251

Gingerbread
(an association for one-parent families)
35 Wellington Street
London
WC2E 7BN
071 240 0953

Haemophilia Society
123 Westminster Bridge Road
London
SE1 7HR
071 928 2020

Health Education Authority
Hamilton House
Mabledon Place
London
WC1H 9TX
071 383 3833

Health Visitor's Association
50 Southwark Street
London
SE1 1UN
071 378 7255

Help the Aged
St James's Walk
London
EC1R 0BE
071 253 0253

Hyperactive Children's Support Group
c/o 71 Whyke Lane
Chichester
Sussex
PO19 2LD
0903 725182
(Tue–Fri, 9.30–3.30)

Institute of Race Relations
2–6 Leek Street
King's Cross Road
London WC1

Invalid Children's Aid Nationwide
Allen Graham House
198 City Road
London
EC1V 2PH
071 608 2462

Kidscape
82 Brook Street
London
W1Y 1YG

PLANTING
BY THE
MOON

A GARDENERS' CALENDAR

2000

Nick Kollerstrom

PROSPECT BOOKS

Published in 1999 by Prospect Books,
Allaleigh House, Blackawton, Totnes, Devon TQ9 7DL, England.

British Library Cataloguing in Publication Data:
A catalogue entry of this book is available from the British Library.

ISBN 0907325 939

Typeset by Tom Jaine.
Layout, illustrations and figures by Philippa Stockley.
Cover design by Philippa Stockley.

Printed by the Cromwell Press, Trowbridge, Wiltshire.

CONTENTS

FIGURES

INTRODUCTION

> To everything there is a season and a time to every purpose under heaven: a time
> to be born and time to die: a time to plant, and a time to pluck up what is planted.
>
> *Ecclesiastes*, 3:1-2

HAVE YOU EVER WONDERED whether your garden vegetables would benefit if
you planted them in synchrony with the phases and the cycles of the Moon?

Since time immemorial, man has held a belief in the efficacy of such a
practice in various guises and according to different traditions which have
developed on this subject. In many countries today lunar calendars are
available for farmers and gardeners. There is now considerable evidence that
crops can benefit from the right use of a lunar gardening guide, as this 1999
issue of *Planting by the Moon* attempts to show.

It must be said, however, that present-day lunar gardening guides do
disagree with each other on just about every recommendation they make. Old
traditions on the subject have grown confused with the passage of time and a
new start has appeared within the twentieth-century organic farming/gardening
movement known as Bio-Dynamics. The guide you are now reading differs
from others in that it spends a few chapters reviewing the subject as a whole,
before coming out with its own calendar structure. Folk-traditions are described, as also is the evidence of modern studies. The book is for readers who
want a practical grower's guide to the cycles of time and for those who would
like to develop more of a perspective on the issues involved.

The aim is to stimulate interest and research in the area as well as to
improve your vegetables. The reader is introduced to various modern studies
concerned with the question of lunar influence, placed within the context of the
burgeoning organic movement. But those who simply wish to apply the
recommended sowing times for 1999 can turn straight to those chapters that
talk about how to use the calendar itself. These recommendations are not the
same as those in other lunar gardening guides but they may have a better
chance of producing dependable crop improvements.

A gardener works with time. He or she has continually to make judgements
of how the seasons are progressing, what the weather may do, and so forth,
while simultaneously considering the limited time available. Gardening and
farming take on an extra dimension if one is aware that, besides these mundane
considerations, there are also basic cycles of the heavens to which animals and
the plant world are very much attuned. Plants receive their energy for growth
from the sun but, in other more subtle ways, they are continually affected by

the Moon's ever-changing rhythms. A decision as to when to plant a tree should take such lunar cycles into account, just as a sailor puts to sea only when the tides are right.

With my colleague Simon Best, I produced earlier versions of *Planting by the Moon* in the 1980s. This new edition is concerned to reaffirm our advice, but has several new features in addition. It has, for example, data from years of racehorse breeding which has not hitherto been published. The book is intended as a 'hardy annual' and future editions may not contain the critique of different schools of thought as is here presented. A more detailed work describing the evidence on which it is based is planned shortly. My collaborator Simon Best has been busy elsewhere but may return as co-author in the future as much has developed from our original synthesis.

The idea that the Moon exerts a determinable influence on plant and crop growth may be as old as agriculture. The idea is found embedded in the folklore of many ancient societies, ranging from the Celts in early Britain to the Maoris in New Zealand. As far as recorded comments on the subject are concerned, Pliny the Elder (AD 23–79), the Roman historian, in his *Natural History*[72] gives many instructions on how to regulate agricultural activities according to the cycles of the Moon.

With the dawn of modern science the Moon was reduced to a lifeless orb which influenced nothing but the tides and marine creatures. Beliefs which until then had been taken for granted, that astronomical factors and the changing Moon were important for the growth of crops, became discredited and lingered on only as superstition and old wives' tales. So it remained until relatively recently.

During the twentieth century, systematic experiments began to determine how the various lunar cycles played a part in plant metabolism, growth and development. Certain keys to understanding the relationship of plant response to lunar influence have now emerged and can be incorporated into a gardener's or farmer's plans as to when best to carry out various tasks, in particular sowing, planting* and harvesting.

This manual is presented more as an invitation to gardeners and others to investigate the time cycles involved in plant growth than as a dogmatic statement of how they work. It is an attempt at a synthesis of time-honoured traditions and twentieth-century research. Except where stated, all the advice and knowledge is based on experimentation. This is cited, with explanatory graphs and diagrams where appropriate. Although we are responsible for all the statements that appear in this manual, we would like to acknowledge the influence of the work of the two women, Lili Kolisko (1889–1976) and Maria

---

*Here and throughout the term 'planting' includes the sowing of seed as well as the planting of seedlings.

Thun (*b.* 1922), on our own research and conclusions. While differing from them on some fundamental issues, we nevertheless recognize them as pioneers in lunar-planting research.

There are various astrological and related concepts used in the calendar. Readers unfamiliar with such things need not worry however. Clear step-by-step explanations are given in separate chapters. A star-calendar useful for gardeners is here presented, composed of two kinds of process: on the one hand there are rhythms of energy that pulse, or ebb and flow, in approximately nine-day cycles which should resonate with the sympathetic worker; and there are specific moments, celestial events, which the gardener should endeavour to catch.

It is our hope that this manual will come to be used not only for its practical advantages but also as an inspiration to gardeners to become more aware of the life-rhythms in nature which mysteriously connect the growth of plants with cosmic time-cycles.

Chapter 1

PERSPECTIVES

Pleiades rising in the dawning sky,
     Harvest is nigh.
Pleiades setting in the waning night,
     Ploughing is right.
Forty days and nights in the turning year
     They disappear.
When they shine again in the morning shade,
     Sharpen your blade.

Hesiod, *Works and Days* (Eighth century BC)

PLANTS ARE ADAPTED to the primary cycles of time – the day, the month and the year. This book focuses on the second of these, on the monthly rhythms which are so important for the plant world. These monthly cycles are lunar, in contrast with the day and the year which are solar. It may be a mystery as to how plants respond to these monthly cycles, but that doesn't stop them from being of practical value in farm and garden.

The sensitivity of plants to minute levels of energy was first systematically studied by the Indian scientist Sir Jagadis Chandra Bose (1858–1937) in the early years of this century.[13] Using carefully designed apparatus, he produced a mass of evidence showing that plants have a far greater capacity to respond to subtle environmental stimuli than had previously been believed.

Plants, small animals and birds seem to be attuned to the natural electric and magnetic fields of the Earth. By altering such fields in a laboratory, scientists have been able to alter the rate and other characteristics of a plant's growth, and the direction in which a bird will fly. Earth's geomagnetic field has a large lunar-monthly component to its variation.

The Biosphere

One of the first lunar-cycle effects to be clearly demonstrated was in rainfall. This was reported in 1962, by two independent groups of researchers, one in the northern and one in the southern hemisphere. Their results appeared in *Science* magazine – in the same issue, for mutual support![14] The Moon pulls on the sea according to a twice-monthly rhythm, so that tides reach their highest twice a month, every 14.7 days. Likewise, the amount of rainfall on average also shows a twice-monthly cycle, peaking three or four days after the Full and New positions. The highest tides, for comparison, appear on average a day after the Full and New positions, they have a lag of one day. The two groups of researchers examined a good half-century of data, and found that the magnitude of the lunar effect they had discovered depended on the level of solar activity.

The Earth is surrounded by a large magnetic field, which acts like a membrane which protects us from solar radiation. This pulsates to a monthly rhythm, becoming strongest on the days following the Full Moon – as was again discovered by another two independent US groups.[7,82] The GMF (geomagnetic field) stays low for the week prior to the Full Moon, then it increases sharply, remaining high for some days afterwards.

Thunderstorms recorded by eastern US weather stations over the years 1942–1965 showed a peak two days after the Full Moon,[61] just as did the geomagnetism data. They decreased for a few days before the Full Moon, followed by a sharp increase. Conversely, there was a definite decrease on days following the New Moon. In contrast, a survey of hurricanes and typhoons in the North Atlantic, from 80 years of data, found they tended to occur twenty per cent more frequently on days following both the Full and New Moons.[21]

So, the biosphere as a whole responds to this fundamental cycle, either in a monthly or a fortnightly rhythm. The effect of this pulsation upon climate is science, not just folklore. The changing Sun-Moon angle causes huge electric and magnetic changes in the upper atmosphere. It is therefore little more than common sense to affirm that a farmer should take notice of it.

Traditional Lore

There is a wide but fragmentary body of folk-knowledge, gleaned from many cultures and various ages, that reflects the age-old belief of farmers and gardeners that the Moon somehow influences the growth of their crops. Hesiod, the Greek astronomer and contemporary of Homer, is considered to have written the first lunar agricultural manual, in the eighth century BC. His poem *Works and Days* advised farmers how to regulate many activities by the phases of the Moon.[43] Later, this emphasis on the lunar phases became particularly important to the Roman farmer. Lunar planting rules were recorded by such writers as Cato and Pliny.[83] The primary rules, many of which have persisted in folklore to this day, focus on the differences between the effects of the waxing and waning Moon.

Basically, whatever required growth or development was started during the waxing phase, and whatever needed to dry, cure or decrease without decay was dealt with in the waning. Just before New Moon, at the dark of the Moon, was said to be especially favourable for the latter activities. Thus, the planting of crops, picking of grapes for wine and shearing of sheep were carried out during the waxing Moon, and the general harvesting of crops, felling of timber and castration of animals during the waning phase.

Pliny was a keen observer of nature, shown by his multi-volume *History of Nature*. He believed he could discern how, 'that tiny creature the ant, at the moon's conjunction keeps quite quiet, but at full moon works busily even in the nights.'[72] If there was a problem with the ground being damp, then Pliny's advice was to sow seeds in the waning half of the lunar cycle so that it might dry out. Seventeenth-century British gardening guides quoted Pliny in this regard.[44]

The various facets of lunar lore were transmitted, both verbally and in scattered writings, down through the ages and across cultures to the present, although modern collections of these adages illustrate markedly the confusion of ideas in this area.[5] Grafting and planting-out operations should be performed during the waxing Moon, because rising sap is said to aid the formation of new shoots or the establishment of a new graft. Lawns are said to benefit from being sown during the waxing phase, a time also propitious for the transplanting of trees and flowers. One of the oldest maxims using the waxing/waning division with respect to planting is as follows: crops which produce their yield above ground should be planted during the waxing Moon, whereas those that produce below ground should be sown during the waning Moon. This idea can be found in many parts of the world, but so can similar ideas which modify or contradict it.

In particular, it is claimed that sowing around the Full or New Moon will improve crop growth. Here again opinions vary: for example, some advocate planting in the days immediately preceding the New Moon so that seeds will have germinated and be ready to grow as the Moon begins to increase. More widespread is the opposite opinion, that crops should be sown just before the Full Moon, the view particularly associated with the work of Lili Kolisko. She came to Britain from Germany in 1936, and the results of her years of study were published in 1938–9[51,52] claiming that seed germination, and especially the unfolding of the first leaves of young shoots, pointed to the days prior to Full Moon as an optimal sowing-time, while those prior to New Moon were the worst, or rather slowest, in growth.

However, as will be discussed in Chapter 4, although Moon phase does affect plant metabolism, there is little reliable evidence that sowing at any particular point in the lunar-phase cycle will influence the final yield. Seedling germination and growth may increase around and especially just before the Full Moon, but such effects may not show up in the final crop yield. Much of the confusion of traditional beliefs may have arisen from such a confounding of different aspects of plant growth.

That crops should be harvested according to the phase of the Moon was widely accepted by farmers of antiquity. Pliny the Elder described the then customary practice of harvesting crops needed for storage near the New Moon, when they would be driest and preserve the best, or gathering those that were to be eaten fresh at Full Moon:

> for it makes a very great difference whether one wants to store the crop or put it on the market, because grain increases in bulk when the Moon is waxing.

The very same view was current in seventeenth-century England:

> he [the farmer] shall gather and carry into his house whatsoever he would have to endure and last long, at such times as the Moone shall decrease.[35]

In more recent times, it used to be a common custom in the west of England to gather in the 'hoard fruit' in the shrinking of the Moon. Apples bruised in the harvesting would then tend to preserve better over the winter. This accords with modern studies showing varying plant water-absorption at the different phases, suggesting that some facets of lunar lore may be vindicated by modern research.

The Four Elements

At the present time, a variety of lunar gardening guides is available but, alas, they disagree over just about every recommendation they give. Despite this, there would seem to be one thing which they have in common: they all use some notion of the fourfold division of the zodiac into periods that each influence a particular element (earth, air, fire and water). This means that they all have a nine-day rhythm for sowing crops – let's explain that.

The scheme here used has developed within the context of Bio-Dynamic farming, which has the longest tradition of organic gardening in the twentieth century.[30] It was founded in 1924 by the Austrian teacher and philosopher Rudolf Steiner (1861–1925), the founder of the Anthroposophist movement. It attempts to use holistic principles, viewing the farm as an integral whole and taking account of the condition of the cosmos.[77]

At the core of the Bio Dynamic calendar is a four-element pattern, generated by the motion of the Moon against the stars. Each month, the Moon moves around the sky against the twelve constellations of the zodiac. This means that every two or three days it enters a new constellation, each of which has its particular affinity with one of the four elements.

The elements are Earth, Water, Air and Fire and these are deemed to influence the growth and performance of a particular sort of plant, respectively root, leaf, flower and fruit or seed. This model is specifically a four-element theory, in which the further division into the twelve signs of the zodiac is very

EARTH ELEMENT: ROOT

Taurus   *Virgo*   *Capricorn*

WATER ELEMENT: LEAF

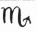

Cancer   *Scorpio*   *Pisces*

AIR ELEMENT: FLOWER

  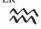

Gemini   *Libra*   *Aquarius*

FIRE ELEMENT: FRUIT OR SEED

Aries   *Leo*   *Sagittarius*

much secondary. It is a modern application of a very ancient idea, that of the four elements. There are parallels in the discovery by scientists that there are twelve types of 'fundamental' particles, or in the description by biochemists of four types of code in the DNA strand, or in physicists' four states of matter – solid, liquid, gas and plasma (hot, and above the atmosphere) – just as Jungian psychology has four temperaments. So this elemental theory underpinning our understanding of plant growth uses four types of 'formative force'. These form-forces link time of sowing to the final condition of the crop when it is harvested.

For readers new to the idea, let's just say: first one builds a house, establishing the foundations and structure – Earth. Then one fits in the water supply (Water). Next one checks out that it will be adequately ventilated (Air) and lastly one fits in the heating and electricity (Fire). It's quite natural: in fact, it's elementary.

The ancient Greeks applied the theory in their four temperaments, much used in their medical practice. The melancholic was pensive and prone to depression (Earth), while a choleric character was impulsive and fiery and of thin and wiry build. A phlegmatic character (Water) was emotionally sensitive but prone to becoming overweight.

The four-element theory was first expressed by Empedocles in the fifth century BC in Sicily (shortly before he jumped into Mount Etna). Mother Nature used the four elements to paint with, he explained, in a long poem, just as an artist uses four colours. He didn't say what the four colours were! In fire and wind, in sea and

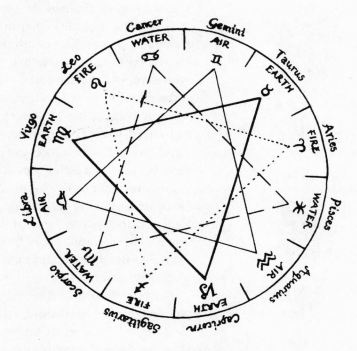

Figure 1. The four-element cycle underlying the zodiac.

stone, Empedocles discerned this fourfold pattern. He would surely have appreciated the new twist to his theory in the twentieth century.

What are here called root-days are the times to sow carrots, potatoes and the like. These days occur, for example, when the Moon passes in front of the stars of Taurus, the Bull, when the Moon is said to be 'in' Taurus. Taurus is viewed as having an 'earth' type of energy, and this earth-type of energy is linked with sowing root-crops – hence, 'root-days'. So, the root-days have an astronomical definition, and are timed by the Moon's motion against the stars.

There are three constellations linked to the Earth element, spaced equally around the circle of the zodiac. Taurus, we have mentioned. The other two are Virgo (the Virgin) and Capricorn (the Goat). Because it takes 27 days for the Moon to go once round (as will be explained in the next chapter), one set of root-days for planting potatoes will turn up every nine days. The diagram shows the sky-triangle that maps the three Earth-signs.

Lettuce or broccoli are sown or planted on leaf-days, these being times when the Moon is in front of the constellations that have traditionally been viewed as 'watery'. The three water constellations of the zodiac are Pisces (the Fish), Cancer (the Crab) and Scorpio (the Scorpion). In exactly the same manner as the constellations that are reckoned to influence the earth element, they form a triangle in the sky. Thus, the 27-day orbit of the moon against the stars produces three periods of the same element. So, if the weather is unsuitable for sowing lettuce, one just waits for the next set of 'leaf-days', nine days later. Flower-days (Air) and fruit-seed days (Fire, or Warmth) complete the picture.

Calendars based upon this four-element structure have been published and acted upon for more than 30 years. Their utility and accuracy are beginning to acquire a time-tested quality. Some reports of long-term trials are described below.

In using this model, our calendar assumes that there are four types of crop:

Root-days
Element: EARTH
Example of crop: carrot, radish, potato
Moon-constellation: Taurus, Virgo, Capricorn

Leaf-days
Element: WATER
Example of crop: lettuce, cabbage
Moon-constellation: Scorpio, Cancer, Pisces

Flower-days
Element: AIR
Example of crop: cauliflower, globe artichoke, broccoli
Moon-constellation: Gemini, Libra, Aquarius

Fruit/seed-days
Element: FIRE
Example of crop: tomato, peas, beans
Moon-constellation: Leo, Aries, Sagittarius

One can visualize this as a sequence of plant development: first the root descends into the soil (Earth), then the leaves unfold, with water flowing up the stem and transpiring out through the leaves (Water). Then come the flowers, emitting their fragrance to attract bees and butterflies to fertilize them (Air). Lastly, the flowers fall away as the heat of the summer shrivels up the plant, drying it into the final stage of the seed (Fire). The tiny seeds contain the essence of the flower, just as fire is the least material or least dense of the four elements. Biologically, one may prefer to view the last stage as Warmth rather than Fire, emphasizing its constructive role in a process of maturation.

As a sequence in time, this goes root-days, flower-days, leaf-days and then fruit/seed-days. This repeats every nine days. The calendar is concerned with the zodiac in terms of this 'elementary' division according to the four elements.

The theory is that in nature there are four kinds of subtle-energy 'formative forces', which work to influence the way a plant will develop, and that these are activated by the Moon's passage through the zodiac-elements, as the seed is sown. This pattern of influence is to do with the stars, the real stars, and not with the zodiac used in modern sun-sign astrology. This is a difficult issue, and readers who wish to grapple with it may do so in Chapter 5.

Using a star-rhythm in a calendar sounds OK, one may say, but does it work? Chapter 4 looks at the evidence but, for now, let's just note that in 1979 the result of eight years of sowing experiments appeared, co-authored by Maria Thun (pronounced 'Toon'), who pioneered the theory back in 1956,[89] and statistician Dr Hans Heinze.[90] Each year, they had sown twelve rows of potatoes per lunar month, and then compared their final yields. These trials showed a zodiac rhythm in weight-yield per row that was highly significant. All of the debate and all of the evidence concerns this very physical thing, the final weight-yield of rows of vegetables. The distant stars are supposed to be doing this, which some readers may find credulity-straining. I did.

Such crop-yield experiments use twelve, or even twenty-four or thirty-six, rows of a given type of vegetable, each grown for the same length of time. It was always a surprise that it was the zodiac rhythm and not a moon-phase effect which showed up in the final yields.[56] That is hardly what traditional lore would predict. But organic growers are concerned with quality rather than mere quantity, and the biggest vegetables may not be the tastiest, so we will also be looking at 'quality' in this context.

This element-cycle (whose framework is 'sidereal' – see next chapter) is one of the two fundamental lunar cycles relevant for a lunar-gardening calendar. The other is the better-known waxing-waning lunar month of 29.5 days, which influences fertility, germination, water absorption and metabolism.[42] (NB, there does not exist any 28-day lunar cycle, contrary to widespread belief.) Chapter 3 looks at the evidence for this primary cycle affecting living things and why a modern grower should take notice of it. The sidereal rhythm is especially relevant to organic gardening. There are indications that it requires a decent 'living' soil for the element-rhythm to work; whereas, in contrast, lunar-phase effects will turn up anywhere!

Belief in the Moon's influence on the fertility of plants was once firmly embedded in the consciousness of ancient peoples. As science comes again to discover these subtle links between earth and sky farmers may again regard the application of lunar cycles as a sensible and valuable practice.

Chapter 2

CYCLES OF THE SKY

Time faire, to sowe or to gather be bold,
  but set or remoove when the weather is cold.
Cut all thing or gather, the Moone in the wane,
  but sowe in encreasing, or give it his bane.

Thomas Tusser, *Five Hundred Points of Good Husbandry* (1573)

As WE LOOK AT the stars scattered across the night sky, and the ever-changing visage of the silvery Moon, we cannot but be struck by a sense of the primal mystery of the Cosmos. Are we linked to it in some fundamental way, or is that only wishful thinking? What of the ancient doctrine, 'as above, so below'? Why does that Moon always face us, and why is it the same apparent size as the Sun? How did it get into that nearly circular path so far away from us, far too large to be a proper satellite of Earth, more like a companion planet?

The Moon's motion can be expressed in terms of four main, monthly cycles. These describe its motion in relation to the Sun (synodic), to the stars (sidereal), to the Earth (apogee-perigee) and to the ecliptic plane (nodal). Let's look at them one by one.

The Synodic or Phase Cycle (Moon-Sun)

As the Moon waxes and wanes each month, it mirrors the Sun's light from different angles – the best known lunar cycle. It takes twenty-nine and a half

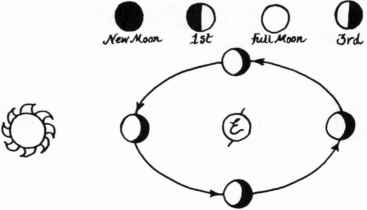

Figure 2. The synodic or phase cycle.

days to do this. When Full, the Moon is opposite to the Sun in the sky, so that as it rises, the Sun sets. The four positions of the Full, New and quarter-moons each month are shown in the calendar.

There are usually twelve Full Moons in a year. The months were originally lunar, and still are in the Jewish and Muslim calendars. To keep them in step with the solar year, a thirteenth month was added in every third year. This is called, intercalation. Muslims don't do this, so their twelve lunar months move round, with respect to the seasons, by eleven or so days every year.

Our two luminaries meet together in the sky at New Moon, when it becomes impossible to see the Moon for several days, because it is close to the Sun. The Greek word *synodos* means meeting. Let us note that this word also signified copulation, pointing to the deep connection this cycle has to germination and fertility. The next chapter will discuss this matter.

The Sidereal Cycle (Moon-Star)

Once in 27.3 days the Moon orbits around the Earth against the fixed stars. In this time, called a sidereal month (from the Latin, *sidera*, star) it returns to the same part of the heavens as seen from Earth. It also revolves on its own axis in this same period, enabling it to keep facing the Earth.

The Moon moves against the same background of star-constellations as do the other planets. It orbits around the Earth in a plane fairly similar to that in which the Earth and planets orbit around the Sun (called the Ecliptic). These constellations against which the Moon and planets are seen to move are therefore of special importance. Since ancient times they have been regarded

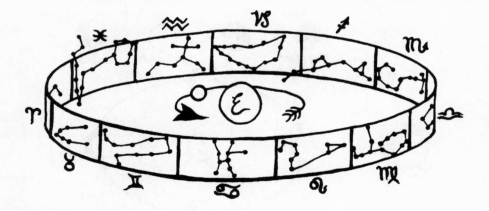

Figure 3. The sidereal cycle.

as divided into twelve, the twelve constellations of the zodiac. The Moon thus spends two to three days in each zodiacal constellation.

Chapter 4 describes how this cycle works in agriculture, then Chapter 5 looks at it from a different viewpoint, that of the 'sidereal' zodiac on which this calendar is based. This cycle has a special link with the four elements described earlier, as these colour the signs of the sidereal zodiac. Sky-triangles are thereby formed, and there is a handy German word, 'trigon,' by which Bio-Dynamic users refer to the three periods in a 'sidereal' month which influence the same element, for example the three sets of leaf-days.

The Apogee-Perigee Cycle (Moon-Earth)

The Moon moves around the Earth in an elliptical orbit, which means its distance from the Earth varies considerably through the month. Every 27.2 days it reaches its apogee, furthest away from the Earth, then at its perigee draws closest. At perigee it appears larger in the sky, pulls on the tides more strongly, and moves faster against the stars. This causes the time which the Moon spends in each of the twelve zodiacal divisions to vary by more than 30 per cent in a single rotation. At perigee, the Moon is moving fastest and it takes only two days to pass through one zodiacal division, whereas at apogee, when moving slowest, it takes almost three.

This cycle cannot be seen in the sky, as the change in size of the Moon's visage is too small to notice. Its effect can be seen in the calendar, however, whereby the Moon spends the least time moving through a sign at perigee, and the longest at apogee.

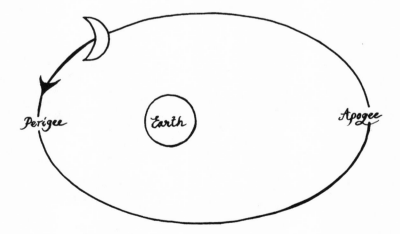

Figure 4. The apogee-perigee cycle.

The Nodal Cycle (Moon-Ecliptic)

The planets revolve around the Sun in approximately the same plane, the ecliptic, and the Moon's orbit is tilted at a slight angle, about five degrees, to this plane . This means that each month it rises above and then sinks below the Ecliptic. The two points at which it crosses the Ecliptic in each 27.5-day period are called nodes. When moving from south to north of the Ecliptic, the Moon reaches its north node and, when moving from north to south, its south node.

Eclipses can occur when the Moon reaches these points, and the ecliptic is so named because eclipses happen when Sun, Moon and Earth are in line and on this plane. When the Moon becomes New or Full close to a node, there will be, respectively, a solar or lunar eclipse. A solar eclipse draws a thin pencil of darkness upon the Earth, and its 'zone of totality' is confined to that line – such as passed over the south-western England on August 11th 1999. A lunar eclipse, in contrast, is a reddish shadow that passes across the Moon, and is visible from one-half of the Earth.

The north and south nodes were called Dragon's Head and Dragon's Tail, respectively, indicating a belief that they were two special power points in the Moon's orbit – as if a menacing dragon were curled round the zodiac liable to swallow the Sun at some unpredictable moment.

A traditional British gardening guide advised readers to avoid sowing seeds 'over the dragon's tail' – the South Node – whereas the dragon's head was an acceptable time for these undertakings. This calendar, in common with Bio-Dynamic calendars, makes no distinction between the two lunar moments, advising avoidance of both of them at sowing time.

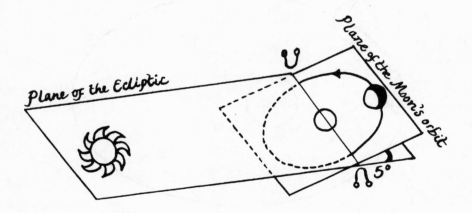

Figure 5. The nodal cycle.

The Moon 'Riding High'

The sidereal, monthly rhythm also expresses the varying height to which the Moon climbs above the horizon. On one day each month it arcs highest across the sky, and remains above the horizon for the longest time, then a fortnight later sinks to its least height above the horizon. American lunar-gardening manuals refer to these two halves of the month as 'riding high' and 'riding low.' The effect is very latitude-dependent, so in Scotland and northern countries one's experience of this cycle is more pronounced. There, the Moon hardly sets at one end of the month, then a fortnight later hardly rises.

Bio-Dynamic calendars allude to the two halves of this cycle as ascending, and descending. This reflects the Moon's monthly journey around the zodiac; the observed variation in its arc is due to the Earth's axis being tilted at an angle to the Ecliptic. It is the 27.3 day sidereal cycle viewed with reference to the Moon's height above the observer's horizon. The cycle gets confused with that of the waxing and waning Moon, and may account for similar recommendations to the above being ascribed to the waxing Moon period by English and American folklore.

This cycle mirrors the annual cycle of the Sun: in midwinter the Sun remains low above the horizon, and is then in front of the zodiac stars of Sagittarius, whereas in midsummer it rises high in the sky and is 'in' the constellation of Gemini. In midwinter, the Full Moon rises highest in the night sky, and it will then be 'in' the Gemini constellation, when the Sun, directly opposite, is in Sagittarius. Conversely, the midsummer Full Moon hangs very low above the horizon, in the constellation of Sagittarius. This cycle fades away near the Equator, then in the southern hemisphere is reversed, with both Sun and Moon rising highest against the stars of Sagittarius.

Bio-Dynamic calendars are characterized by their use of this cycle. They take the view that the planting-out of seedlings should be done in its 'descending' half.

The Harvest Moon

Each September a Full Moon appears, of special importance to farmers: the Harvest Moon. It rises for a week or so just around sunset, providing those extra few hours of illumination that can be so valuable at this time of year. Hanging large and low in the evening sky it often seems especially bright.

At the Autumnal equinox (about September 23rd) as the Sun crosses the equator into the southern hemisphere, the Ecliptic (the path of the Sun) is tilted at its lowest angle to the horizon. So the zodiac belt, containing the orbits of the Moon and planets, runs low above the horizon. For this astronomical reason, the Moon at this time rises only about 12 minutes later each day – whereas on average throughout the year it rises about 50 minutes later each day. Thus, at this time of harvesting, the Moon continues to rise soon after sunset for a number of successive evenings.

The Harvest Moon was held to be responsible for the ripening of produce, and, to the Romans, Diana's day fell at the time of the Harvest Full Moon, when offerings were made to her to ensure the ripening of their fruits. Seen through autumnal mists, the Moon often assumes a yellow hue. It then appears large in the sky due to its remaining close to the horizon, just as the Sun appears larger at sunset. The following Full Moon in October is called Hunter's Moon.

Use of a star-calendar has the advantage that it gives one a motivation for looking at the heavens. Anyone can recognize Orion and the Plough, but what about Taurus and Gemini? The ecliptic is that path through the constellations, along which the heavenly bodies move. In the afterglow of sunset, if the Moon and one or two planets are visible, one can trace its path as a line through the sky along which the Sun, Moon and planets all travel. Most of what is used in this calendar is visible to the naked eye in the sky above your garden.

Chapter 3

THE MOON AND FERTILITY

The thirteenth of the waxing month
Is a bad day to start seeding
But the best for transplanting.

Hesiod, *Works and Days.*

Figs, olives, apples, pears, vines can be planted at new moon, in the afternoon,
when there is no south wind.

Cato, *On Farming*

In bringing together this gardening guide, we take the view that modern
research gives sufficient basis to begin to sift the wheat from the chaff in these
old traditions. This is in itself a fairly new situation. For long it has appeared
that scientific belief and old lunar lore clashed completely, the former invali-
dating the latter.[7] But in recent decades a distinct change can be noted.[10]
Scientists are prepared to discuss how subtle changes in the Earth's magnetic
field are detected by organisms, investigate how birds use the lines of the
magnetic field for navigation and how they use certain star-constellations for
orientating themselves at night-time on their long migrations.[20] The germination of seeds has been found to depend upon the direction in which they are
aligned with respect to the magnetic field of the Earth. In this climate of
thought it no longer seems sheer moonshine to say that rhythms astronomical
in origin are important to a gardener.

'There seems little doubt that the lunar cycle influences the life processes
of plants,' wrote Dr Bernard Dixon, former editor of the *New Scientist*.[29] Dr
Dixon was referring to the Moon-phase cycle which affects many of the
growth-processes in a plant: its metabolic rate, absorption of water and
nutrients, rate of growth and its electrical activity have all been observed to
fluctuate in accordance with this rhythm.[18,54] This is of enormous significance
to farmers and gardeners.

The Phase Cycle and Plant Growth

The rate at which seeds germinate in relation to lunar phases was first studied
systematically in the 1930s by Kolisko, who concluded that wheat germinated
faster when sown at Full Moon than at New Moon.[51] Confirmation of this
result appeared in studies by M. Maw, funded by Canada's Department of
Agriculture, on the rate at which cress germinated. Over a six-month period,

25

batches of cress grown in water usually germinated quickest at Full Moon and slowest at New Moon, the difference in rate being very marked.[66]

Lunar-phase rhythms also appear in the rate at which plants grow, as was shown by Giorgio Abrami at the botanical gardens of Padua University.[3] Using several different species of herbaceous plants, taking a measure of their stem lengths every few days, he found, after applying a correction for daily temperature variations, that there were growth rhythms which, although different from one species to another, were phased according to Full and New Moon positions. Growth rates tended to be maximal at either the Full or New Moon positions.

Traditionally, it has always been assumed that sap in plants and trees rose most markedly during the Full Moon. Therefore, activities such as tree-felling should be performed at New Moon, and crops would preserve best if harvested at New Moon due to minimal water content. While direct evidence from studies of sap in trees and shrubs is scant, a study by Professor Frank Brown and Carol Chow investigated day-to-day variations in the absorption of water by bean seeds, under temperature-controlled conditions at their laboratory in North-western University, Illinois.[17] Each day, the amount of water the seeds absorbed over a four-hour period was measured. Large maxima were found to occur just before the Full Moon, absorption being on average 35 per cent higher than at New Moon.

Using wheat and pinto beans as her focus, a three-year study by Dr Jane Panzer, a biologist at Tulane University in the USA, confirmed the Brown and Chow findings regarding water absorption.[70] She found distinct lunar-related rhythms in water uptake, comparable to those Brown and his colleagues had

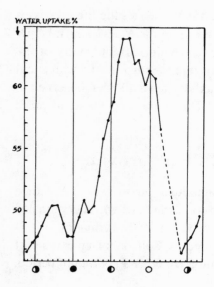

Figure 6. Water uptake by bean seeds (after Brown and Chow, 1973).

demonstrated, also a smaller effect observed with pinto beans which had been sterilized: The lunar link persisted, although to a lesser degree, even using pinto beans that had first been pasteurized or sterilized. She identified seasonal variations in this cycle of water uptake, as well as a rhythm in seed germination that mirrored the monthly patterns found for water absorption.

Biochemist Dr Harry Rounds at Wichita State University in the US reported that stress hormones in the blood of mice and men decreased sharply at Full and New Moon. He then extracted similar stress-related, 'cardio-acceleratory' substances from the leaves of various plants, especially geraniums, and found that their potency changed sharply for a short period following the Full and New Moon.[76] His research is relevant to the traditional advice that medicinal herbs should be picked at such times.

An important biochemical study was reported in 1989 from the University of Paris. It concerned a lunar pulse in plant DNA.[75] Plant chromosomes, inside the nucleus of every cell, are large, much bigger than in animal cells. Two different types of structure were reported from X-ray studies. One, whose function is more related to storage of carbohydrates, was more developed at New Moon. Another type, more closely related to flowering and growth functions, was more developed at the Full Moon. This DNA response in plants is relevant to the traditional connection of the lunar cycle with fertility and growth.

A plant's metabolism can be assessed by how much oxygen it absorbs from the air. This was investigated in the classic experiments of Professor Frank Brown in which potatoes and carrots were maintained in the dark over quite long periods, with the ambient conditions of temperature, humidity and pressure held constant.[16] Through the years, he patiently charted over a million hours of potato time! From this, it emerged that the potatoes, although sealed from all light, were not at all in the dark about the cycles of the Sun and Moon. The Moon's daily rising and culmination (reaching its highest point in the sky) appeared as the hours of maximum metabolic rate for these root vegetables. In addition, their metabolic rate waxed and waned with the monthly lunar cycle: potato metabolism over the two weeks around the Full Moon was on average fifteen per cent higher than that around the New Moon. For carrots the figure was eleven per cent.

Specific aspects of plant growth may respond to different parts of the phase cycle. An experiment by T.M. Lai, looking at nutrient absorption by corn seedlings according to lunar phase, was reported in the US journal *Bio-dynamics*.[59] The amounts of potassium and phosphorus, two nutrients vitally important for plant growth, absorbed over a one-week growth period, were measured for six months. The amount of phosphorus which the plants were absorbing peaked at Full Moons and was least during the New Moons. For potassium, this was the other way around. Phosphorus is acidic and root-nourishing, while potassium is required more by flowers and is alkaline (a higher pH), so there is an interesting polarity here.

A growing plant builds up an electrical field around it, in which the electrical potential at its top differs from that at the ground. This was investigated by Harold Burr, a professor at the Yale University School of Medicine. Burr found that measuring such weak electrical fields in humans could lead to better prediction of the time of ovulation in women and an enhanced ability to diagnose the early stage of cancers.[20]

Burr decided to record the electrical potentials of trees by placing electrodes in their trunks.[19] The first thing he discovered was that fluctuations in potential were the same for all trees he investigated over a large area. Surprisingly, these were apparently unrelated to fluctuations in barometric pressure, humidity, or the weather. He then monitored the potential of a single beech tree over a nine-year period, and this clearly showed that the dominant rhythm was tidal, i.e. of 14.7 days, and that it peaked at the Full and New positions. A further analysis of this nine-year experiment was performed by his student Ralph Markson, which showed that the tree's electrical activity was also responding to the level of solar activity (sunspots) but that the lunar cycles were stronger than these solar effects.[20]

Bees are well adapted to the lunar month in their flight activity. Counters were fixed to beehive entrances by M. Oehmke, a biologist at the Goethe University, Frankfurt. Through the course of the year, these showed a huge lunar fluctuation in bee activity.[69] This varied a bit between species, one being at least twice as busy at New Moon as at the Full. Bee activity fertilizes flowers, reminding us of the connection between the synodic cycle and fertility. Surely this matter is just as fascinating as the bee-dance, whereby bees communicate directions for finding flowers to their fellows, even on cloudy days, using the vector of plane-polarized sunlight

At Lyons University, botanist Dr E. Graviou measured the small amount of oxygen which seeds use in respiration when kept in darkness at a constant temperature, when apparently they are quite dormant.[42] With tomato and other seeds she found that maximum oxygen absorption tended to occur bimonthly, at Full and New Moon.

Nowadays, when we speak of a month we forget the lunar origin of this term, and do not consider the life-rhythms in all living things linked to this monthly cycle. No doubt man, in his mechanical environment, responds less to it than do other living things.[30] 'On the days of the Full Moon, something colossal is taking place on Earth,' averred Rudolf Steiner in his 'Agriculture' lectures of 1924, adding the important corollary, 'these forces spring up and shoot into all the growth of plants, but they are unable to do so unless rainy days have gone before.[80] Plants, in spite of man-made changes, still live and grow attuned to this primary cosmic rhythm. The various results reported here show that there operates in plant growth a complex of different rhythms related to the Moon's synodic cycle and that the time of Full Moon is especially important for them. Around this time a plant's metabolic rate and water absorption are at their greatest.

We have seen how laboratory studies indicate that a higher rate and speed of germination is attained if seeds are sown just before or around the Full Moon and, to a lesser degree, if sown over the New Moon; also that seeds and plants absorb water optimally around this part of the lunar month. In countries where drought is endemic this would have some bearing on the success of a crop and may have reinforced the idea that all plants should be sown around Full Moon.

Female Fertility

Many ancient and modern societies believe that women and their biological functions are intimately connected with the cycles of the Moon. The period of human gestation which, from conception to birth averages 266 days, is precisely nine lunar months, reminding us of the mysterious connection which this cycle has with fertility.[25]

The average length of the female menstrual cycle is 29.5 days, i.e. the lunar month, not 28 days as is normally averred. The most common period length is indeed around 27 days but, overall, large-scale surveys have shown the mean to be indistinguishable from the lunar month.[94,97] This is notably so during the peak childbearing years, when the subjects were in their twenties, whereas the mean period length becomes much longer for girls under twenty and is a couple of days shorter for women in their forties.

In general, women with cycle lengths near to the lunar month period of 29.5 days tend to be the most fertile.[26] Also, women tend unconsciously to synchronize their periods when living together.[68] Selecting the sub-group of women with cycles near to the lunar length, between 28–31 days (about one-third of the total), it was apparent that they had a tendency to ovulate at one or other end of the lunar cycle, in other words to have a link either to the Full or New Moons.[25] All these things could imply that the cycle of womankind once had some large degree of synchrony and moved in accordance with the waxing and waning Moon. Then, indeed, the Moon would have been experienced as a fertility goddess. Whether or not this was so, it is a fact that, in ancient societies, agricultural practice did move in tune to the monthly cycle of the Moon[83] and that belief in the power of the Moon to induce fertility and growth was very widespread.

Such findings, and the ancient association of the New Moon with menstruation and the Full Moon with ovulation, led to the expectation that more babies would be born around the Full Moon phase of the cycle, which some modern research has confirmed.[62] After all, ancient traditions linking the Moon with fertility find some support from modern evidence. Such traditions apply equally to the sowing of seed and the fertility of the soil.

Full Moon and Animal Husbandry

> Geld hogs, steers, rams and kids when the Moon is waning.
> Pliny, *History of Nature.*

It seems that even nowadays many farmers who have never heard of Pliny's recommendations still follow them regarding castration and other surgery on animals, fearing complications due to excessive bleeding at Full Moon. There is some medical evidence to support this practice. Some years ago a doctor in the United States investigated a group of 1,000 operations which had been performed in his hospital.[4] For all the operations in which complications from bleeding occurred he noted the Moon's phase at the time they had been performed. To his surprise he found that at least four times more occurred at Full Moon than at New Moon. He analysed other groups of operations and obtained the same striking result. From this data it appears that the period around the New Moon is indeed the optimal time for such operations, and that the Full Moon period should definitely be avoided.

Horse breeding

> [Farmers] notice the aspects of the Moon, when at full, in order to direct the copulation of their herds and flocks, and the setting of plants or sowing of seeds: and there is not an individual who considers these general precautions as impossible or unprofitable.
> Ptolemy, *Tetrabiblos*, Ch. III

In the Middle Ages, the Arabs were the finest horse breeders in Europe and the Near East. Their subtle understanding of astrology may well have helped them in this breeding process. Then, in the eighteenth-century, Britain out-bred the Arabs, creating the finest racehorses in the world. The UK is presently slowly losing this edge, partly because, with the price of top stallions at several million pounds apiece, they are falling to Japanese and American buyers.

The sex life of racehorses is uniquely documented and published. Nine years of such data were acquired by the author from a thoroughbred studfarm with a throughput of several hundred matings a year. Each mare is covered several times per season until it conceives, though a few per cent remain barren.

Like cows, horses ovulate every three weeks through the breeding season. Veterinary surgeons can tell within 48 hours or so if conception has occurred,

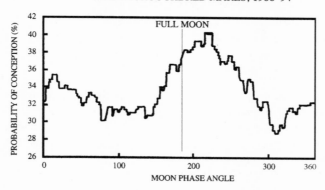

HORSE FERTILITY: FIRST COVERING ONLY
1592 THOROUGHBRED MARES, 1986–94

Figure 7.

therefore the record of mare coverings is a record of their times of ovulation. There is a tendency for horses to become synchronized in their ovulation, hence a studfarm tends to become more busy at three-week intervals. In this horses resemble many creatures in the wild where the females of a species tend to ovulate in synchrony.

Using hormones, vets have unnaturally shifted the season of œstrus (coming on heat) so that it begins in February. Gestation in horses takes eleven months and in the wild they would not foal until May, only dropping their young when the frosts were over. Normally they would be on heat in the summertime.

To analyse this data by Moon phase, only the first covering per mare per season was used, and scored by whether or not conception occurred. The probability of conception is less than 40 per cent at this first covering. The diagram plots this probability around the lunar cycle (a 'moving average' has been put through the data). It clearly peaks just after the Full Moon.

Thus, three- and four-week rhythms of fertility interact in a horse population, as the mares come on heat in the spring. The former expresses a biochemical cycle within the horses, while the latter responds to the opposition of the two luminaries in the sky. There was also a tendency for horse œstrus to peak somewhere around Full Moon, being then in the region of ten per cent more than at New Moon.

There is a seasonal trend in horse fertility, which makes the Full Moon in June the most fertile time of the year for thoroughbreds. One appreciates that not many readers may have such creatures to breed, but for one's pet gerbil or whatever the same principle should apply.

Harvest Time

Traditions link the time of harvesting crops to the Full or New Moons. One may believe that water and metabolic rhythms connected to this cycle should affect the final condition of a crop. Roman and Greek beliefs on this have already been touched upon. As an instance of modern awareness of lunar rhythms, here is the account of a Sydney-based company on the subject of their tomato harvests (personal communication):

> We are growers of tomatoes, on a relatively large acreage, and found throughout the years that, during the period of the Full Moon, a noticeable change takes place in the maturing and colouring of tomatoes. This quickening maturity, irrespective of temperature, only takes place two or three days before and after the Moon has reached its fullness.
>
> During this period, market places on the east and south coastal states have an influx of coloured fruit where in normal times there is a high percentage of green and semi-coloured fruit. We have tested this out on many occasions and our statistics over many years have shown more fruit passing through our packing house through these periods and that the fruit is much more forward in colour. These conclusions may well echo the experience of many growers.

Such a clearly perceived effect surely reflects the more regular and predictable climate of Australia: one tends not to find so definite a view expressed by British tomato growers.

For crops that are to be dried, where juiciness and high water content is not required, at or just before New Moon seems the appropriate time for harvesting. Thus, the great French herbalist Maurice Messeng always picked his herbs at this time.[67] He dried the herbs before use and believed that their virtue would preserve best if picked then.

Moonstamp for Timber

A related practice which can be traced back to antiquity is that of felling timber at the New Moon. The founder of the US Cycles Foundation in Pittsburgh described how in South America the Moon phase at which timber is felled was stamped on the wood, the idea being that New Moon timber preserves better and cuts more easily than that felled at Full Moon.[28] French law from 1669 until the Revolution specifically required that timber be felled only during a waning Moon, a practice directly echoing the words of the Roman historian, Plutarch:

> The Moon showeth her power most evidently in those bodies which have neither sense nor lively breath; for carpenters reject the timber of trees fallen in the Full Moon as being soft and tender, subject also to the worm and putrefaction, and that quickly by means of excessive moisture.

Accounts of this practice (discussed in Kolisko's *Agriculture of Tomorrow*) give the impression that the effect is more evident in tropical or near-tropical regions. The experience of the Australian Bio-Dynamic farmer, Alex Podolinsky, is relevant:

> There is more water in trees and grass and all plants towards full moon than towards new moon. In the old days good timber cutters chopping down valuable timber would never cut other than towards the new moon. They would not cut towards full moon, the timber was not as good. If we cut hay we also cut as much as possible towards new moon and not towards full moon. We get much better quality hay that way.[73]

On the Trout Farm

It isn't just plants that have their fortnightly rhythms of growth. Trout in an aquarium grow to a rhythm whereby their weight peaks just before the Full and New positions.[37] This was shown using several hundred small trout, and weighing them every four days, as they grew – a commendably simple experiment.

Fish respond biochemically to the lunar cycle. Salmon and some species of trout hatch in fresh water and at a certain stage of their lives transform to become ocean-dwelling salt-water fish. Salmon fisheries need to be able to predict this event, as they have to release hatchery-reared fish into the river shortly before it occurs. The thyroid hormone thyroxine triggers this big moment in the salmon's life and there is a specific New Moon in the spring which precipitates this hormone surge.[41] If the salmon wish to swim down the river without being seen by predators then a New Moon is the optimal time of month for them. This was discovered by zoologists at the University of California who concluded that a lunar calendar was essential for efficient culture of this economically valuable resource.

Back in the 1920s, an American called John Knight developed his theory about when to fish.[58] He posited that fish feed only twice a day when the Moon either culminates (reaches its highest point) or reaches its nadir (lowest point below the horizon). For avid Izaak Waltons, the correct time to indulge their art can be calculated from the calendar below. The time of moonrise each day is given and, very roughly, the zenith and nadir can be found by adding or subtracting six hours from them. Nifty footwork is required to make sure the correct local times are worked out as our calendar is based on GMT.

Knight's theory didn't just apply to fish, he explained. Animals, including humans, would become more active and have more energy at these times than at any other time of day. A recent review of this theory by Michael Theroux concluded that:

As you become familiar with these Solunar periods [Knight's term for daily moonrise and culmination] you will also begin to notice how many other daily events are directed by the moon's influence. Once the connection has been made, there is no turning back.[86]

Power of the Nodes

To remind the reader, the lunar nodes are the two places where the moon crosses the ecliptic each month. We see the ecliptic as a line through the night sky along which the planets move and the Moon's serpent path swings from side to side of this, crossing over it at a node.

Traditionally, the nodes were regarded as powerful energy-points in the Moon's cycle, and large-scale American investigations have confirmed this clearly . At the Washington Weather Bureau, the same team of investigators who discovered the Full Moon peak in rainfall (Chapter 1) also found that the magnitude of the effect varied greatly and depended upon how close the Moon was to a node.[15] The effect was strongest for the Full Moons which happened near to the nodes, and weakest for those farthest away.

A comparable effect on the Earth's magnetic field was found by Bell and Defouw at the Massachusetts Institute of Technology.[9] We all know that the Earth's magnetism points towards the North Pole but, in addition, it fluctuates in magnitude a great deal from day to day; it's a very mutable thing. We have already looked at how it intensified on days after the Full Moon. These

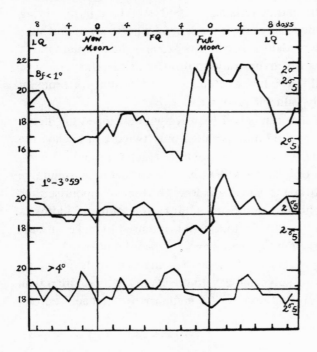

Figure 8. The index of geomagnetic activity according to the lunar phase and the celestial latitude of the Full Moon (after Bell and Defouw, 1966). The three graphs show how far geomagnetic activity peaks at the Full Moon. At zero latitude, the top graph, the variation is greatest. The bottom graph shows the least activity at maximum latitude, i.e. furthest from the nodes.

researchers found that much bigger changes in geomagnetism over the Full Moon occurred when it took place at a node, whereas the effect was hardly present when the Full Moon was furthest from the two nodes. This clearly shows that the nodes affect the power of a Full Moon.

The figure based on their research shows how the GMF (geomagnetic field) peaks at the Full Moon when the latter occurs close to the nodes. There is a disturbance of the Earth's magnetic field of around 30 per cent at this time. This reinforces the idea that the nodes are important power points as well as possibly explaining why the Full Moon is such an energizing time for plants and other organic systems. The effect was much weaker away from the nodes.

There is growing evidence that plants are highly sensitive to changes in the Earth's magnetic field.[31] The biologist Professor Frank Brown found that organisms could detect and respond to small changes in the Earth's magnetic field of a magnitude comparable to those linked to the motions of the Sun and Moon.[18]

Chapter 4

THE MOON AND CROP YIELD

To speake then of the outward and active knowledges which belong to our English Hous-wife.... Shee shall also know the time of the yeere, moneth and moone, in which all hearbes are to be sowne; and when they are in their best flourishing, that gathering all hearbes in their height of goodnesse, shee may have the prime use of the same.... In February in the new of the Moone shee may sow Spyke, Garlicke, Borage, Buglose, Chervyle, Coriander, Gourds, Cresses, Marjoram, Palma Christi, Flower-gentle, white Poppy, Purslan, Radish, Rocket, Rosemary, Sorrell, Double Marigolds and Time. The moone full shee may sow Anisseedes musked, Violets, Bleets, Skyrrits, White Succory, Fennell, and Parslie. The moone old sow Holy Thystell, Cole Cabadge, white Cole, greene Cole, Cucumbers, Harts Horne, Diers Grayne, Cabadge, Lettice, Mellons, Onions, Parsnips, Larkes Heele, Burnet and Leekes.

Gervase Markham, *The English Hous-wife* (1615)

IN EARLIER CHAPTERS we have looked at many of the influences of the phase of the moon on plants and animal life. Most of the experiments we have reported have related a Full or New Moon to some perceived change in metabolic rate or physical performance. Alternatively, they have investigated the consequences of the relationship of the moon's orbit to that of the Sun, for instance when it crosses the nodes. The moment has come, however, for us to move forwards: to evaluate the importance of the relationship of the moon to the zodiac. This, you will recall, was touched on in our description of the four elements and the sidereal cycle in the first two chapters.

Whereas the phase or synodic cycle is related to the general growth of a plant, it is the sidereal cycle that is mainly linked to the final crop yield. A sidereally-based rhythm applies to one instant in a plant's life, when the seed is sown on moist ground and growth begins. At this critical moment it is the Moon's position against the zodiac which influences the overall development – that is, how the seed's potential will come to fruition.

Systematic investigation of how the time of sowing affects final growth really started with the experiments of Maria Thun in Germany. In 1956, she developed her theory using the procedure of sowing twelve rows of a crop over one sidereal lunar month, usually in May. This method had been followed in investigations within Steiner's Anthroposophical Society since the 1930s, but it was Thun who had the idea of picking out the element-rhythm rather than the separate Moon-zodiac constellations.

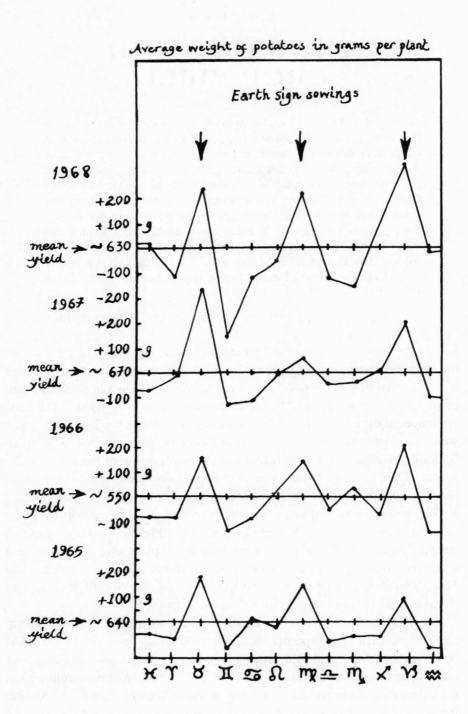

Figure 9. Potato yields according to the experiments of Maria Thun (1979).

One row of seeds was sown every few days, each time the Moon reached the middle of a new zodiac constellation, so that twelve rows were sown in the course of one revolution of the Moon around the zodiac. Each of these rows was allowed to grow for the same period of time and, after harvesting, the weights of the crops from each row were compared. Results for potatoes have been published since 1972 (co-authored with statistician Dr Hans Heinze). Maria Thun has subjected many other crops to the same type of experiment.

Her research garden in a small, tranquil village surrounded by hills near Marberg, Germany, carries on this work. Over the decades she has developed a remarkable insight into the way in which cosmic influences affect crop yield. This may be the only place in the world where systematic research into the link between crop yield and the Moon's position is ongoing. The work was initially funded by a 'research-ring' of German Bio-Dynamic farmers.

The dominant effect emerging from her trials related to a fourfold pattern in the zodiac which allocates each of the twelve constellations to the four elements – Earth (influencing root plants), Water (leaf plants), Air (flowering plants), and Fire (fruit- and seed-bearing plants) – as described in an earlier chapter. For potatoes, maximum yields occurred in the three rows which were sown on root days, that is when the Moon was standing in front of one of the three zodiac constellations traditionally associated with the element Earth, while minimum yields tended to occur when the Moon was standing in one of the Water constellations, in between those of Earth. This pattern indicated the worst as well as the best times of the month for sowing potatoes. There began to appear in the data a basic wave pattern related to the kind of plant sown. The yield increases obtained were in the region of 30 per cent for the three Earth-element sign sowings as distinct from the other nine.

Figure 9 shows the results of the Thun-Heinze potato experiments over 1965–68.[90] Clear maximum yields can be seen over earth-element sign sowings (root days) and minima over water-element sign sowings (leaf days). The results were tested for statistical significance by comparing the mean of the three root-day yields with that of the nine other sowings. Clearly, such a test shows a very high significance level for the yield-excess of the root-day sowings compared to others.

Other studies using a similar experimental procedure as Thun have, in general, confirmed this four-element theory. Ulf Abele at Giessen University, as part of a doctoral study of Bio-Dynamic farming methods, tested barley, oats, carrots and radish over the years 1970–74, sowing twelve rows over the course of a month for each year. His barley and oats gave yields which increased by seven per cent overall when sowings were made on seed days (see Figure 10 overleaf), while his carrots and radish averaged a 21 per cent yield increase on the root-day sowings.[1,2]

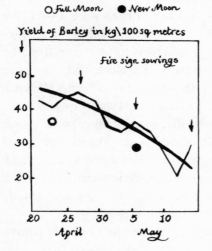

Figure 10. Barley yields according to Abele (1973).

A German study by Ursula Graf investigated the Moon-zodiac rhythm for different soils.[40] Over the three years, 1973–75, potato and radish crops were investigated and yield increases were usually found for root-day sowings as the theory predicted. However, this occurred only in crops grown on organically cultivated soil, to which no chemicals had been applied, and not in crops grown on soil treated with synthetic fertilizer. Graf's conclusion was, 'the soil seems to be a decisive factor in the occurrence of connections between Moon-zodiac constellations and crop yields,' a view which directly echoes Thun's comment in 1964:

> I came to the conclusion that mineralized soils hardly reacted to these cosmic rhythms and their fine influences, whereas a humus-filled soil of whatever soil type was a good mediator for these forces.

In other words, organic gardeners are the only ones who are going to reap important benefits from the calendar and method of working I offer in this book. Soil quality appears very relevant to the way lunar influence will show up and may account for variations in results achieved.

In Britain in 1976, the author and Reg Muntz, a market gardener in Sussex, planted 24 rows of potatoes over two sidereal months.[53] The results showed a mean yield increase of 25 per cent for rows sown on root days as compared to other sowings. Other trials by Muntz involved beans, carrots and lettuce. Maximum yields consistently showed up in the element-trigons predicted by the Thun theory, whereas there was little indication of a lunar phase effect.

Some quite thorough experiments were done in Wales over three years by Colin Bishop, an amateur gardener and astrologer.[12] In 1976, he planted 36 rows of lettuce over three months and achieved the results shown in Figure 11. The average weight of the lettuce tops increased by approximately 50 per cent

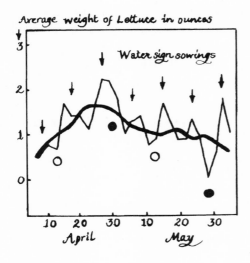

Figure 11. Lettuce yields according to Bishop (1976).

for those rows sown on leaf-days when compared with sowings made on other days. This surprised him. A repeat of the experiment in 1977 produced substantially the same results. In 1978, Bishop experimented with daily sowings of radish and again found that the relevant days, in this case root-days, produced the highest yield by 45 per cent.[55] None of these data-sets showed a Moon-phase effect on crop yields.

There is skill involved in growing rows of vegetables uniformly so that they aren't consumed by birds or slugs and that lettuce form their hearts without bolting. Such uniform conditions of growth are vital for the data to mean anything. Overall, between the years 1975 and 1986, Muntz and Bishop grew some four hundred rows of different vegetables in such trials and, overall, the net yield increase from sowing in the predicted trigons was 22 per cent. The soil used was not especially rich. These British results formed the groundwork for putting forward the calendar you are about to read.

In 1980, J. Lücke sowed four different plots of potatoes, with twelve rows per plot, as part of another doctoral thesis at the University of Giessen, one per Moon-constellation as usual, i.e. 48 rows in all.[63] Overall, his root-day yields were very significantly in excess of the others, just as yields from the leaf-day sowings (opposite to the root-days, as being Water rather than Earth) were the least.

Sometimes a low-amplitude effect is observed, as in the extensive trials designed by Dr Hartmut Spiess.[79] In three years of carrot trials in 1979–81 at Dottenfelder farm near Frankfurt his yields averaged eight percent more on root days, which is not much, but was significant as he undertook many sowings. The plot used was in an industrialized region of Germany where one might expect any sidereal-rhythm effects to become diluted. Some degree of scepticism has developed in Germany over the Thun model, amongst Bio-Dynamic experts, which has focussed on the Spiess results as if they had failed to confirm the sidereal rhythms. I suggest, however, that they are low-amplitude effects rather than null results. Spiess concluded that, 'the magnitude of the yield deviations that were associated with lunar factors was of practical significance.'[78]

For a practical, Australian view of how to use the sidereal rhythms we may quote from the lectures of Alex Podolinsky:

> The market gardeners may have noticed the best beans you have ever picked are on plants that are not huge and have not all that many leaves.... Now if you sow beans under a 'leaf' zodiac sign, then they turn out such huge plants and they have very poor fruit. When you sow under a 'seed' sign, you don't have all that much foliage (the plants don't need it, anyway) but they do have a lot of fruit. For pumpkins, in our experience, sowing under Leo is the most desirable.... We have run such trials and we have had roughly four times as many pumpkins in roughly the same acreage sowing them under 'fruit' rather than under 'leaf'.[73]

A Quality Test

Is the taste of a crop affected by the trigons as well as the yield? Organic growing is about improved quality, after all. Jack Temple, the *Here's Health* organic gardening correspondent, performed such a test in the spring of 1982, using the Thun sowing calendar:

> Every time a leaf-sowing date turned up I sowed a row of lettuce and a row of radishes, and every time a root sowing day featured in her calendar we also sowed both lettuce and radish again. Then, when the directors and students from the Henry Doubleday Research Association dropped in on their yearly visit, we put the trial to the test.

Initially, Jack's visitors were shocked by the outlandish notion so that his reputation with them appeared to be at stake:

> However, all that disappeared as I put my knife through two radishes. One was juicy and the other had the texture of cotton wool. The juicy one had been sown on the correct day, a root-day, and the pithy radish had been sown on a leaf-day. That was not all: the juicy radish was ten weeks old while the pithy one was only eight weeks old. Both radishes were also tasted for quality and flavour.
> Subsequently further sowings were tested. Each time we had the same result. Radishes sown on leaf-days were pithy and radishes sown on root-days were firm and fleshy. The lettuce trials did not produce quite such clear evidence, but lettuce sown on leaf days were slower to bolt than those sown on root days.[85]

So, it was shown that the root-day radish had better texture and the leaf-day lettuce were slower to bolt, in front of some fairly critical witnesses.

To date the evidence from such sowing trials demonstrates an effect caused by the primary element-rhythms of the zodiac, but not for specific signs, as if plants, being simpler in their organization than man, respond to this less-differentiated rhythm embodied in the zodiac. The weight of evidence to date indicates that the Thun model is valid and that the final yield of crops, when sown in good, organic soil, is related to the Moon's position according to the sidereal zodiac sign-element at the time of sowing.

Maria Thun has been publishing a calendar to guide organic growers and gardeners for several years. This is translated into several languages, including English. However, it is not able to shake off imitators and plagiarists. In Germany, some half-dozen clones appear in the bookshops each year with a substantially identical calendar and sowing advice to the Thun publication but in glossier covers. 1998 was the first year that one of these imitations appeared, translated into English. These may show that the idea is spreading and help its wider acceptance nonetheless, ethical issues are raised by such copying. I would point out, for the comfort of readers anxious about the abuse of copyright, that the calendar developed for this book is substantially different from Thun's. The reasons for our variations are explained at length below.

There is at present less evidence for the effects of the lunar nodes on plants. According to Thun, the influence of the two nodes is liable to interfere with plant growth and to weaken the viability of seeds from plants sown at these times.[91] The 1977 lettuce experiment by Bishop shows that the three or four rows sown over the Moon nodes failed to germinate. Yields from the leaf-day sowings were on average 54 per cent higher than the others, but the one leaf-day sowing that coincided with a Moon node (14th May) was comparatively inhibited and resulted in a reduced yield.

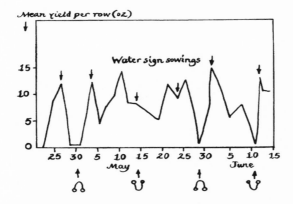

Figure 12. Lettuce yields according to Bishop (1978), with indications of Water (leaf) element days and lunar nodes.

43

THE RAW
DATA:
RADISH
YIELDS

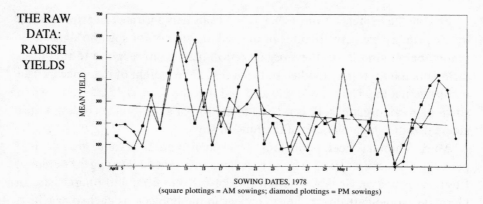

SOWING DATES, 1978
(square plottings = AM sowings; diamond plottings = PM sowings)

Figure 13. The Bishop radish trial. The root days in this period were April 11–13, April 20–22, April 28 – May 1, and May 9–11.

THE
SIDEREAL
LUNAR
MONTH

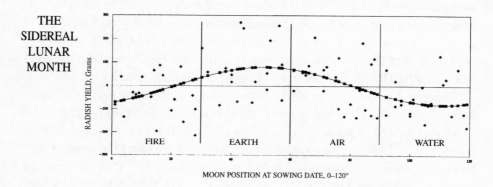

MOON POSITION AT SOWING DATE, 0–120°

Figure 14. The Bishop radish trial. Here the yield data are plotted against the sidereal lunar longitude (0–120°) at sowing time. The element signs are shown, and a best-fit waveform has been added to make clear the tendency in yields.

THE
LUNAR
DAY

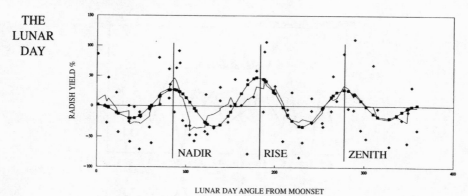

LUNAR DAY ANGLE FROM MOONSET

Figure 15. The Bishop radish trial. Here the yields are plotted against the passing of the lunar day. The individual readings have been translated into a waveform and a moving average to better demonstrate the variation in yield according to the time of lunar day of sowing.

At perigee, when the Moon draws nearest to the Earth each month, the tides are pulled higher, some 30 per cent more than at apogee. It has been claimed that perigee is linked with stress.[62] In the 1976 lettuce experiment by Bishop it was found that the highest yield over a three-month period came from a row sown at apogee. Thun has claimed that the apogee position causes sowings to sprout up rather quickly – which may not necessarily be beneficial for fruit formation – whereas the perigee position tends to inhibit growth. Evidence for the supposed adverse effect upon growth of perigee remains scant.

Sowing and Harvesting in the Phase Cycle

Does sowing at some point in the lunar phase cycle (i.e. when the Moon is Full or New, or at a quarter position) produce better crops? Widespread folk traditions have affirmed it, as Moon-gardening almanacs have for centuries recommended diverse Moon-phase rules for the sowing of crops: note, for instance, the suggestions by Gervase Markham quoted at the head of this chapter. Modern experiments have been equivocal, though field experiments by Mather at the John Innes Horticultural Foundation in 1940[64] showed a consistent fifteen per cent yield increase for maize and tomatoes sown in the second lunar quarter, confirming the hypothesis which this gardener had wished to test – that Kolisko had just published in her 1939 *Agriculture of Tomorrow*. Despite this confirmation, the author of the report was quite dismissive of his results, and subsequently a review in *Nature* by Beeson echoed his sceptical tone.[7] Crop-yield sowing trials which Simon Best or myself have seen or been involved in have failed to detect much by way of any Moon-phase effects on yield. A comment by Thun on this issue is of interest, indeed possibly crucial:

> The influence of the Full Moon, throughout all the years of our research, only brought higher yields when these had been forced by mineral fertilizers or unrotted organic manures.

Moonrise

Perhaps the most thorough lunar-gardening experiment ever performed was that by Colin Bishop in 1978, using radish. He sowed two rows in the morning and another two in the afternoon for 38 consecutive days with no gaps. The data is shown broken down by the four elements, the sidereal lunar month, with peaks as predicted on root-days. A waveform has been put through the data to show the star-rhythm. Its amplitude is around 30 percent. Lastly the lunar day angle is shown, centred on moonrise. This graph was possible because Colin Bishop noted the time of each sowing. It shows a large peak over the hour of moonrise. He watered each row before inserting the seed on his way to work each morning and then each afternoon as he returned home. This meant that the seed started growing as soon as it was inserted into the soil. This is important if we are to take seriously the notion that the hour of moonrise showed up as the largest-amplitude effect in this data-set, as here appears.

In the nineteenth century, there was a regular gardening column in *The Astrologer*, a London-based monthly, which always gave the time of moonrise, and recommended it be used for important gardening operations. The calendar we have printed here for you also records the hour of moonrise, even when it is in the middle of the night. My own opinion is that it is a very significant moment in the day when contemplating seed sowing or planting.

Chapter 5

USING THE STAR-ZODIAC

A Doctor too emerged as we proceeded;
No one alive could talk as well as he did
On points of medicine and of surgery,
For, being grounded in astronomy,
He watched his patient's favourable star
And, by his Naturall Magic, knew what are
The lucky hours and planetary degrees
For making charms and magic effigies.

Chaucer, *The Canterbury Tales* (trans. N. Coghill)

Lᴇᴛ's ᴛʀʏ ᴛᴏ ᴛɪɢʜᴛᴇɴ ᴜᴘ the use of the terms 'sign' and 'constellation'. The zodiacal signs are all of 30° length, whereas the constellations associated with them vary greatly, from 46° (Virgo) to a mere 18° or so (little Libra, the Balance, next to Virgo). The calendar here used always employs the equal sign divisions. However, the earlier chapters alluded to the constellations because Bio-Dynamic research always uses them, never an equal zodiac.

In the debates that go on amongst users of Bio-Dynamic calendars, it is generally appreciated that sowing is not advised near the ingress times, so that 'border disputes' over just where a constellation begins and ends are not very important. The irregular constellation divisions used by Bio-Dynamic calendars differ from those here used for one-sixth of the time. That is, some sixty degrees in the circle of the zodiac. This chapter looks at the 'glorious heritage' of the star-zodiac, and argues that the splintered traditions of the twentieth-century calendars can be resolved by an historical view.

The sidereal zodiac, or zodiac of the stars, is composed of twelve equal thirty-degree divisions.[74] It is a kind of 'best-fit' of such a regular structure upon the irregular constellations of the ecliptic. It is called 'sidereal' to differentiate it from the 'tropical' zodiac that astrologers use nowadays. It derives from antiquity, and as such would have been used by the three Magi or 'wise men' of the New Testament: the Magi were astrologer-astronomers of the Near East, chiefly Chaldea, renowned for their star-lore.

In the fifth century ʙᴄ, the Greek historian Herodotus went to visit the Chaldeans of Mesopotamia. He was mainly impressed by the sheer abundance of their harvests: of grain, figs, olives and vines. Indeed, he was concerned that the account he gave of these things, and of how tall their millet and sesame grew, would strain the credulity of his readers. The Babylonians built an extensive irrigation system using underground piping for their gardens.

Herodotus must have gazed upon the fabled hanging gardens of Babylon, where now is only the dusty desert.

In that period, 25 centuries ago, the Chaldeans began using the zodiac divisions,[98] dividing the sky into twelve equal sectors, to mirror a division of their year into twelve thirty-day months. Did the star-wisdom, for which the Chaldeans became renowned in antiquity, help them in their harvests? Whereas the modern zodiac is anchored to the seasons of the year, with its start at zero degrees of Aries always at the 'Vernal point', for the Chaldeans of old it was fixed by various bright stars.[57]

The Chaldeans were never interested in the Vernal point's position against their zodiac. That was more a Greek notion, and used more for purely astronomical purposes. Rather, the Chaldeans were concerned with what they experienced of the night sky, for example they recorded each time Venus appeared and disappeared from the sky, and perhaps their more experiential attitude could be of value today.

Debates over the star-zodiac's position are over a degree or so.[36] It is important in some contexts but immaterial for a lunar gardening calendar. There were certain stars that fixed the zodiac position, in particular Spica the bright star signifying the sheaf of corn held by the Virgin, around 29° of Virgo. The Chaldean star-zodiac was used by the astrologers of antiquity around the Mediterranean – Greece and Rome, Syria and Egypt – until the fifth century AD. A different tradition then developed in the Muslim Arab world using the tropical zodiac. The two zodiac systems were then only a few degrees apart.

The four elements – Earth, Air, Fire and Water – had been used in Greek medicine and philosophy for seven centuries until, in the second century AD, after Claudius Ptolemy's time, they were absorbed into the fabric of the zodiac. Thenceforth the Lion, the Archer, and the Ram all had one element in common: fire! And, indeed, these three images do seem to have that fiery quality in common. The sky-triangles (trigons) were thus established, linking the four elements. This happened in Syria, where Vettius Valens first recorded it. They entered into the sidereal zodiac and not into the irregularly shaped constellations.

Memory of the sidereal zodiac became lost in Europe but continued in India: the zodiac used there is much the same as that understood by the ancient world. Thus, the primal star-zodiac, from which the modern tropical zodiac evolved, has been in continuous use for over two millennia. It was rediscovered at the end of the nineteenth century, when clay tablets dug up from the banks of the Tigris were deciphered. A sidereal ephemeris was published in 1981 by Neil Michelson of the US Astro-Computing Services. The present calendar uses the same reference as did Michelson, taking the 'Bull's Eye' star Aldebaran as being 15° of Taurus.

In the twentieth century, two incompatible lunar-gardening traditions burgeoned, both ignoring the sidereal zodiac. They offered a choice, of *either* using the tropical zodiac, as used nowadays by astrologers, *or* using twelve unequal constellations, as used in Bio-Dynamic calendars. The former sells about two orders of magnitude more calendars each year (chiefly in the US) than does the latter (chiefly in Europe).

Use of the Tropical Zodiac

The tropical zodiac denotes the Sun's course through the year, that is to say: the Sun will always enter Aries on March 20th or 21st, the Spring Equinox. This zodiac has no connection with the stars! It is related primarily to the seasons. Its only connection to the stars is historical: a long time ago, it was aligned with the constellations. It is the one used in Sun-sign columns in newspapers and by most practising astrologers. It is slowly moving away from the star-zodiac, due to what astronomers call, 'precession'. As I write, it has moved 25 degrees away from the star-zodiac that gave it birth.

In the early 1980s, previous editions of *Planting by the Moon* took a diplomatic view of the way the tropical zodiac might be appropriate for human fate, while emphasizing that evidence pointed to the sidereal as the right one to use for plant growth:

> Incidentally, we are not implying that astrologers should be using the sidereal zodiac for their work. Rather, it seems that different phenomena may be attuned to different systems. The tropical zodiac is a moving zodiac, moving around once every 72 years against the fixed stars, and this evolving system may be valid for man. However, plants are simpler in their organization than man, and have a far longer history, two factors which seem to have inclined their response to the Moon in terms of the more primal and unchanging sidereal zodiac. The position of the Moon in the tropical zodiac requires calculation, whereas its position in the sidereal zodiac can be observed in the sky. Although plants do not respond to the tropical zodiac divisions, it may well be that man's being is more in tune with the special mathematical treatment of time and space on which the tropical system depends..

To put that in simple terms: without an ephemeris (a prepared, printed table giving star times and calculations) could one discern when the Moon was entering into a tropical zodiac sign? Assuredly one could not without a most difficult calculation. If we cannot do it, how could one expect the much simpler plant realm to respond to a tropical ingress? In contrast, growers using the calendar we offer here have the advantage of being able to see in the sky what is happening in the book.

In terms of agriculture, the tropical zodiac reflects the seasons of the year, at least in the northern hemisphere. Thus, the glyph or sign for Aries signifies the young seedling emerging in spring, then the next sign Taurus, the Bull, signifies the vigour of springtime. The Sun's entry into Leo at the height of summer indicates its strength there, followed in September by the Virgin as a Ceres-figure signifying the harvest. After that comes Libra, the Balance, as the harvest is measured out; and then the Scorpion signifies the dying and decomposition of nature.

Interpreting the evidence of field experiments in terms of a zodiac framework depends entirely on the symbolism of the four elements. Thus, experiments show that root crops such as potato or radish grow better when the Moon is in front of one of the three 'Earth' sectors of the sidereal zodiac. In terms of the tropical zodiac, one would have to say that they were growing best when the Moon was in front of one of the three 'Air' signs, because the shift between the two systems is nowadays almost one sign, or 24°-25°. This would not have the same symbolic significance as associating them with the Earth signs. Likewise it makes more sense to associate leaf crops such as lettuce with Water (sidereal) than with Fire (tropical). The four stages of plant growth – root, leaf, flower and fruit/seed – are associated with the four elements, earth, water, air and fire, *only* if a sidereal reference system is used.

Users of this 'zodiac of the seasons', i.e. the tropical, tend to advocate that the three Water signs are fruitful while the three Fire signs are barren, based on straightforward analogy or symbolism. It amounts to viewing only one-quarter of the zodiac as fertile. Sometimes the Earth signs are also admitted to be fertile. Experimental work supporting this view was published by Timmins,[85] which involved sowing only two rows, one supposedly at the right time and the other outside it. This was viewed by Simon Best and this writer as being of doubtful value, on the grounds that one's attitude is too likely to affect the outcome of such a simple and short-term experiment.

Use of the Constellations

Bio-Dynamics developed within the Anthroposophical movement founded by Rudolf Steiner which had drawn up its own twelvefold division of the heavens, loosely based upon the divisions made by the International Astronomical Union in 1928. The astronomers then decided to map out thirteen constellations as lying on the ecliptic (Ophiucus, the Serpent-Bearer, being the thirteenth). The Anthroposophists wanted no truck with this, however, and reconstructed a zodiac of just twelve constellations. Whereas the astronomers saw Libra as being 23° in length along the ecliptic, the Anthroposophists gave it merely 18°, making it even shorter.

The divisions imposed on the heavens by the Anthroposophists had little connection with earlier zodiacs. Whereas both sidereal and tropical zodiacs allocate an equal space to each sign, Steiner and his followers attempted to reflect more closely astronomical reality. The constellations (which is how they divided their calendar) are by their very nature unequal in size.

There was no great harm in any of this, indeed it was quite audacious. The trouble began when Maria Thun stuck the four elements into this irregular setup in the 1950s. Her use of these divisions made for a radical imbalance in the four elements. Root days (Earth) were assigned over 50 per cent more of the month than the flower days (Air). The Air-constellation Libra is very short, while the Earth-constellation Virgo is 46°, two and a half times longer. The system was badly out of kilter, but nobody seemed to mind.

The Sidereal Zodiac

I would ask the reader to put all thoughts of the tropical zodiac, and the variations worked upon it as described in earlier paragraphs, to one side. The present calendar is based upon the sidereal zodiac as being the correct and optimal reference that does really work in an organic gardening setup. Its basis is thus very traditional, tried and tested over millennia. The element-rhythm of the star-zodiac is a simple thing, which is why plants respond to it.

Just as investigation of lunar influence on plants is a recent phenomenon, so also is the rediscovery of the sidereal zodiac in the West. Traditional gardening manuals have used the tropical zodiac without question, largely because it was the only one known to them. With the steady accumulation of evidence supporting the sidereal zodiac framework the practice of lunar planting can now be established on a firm foundation.

Let's check out two sets of evidence for preferring it. First compare the results of the radish experiment by Colin Bishop that was described in the previous chapter, with three graphs to illustrate it. If you recalculate the findings according to the Bio-Dynamic zodiac calendar on the one hand, and the sidereal zodiac on the other, the yields reported by Bishop are as follows (mean weight in grams per radish per row).

	Root days	*Others*
Sidereal:	3.1g (n=18)	2.11±1.5g (n=60)
Bio-Dynamic:	2.8g (n=23)	2.15±1.5g (n=55)

Each of the zodiacs in question is divided into the four elements that we have already discussed, but the unequal division of the Bio-Dynamic tropical zodiac means there are quite a few more sowings on 'root-days' according to their calendar because their three Earth element (Roots) constellations, Bull (Taurus), Virgin (Virgo) and Ram (Aries), are more than 30° in length.

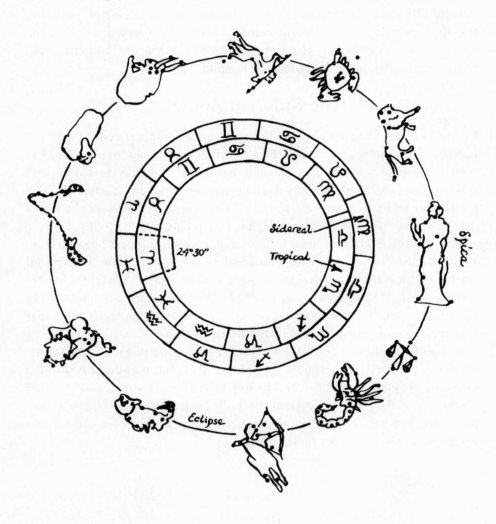

Figure 16. The relationship of the sidereal and tropical zodiacs against the constellations.

Whichever calendar one prefers, the mean yield excess of root day sowings over sowings in other element-signs was over 30 per cent.

A second trial that may be useful for comparing the impact of the two zodiacs concerns goats. One is sometimes asked, did not Maria Thun perform trials herself to check out the validity of the Bio-Dynamic movement's zodiacal divisions? She did perform and write up a fine experiment with goats she milked each morning.[92] For two months, she measured the milk they gave, and then weighed the butter she made from it every afternoon. The goats produced about a quarter of a kilogram of butter each day. A large excess of butter (nearly 20 per cent more) was made on the 'warmth-days', i.e. what the present calendar calls fruit-seed days. This experiment looked at milk quality, not quantity. The total amount of daily milk did not vary greatly, but the amount of butter extractable therefrom varied with the Moon-trigons. Analysing these yields using the sidereal zodiac instead of the constellations (as there are a few days which fall out differently) gave a slightly greater excess of butter yields on the warmth-days than was obtained by the constellations.

If this result turned out to be repeatable then *Planting by the Moon* could start including milking in the calendar recommendations. Readers will appreciate that it would presently be inappropriate to do this – indeed it would be mere intellectual theft (as does happen in certain quarters, but not here).

Seeds of Confusion?

As an example of how the different divisions work, let's consider the figure of Leo the Lion. Tropically, he spans the 30° of 120°–150° (measuring from zero as the start of Aries). Adding on 25° gives sidereal Leo, 145°–175°. Simple, isn't it? For comparison, the *constellation* of Leo is larger, reaching from about 138° to 173°. It can be seen that there is a day when Tropical Leo overlaps the constellation of Leo, bearing in mind that the Moon moves 13° a day.

An American writer and gardening advisor called Llewellyn finds Moon in Leo to be the most barren sign, used only for destroying weeds.' Thun's advice is quite contrary to this. To quote from the US *Kimberton Hills* calendar, Moon in Leo 'enhances the power of regeneration', and is a time for 'sowing crops whose seeds will be saved.' This is the day in each month which one tradition finds to be the most barren and worst for seed quality, while another recommends that, *au contraire*, sowing will produce the most fertile seeds for the future. Days in the calendar with the Leo ingress (boundary) marked in the daytime, for example June 7th 2000, fits the bill. One should cultivate a mood of ironic reflection on such days.

Chapter 6

GARDENING ASPECTS

To the better furthering of the gardener's travails, he ought afore to consider, that the Garden earth be apt and good, wel turned in with dung, at a due time of the year, in the increase of the Moon, she occupying an apt place in the Zodiack, in agreeable aspect of Saturn, & well-placed in the sight of heaven ... for otherwise his care and pains bestowed about the seeds and plants, nothing availeth the Garden.

Thomas Hill, *The Gardener's Labyrinth* (1577)

As viewed from the Earth at Full Moon, the two luminaries, the Sun and the Moon, are said to be in 'opposition,' then two weeks later at New Moon, when they have drawn together in the sky, they form the aspect called 'conjunction'. An aspect is an angle, measured around the ecliptic from the centre of the Earth, expressing some kind of symmetry within the zodiac. Traditionally there were always five of them and, in order of decreasing strength, these are:

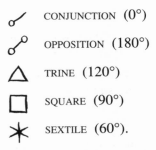

       CONJUNCTION (0°)

       OPPOSITION (180°)

       TRINE (120°)

       SQUARE (90°)

       SEXTILE (60°).

The conjunction, square and opposition are usually considered inhibiting and stressful, whereas the sextile and, in particular, the trine are thought to be beneficial and harmonious.

Each month, the Moon forms similar angles or aspects with Saturn and with the other planets. The relationship thus expressed with Saturn seems to have particular importance to agriculture and the life of plants. The present calendar indicates most of the Moon/Saturn aspects as they occur, a certain number of Moon/Sun aspects where they are relevant and all the aspects between the Moon and Venus when they fall on Flower days. The Venus aspects are here being recommended for working with flowers – sowing, planting-out and grafting.

Aspects to Saturn

The planet Saturn was traditionally viewed as important for farmers. The Roman god Saturn presided over agriculture (his name is thought to derive from the Latin *sator,* sower) and the Saturnalia, held just before the winter solstice, was a week-long agricultural festival of merry-making, in memory of the Golden Age. Indeed, classical writers have mentioned no other planet in this regard. In his agricultural poem *Georgics*, Virgil advised, 'Watch the transit of the cold star Saturn.' Saturn's sickle had a more rustic meaning before it came to denote the limitations of time.

As an example of this traditional view, the sixteenth-century work on gardening lore, *The Gardener's Labyrinth*, explained about sextile aspects between Saturn and the Moon: 'it is then commended to labour the earth, sow, and plant,' whereas, during the square aspect between these two, it was 'denied utterly to deal in such matters'. The trine was also approved, but the opposition was not.[44]

Much the same advice featured in seventeenth-century British works, for example *The Whole Art of Husbandry*,[65] while *Dariotus Redivivus* advised that farmers:

> ought to have a special respect to the state and condition of Saturn, that he be not
> ... afflicted, because he hath chief dominion over husbandry and the commodities
> of the Earth; let him therefore (if you can so fit it) be in good aspect ... to the
> Moon.[27]

For planting crops, the general advice was, 'Plant what you intend, the Moon being either in conjunction, sextile or trine of Saturn.'

In modern times, Bio-Dynamic farmers have considered the lunar opposition to Saturn to be important, so that it was for long the only celestial aspect to feature in their calendar.[11] It is here interesting to note that the Foundation for the Study of Cycles, based in Pittsburgh, has found a 29.8 year cycle in famines,[28] a periodicity which corresponds almost exactly with the average time it takes Saturn to make one complete revolution through the zodiac. (Incidentally, there are no other planetary revolutionary periods near this time-period; the two closest to Saturn, Jupiter and Uranus, having periods of 11 years and 84 years respectively.)

In astrological terms, Saturn represents life's challenging, defining and shaping principle. It can be depicted as *Chronos*, 'Old Father Time'. The present calendar gives the lunar aspects of conjunction, opposition, trine and sextile to Saturn. For those who wish to test these aspects, the traditional advice would be that the harmonious times are suitable for the sowing of perennials and trees, through Saturn's association with long-term cycles, and for increasing the hardiness of plants. Stressful times (conjunction, opposition and square) should be avoided but readers may wish to test the particular belief of Bio-Dynamic farmers that the opposition is the best Saturn aspect to use. All aspects are given to the nearest ten minutes GMT.

One should sow or plant between one hour before and half an hour after the aspect occurs. That was what *Planting by the Moon* has earlier advised. If that seems unduly strenuous, one could quote Adele Barger's view, in *Gardening Success with Lunar Aspects*, 'sow within the six hours prior to exactitude, taking care to sow before and not after the event.'[6] The present calendar gives Saturn aspects for leaf, flower and fruit/seed days, but not for root days, as there would be little point in sowing trees and perennial crops on root days.

In his ever-popular herbal, Culpeper gave some advice about when to pick herbs in terms of finding the right celestial aspects, adding:

> Let them be full ripe when they are gathered, and forget not the celestial harmony before mentioned; for I have found from experience that their virtues are twice as great at such times as others.[22]

Vines and the Sun

Readers with a warm and sunny spot in the garden may wish to try growing vines; with all this global warming, why not? For the ancients and for traditional astrological-rustic books the vine had a *solar* rulership. The US biologist-astrologer Lee Lehman compared rulerships of all sorts of herbs and trees from a variety of traditional sources and she found a nucleus for which all of her sources agreed. The vine was one of these. Most of these don't concern us as planetary events are not given in the calendar which follows in this book (it would be too complicated). However, the main Sun-Moon aspects are given and these are the important options for choosing when to establish a vine, particularly cutting the scion in the autumn and then grafting it in the spring. Such times should also be a fruit-day. Such days occur on February 15th and February 24th.

The ancients also related wine quality to the movement of Jupiter around the zodiac. As it orbits once in twelve years, it will enter a new zodiac sign each year. Various astrologers that I consulted expressed surprise about the solar rulership of the vine. They never guessed it, expecting it to be ruled by Jupiter. The words jolly, jovial, joy and so forth derive mysteriously from that sphere in the sky: Jove. This is something to mull over. One might also seek for solar aspects to Jupiter or Venus (not given in this calendar) for the important and career-determining event of setting up a vineyard. As not many readers are likely to be doing this it is a somewhat theoretical issue.

To help understand this idea, let's quote from a recent book on plant rulerships by Jean Elliott[33] which brought Culpeper's *Herbal* up to date. She gave the grapevine as solar in its rulership and summarized solar qualities as follows:

> The Sun: Core essence, integrated conscious self, playful self, vitality. Play, children; palaces and mansions; day; gold. The Sun rules Leo. Colour: yellow, orange, gold
>
> Grapevine: (*Vitis Vinifera*). Lilly, Culpeper [referring here to the two seventeenth-century astrologers who gave rulerships]. Either grows as a long-lived climber or in bush form for wine. Green/white flowers from early to midsummer. Grapes in Autumn. Under 'Vine' in *Herbal*. Brought to Britain by the Romans.

Fifteen years ago, one of the most respected French wine estates, Clos de la Coulée de Serrant in Savennières, owned by Nicholas Joly, went Bio-Dynamic.[45] Under azure skies in the Loire valley, there are two wines now produced using a lunar calendar: Joly's and Noel Pinguit's Le Haut Lieu. This last has won every award going (described as 'a stunningly intense, joyful wine' – solar qualities, perhaps?). One per cent of French wine is presently produced according to a Bio-Dynamic regime.

Joly expresses his views in rather solar terms:

> When we look at a flower or fruit, it becomes perfectly clear that they owe their beauty, their colour, their fragrance, their variety of shapes and flavours to the sun. And it is precisely this power of expression, which manifests itself in constantly new variations that must again be allowed to flourish in wine – and in every foodstuff.

Readers tired of Euro-plonk will surely appreciate this comment:

> Our apparently progressive agriculture has largely destroyed the soil as a living entity. As a result, the soil is now hardly capable of sustaining growth. It has consequently become dependent on chemical fertilizers, which are inevitably absorbed into the vine itself… In the past, wine growers enriched the soil whereas nowadays, they feed the vines directly. This amply explains the ever-increasing uniformity of wines available from the retailer.[30]

As the grapes ripen a critical situation develops in the last few weeks, crucial for final quality. The grapes have to be collected at their optimal stage of ripeness. As acidity gradually decreases the sugar content rises. After harvesting they are crushed and the mix poured into barrels. That moment needs careful choosing, being the 'birth-moment' of what will mature into wine, so make sure it's a fruit-day.

Maria Thun is collaborating with a wine-grower in the south of France. When I went to visit, her research plot of vines was being treated with various sprays of different copper concentrations. Copper sulphate is regularly sprayed as an insecticide, but she was using higher dilutions of copper, in other words much weaker concentrations along the lines of homeopathic medicines, to investigate their efficacy in the battle against infestation.

In 1988, the Domaine de la Romanée-Conti, producing the most famous red Burgundy of all, announced its decision to go organic, which caused a sensation. In 1995 they formed an association for compost production in an endeavour to revitalize the soil.

1990, the last sunspot maximum, is regarded as a classic wine-year. We will shortly reach a new sunspot maximum. As the Sun expands, with solar flares extending further out from its surface and aurorae maximizing at Earth's poles, are the best wines then formed? To quote from Gauquelin's classic, *The Cosmic Clocks*:

> According to the French Astronomical Bulletin, years in which the number of sun-spots is highest are great vintage years for Burgundy wines; in years with few sun-spots poor vintages are produced. The Swiss statistician A. Rima found similar results when he analysed the production of Rhine wines for the past two hundred years .

Karen's Pear Tree

The great astronomer Johannes Kepler composed calendars that prognosticated for the year ahead and in one of them (1602) he explained how it all worked.[39] He described an early version of the 'Gaia' theory, whereby 'the earth has a vegetable-animal force, having some sense of geometry.' This sense of geometry, he explained, enabled it to respond to the celestial aspects, in terms of climate, harvests, good wine years and political stability. Kepler gave an analogy to explain how this worked: just as a peasant could take delight in the piping of a flute, without knowing anything about the theory of musical harmony, so likewise did Earth respond in an unconscious manner to the changing geometry of the heavens. Earth more or less shuddered during an eclipse, he wrote:

> eclipses ... are so important as omens because the sudden animal faculty of the Earth is violently disturbed by the sudden intermission of light, experiencing something like emotion and persisting in it for some time.

Early tablets from ancient Babylon testified to the belief in the infertility of the land around the time of an eclipse. As a belief, it has endured longer than most. The early Bio-Dynamic sowing-calendars by Franz Rulni advocated not sowing anything important for several days after an eclipse, while its sucessor, the modern Thun calendar, gives just the day of an eclipse as no-planting.

In Holland, there is a garden with a few ragged pear trees which only started to bear small, bitter fruit nine years after they were planted. They were planted under a solar eclipse by Karen Hamaker-Zontag, the eminent Dutch astrologer. As a test, she planted them at this inauspicious moment. One would like to see an agricultural college sowing some fruit trees over a solar eclipse, with others growing on adjacent ground for comparison's sake that were planted at some more favourable time.

That eclipses do in fact diminish seed quality was shown a few decades ago in a series of seed-germination experiments by Theodor Schwenck summarized in his book, *Sensitive Chaos*. Readers unfamiliar with this work have a treat in store.

Chapter 7
THE RHYTHM OF THE SUN

THE SUN IS DUE to reach its next peak of sunspot activity in March of the year 2000. This is expected to damage or knock out all sorts of satellite communication equipment and to overload power grids, causing several billion dollars worth of damage. Experts are predicting that it will be one of the worst (or best, depending on your viewpoint) ever. It will cause Earth's upper atmosphere to expand as it is heated up, affecting low-orbiting satellites…but, our concern is with a very different field, namely its effect upon living things.

If you look at rings in an old tree trunk sawn across, you will notice that some are wider than others, a measure of increased growth during certain years. Usually, it can be seen that these widest bands happen every eleven years or so. The beat to which they and a host of other life forms keep time is that of the changing level of solar activity, as indicated by the number of sunspots visible on the surface of the Sun.[68] The sunspot cycle peaks on the average every eleven years, though it can vary. The solar magnetic field, north-south of the ecliptic, reverses every twenty-two years. This longer period comprises the complete solar cycle.

The cause of these thicker rings is something many millions of miles away: a heartbeat inside the Sun itself. The origin of this pulse remains a mystery, but its cycles are carefully followed by counting the spots and flares observed on the Sun's surface. Sunspots are a barometer of solar activity. Figure 17 shows recent cycles with 1959 and 1980 the highest on record.

While lunar rhythms define optimal sowing days within one season, this grand pulse of the Sun determines the years of peak production and also lean years, linked with times of famine. This expansion and contraction within the Sun affects rhythms of total crop production and much else besides. Experts

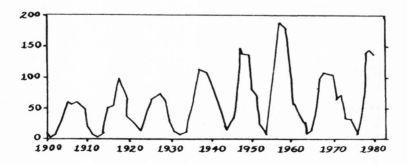

Figure 17. The solar cycle, sunspot activity 1900–1980.

generally assume the influence is indirect via the Sun's effect on climate: electrical and magnetic changes in the upper atmosphere are caused by solar radiation, these affect the climate, which in turn affects crop yield. The subject has implications for economic forecasting and may eventually come to be used for this.[47]

Ever since the astronomer William Herschel stated, two centuries ago, that the price of wheat varied with the sunspot cycle, scientists have been arguing whether the effect is really present. Meteorologists at the Appleton Laboratories at Slough are one group to have researched the subject, and their conclusions were quite positive. Led by Dr J.W. King, they found that, in Britain, yields of potato, turnip and swede tended to peak at years of sunspot maxima and also that rainfall tended to increase during these years.[48]

The scientists further found that the number of days per growing season (defined, somewhat arbitrarily, as days whose mean temperature was above 6°C) increased markedly during years of peak activity.[49] This confirms the observations of an English farmer, Mr Farrar, reported in *Farmers Weekly* in 1975, that the length of his cows' annual grazing season varied with the sunspot cycle. From his family records, he found that over the decades his cows stayed out to graze longest in years of peak sunspot activity, presumably when grass was blessed with an extended period of growth.[38]

The effect of the sunspot cycle on temperature was also found for the US states Maryland, Delaware and Virginia during the years 1900–60. Mean variations of two to three degrees centigrade linked with the solar rhythm – although this correlated primarily with the complete 22-year cycle rather than that of eleven years. This has obvious relevance, Dr King argued, for energy budgeting.

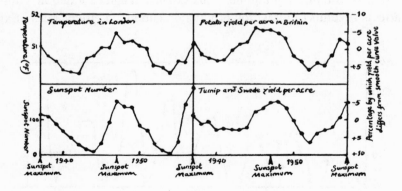

Figure 18. Variations in temperature, sunspot activity, and yields of potatoes, turnips and swedes through two complete sunspot cycles. (After King et al., 1974.)

Rainfall is also linked to the sunspot cycle. Dr R.G. Vines in Australia found that years of drought in certain countries are linked to troughs in the sunspot cycle, and large forest and prairie fires occur more often in these years.[96] He counted bad fire years as those in which losses overall due to fires were of one million acres or more. It is perhaps not surprising that fires on Earth should be linked to rhythms in the fiery energy of the Sun. Major US droughts seem to remain in step with the 22-year rather than the 11-year cycle.

Can farmers expect bumper harvests in years of sunspot maxima and more meagre yields in years when the Sun is quiet? Quite a lot more research needs to be done on Sun-Earth links before such recommendations are likely to be made by agricultural scientists, but it may not be long before farmers take account of this solar pulse when planning ahead.

The effect is geographically dependent, with wheat prices shown to correlate strongly with this cycle in some parts of the world, whereas in others such a correlation is lacking. In countries in the southern hemisphere the cycle is clearly reversed, with least growth in years of sunspot maxima. In general, Dr King and his colleagues found wheat yields in the northern hemisphere increased in years of peak sunspot activity, causing global wheat prices to be lower then because most wheat is grown in this region. Their research indicated that: 'Modulations of 10% to 50% of the wheat production in China, the United States and the Soviet Union seem to be correlate with the solar cycle.' Dr King suggested, as others have done before him, that this could be used as a basis for global economic planning.

Other phenomena have been shown to vary with the Sun's cycle, for example, years of peak activity seem to produce good wines. This appears both for French Burgundy and for German Rhine wines. The Russian expert, Professor Alexsander Chizhevsky, studied this cycle in human history, claiming that more political upheavals, unrest and warfare took place in years of peak activity. Russians regard him as the founder of Heliobiology.

Nowadays, the people having a practical interest in the cycles of the Sun are radio and electrical communication companies. This is because they get more disturbance and interruption during times of solar storms. RCA employs experts to monitor the Sun's activity. Farmers too, let us hope, will find it to their advantage to take account of this mighty pulse at our system's centre.

As long ago as 1937, anthroposophist J.W. Stein postulated 'the solar and planetary influences on weather and climate as the foundation of harvest and prices'.[52] He discussed such phenomena as temperature and rainfall linked to this cycle, emphasizing how much the effects were geographically differentiated. Further studies have confirmed what Gauquelin wrote in 1964, that, 'the relation between the sun and the atmosphere is as complex as that between the two main characters of a psychological novel'.

When the Moon blots out the Sun during a total eclipse, and the sky grows dark, then the red rim of the solar chromosphere appears around the edge. This chromosphere, in years of sunspot maxima, will glow all around the Moon, during a total eclipse, whereas in quiet years of sunspot minima it is seen to glow only at low solar latitudes, each side of the Moon's black rim. This means that the Sun's chromosphere expands and contracts over the 11-year cycle, though normally it is invisible, and only seen during total eclipses. Over the August solar eclipse of 1999, near to the sunspot maximum, astronomers were keen to check out by what degree the deep-red solar chromosphere has expanded.

The Nutation Cycle and Long-Term Planning

Long-term rhythms and recurrent patterns are not confined to the Sun. Every planet will have some kind of cyclical relationship with the Earth. In the 1980s, reports started appearing of the 18.6-year lunar-node cycle being identifiable from climate and agriculture records. It is now viewed as being at least as influential as the solar pulse. The word 'nutation' means a wobble, as this cycle causes Earth's axis to move. The axis of the earth takes many thousands of years to move round against the stars, and added onto this is this relatively small gyrating movement every 18.6 years, which astronomers call 'nutation'. This may help us understand the huge effects which this cycle exerts upon Earth's biosphere, at least as strong as the solar cycle: it moves the axis of the Earth. The solar cycle may be more evident in northerly countries, where a greater flux of energized solar particles, as shown for example in the aurora borealis, can funnel down from the Van Allen belts into the atmosphere. Rainfall or drought are linked with this node or 'nutation cycle' in several parts of the world. The monsoons of India, tidal waves – aqueous or atmospheric – and the nineteen year cycle of flooding of the River Nile are instances that may be cited.

The US cycles expert, Dr R. Currie, has found that droughts in midwestern states seem to follow the 18.6-year node cycle.[23] It affects atmospheric tides which in turn influence the flow of rain-bearing air. This region, where much of the world's grain is grown, is known to suffer severe droughts approximately every 20 years. High-yield periods in the US, nearly free of drought, tend to occur near minimum declination. The 'El Nino' weather pattern, a global reverberation affecting atmospheric perturbation, droughts and many other climatic factors, appears strongly linked to this same nodal cycle.[45] Currie has found both lunar and solar cycles, that is to say of 18.6 and 11 years, present in the atmosphere, the lunar signal being stronger than the solar.[24] For example, he has traced the 18.6-year lunar node cycle through floods and droughts in China for the past five centuries and these measurements and his conclusions have serious implications for food production worldwide.

In times to come, these two long-term cycles will come to be used in economic forecasting: the nutation cycle of 18.6 years and the 22-year solar cycle. In both cases, one-half of the cycle can often appear as the effective length. For comparison, the cycle of the lunar month causes a fortnightly peak in the tides. Astronomically, the lunar 'declination', which relates to how high the Moon rises in the sky, varies with the 18.6-year nutation cycle, while half of this cycle is 9.3 years, in which eclipses revolve around the seasons of the year, as there is no difference between the north and south nodes in this regard. A 9.3 year cycle in US grain production and prices was discussed by Thompson, with high yields occurring in years of minimum declination.[87] In the US, lowest agricultural prices tended to occur every 18.6 years.[88] Currie has also argued that a crop production cycle of 18.6 years exists. This confirms the conclusions of Dewey and his Cycles Foundation who identified cycles in wheat prices that ran for either nine years or 18–19 years.[28] US pig, chicken and egg production also varies with the node-cycle: 100,000,000 more US chickens are produced at the peak than at the trough[24] – the largest lunar influence yet identified! The study was extended over the half century 1910–60. [87] Herschel's original comment on corn prices and the rhythm of the Sun, therefore, may today be adjusted to match a lunar, not solar rhythm.

Chapter 8
THE ORGANIC WAY

Clear the sheds of dung, but not at new moon or half moon.

Cato, *On Farming*

THIS CHAPTER IS LESS an explanation of the beauties of lunar gardening, more by way of a call to all readers to embrace plant and food production along organic lines. I may be preaching to the long-since converted who may wish to skip to the next chapter. But many pay lip-service while dipping the knee to another master. These may care to listen again to a rehearsal of the arguments.

Organic farming took off during the 1980s, during which period the number of UK organic farms increased sevenfold. There are presently in excess of 700 farms certified organic and rather less than ten per cent of these are Bio-Dynamic. The movement has appeared as a largely northern and middle-European phenomenon. Nearly ten per cent of Austria's cultivated acreage is organic; Denmark and Sweden are not far behind. In Germany, over two per cent of farmland is designated organic and France comes a close second with just under two per cent. By contrast, the UK has only one-third of one per cent of its cultivated area classified as organic! However, if measured by the number of farms or the total acreage, the UK is fifth in the European league table.

At last, official support is being voiced for the organic movement. In May 1988, the Minister of Agriculture admitted in a parliamentary statement that,

> I am keen to encourage organic farming as a sustainable farming system that can contribute to environmental objectives and can, in particular, deliver real benefits to bio-diversity, while producing a product that the consumer wants and is prepared to pay a premium for.

It is an indication of the swing in public opinion that the Ministry of Agriculture, Food and Fisheries (MAFF) now makes available grants to assist farmers during the difficult two- or three-year conversion process, before an official seal of approval (usually from the Soil Association) enables crops to be sold as 'organic'. That said, the grant is little more than token. MAFF also funds research into organic systems at Elm Farm, Berkshire. Every week now *Farmers Weekly* has an organic grower's column, and that is quite a change.

In 1993, an EU regulation established a legally-binding definition of organic food. Let's hope this will suffice to block dire new US legislation of 1998, permitting such things as genetically-modified, additive-treated and irradiated materials which would negate the meaning of the word organic. 1998 was also the first year in which food generally available in supermarkets contained genetically-modified foodstuffs *without* consumers being informed. Sixty per cent of processed food contains soya products, two percent of which comprises the new US genetically-modified soya.

Genetically-modified tomatoes last longer on the shelf, and no doubt genetically-modified vegetables will be more resistant to the poisons which farmers spray so liberally upon the land. However, it is far from evident that such developments will have *any* benefit to the consumer. For US agribusiness to railroad the use of genetically-modified soya without even having to label the package is a frightening indication of the shape of things to come were they to have their way. 1999 saw many instances of direct action by consumers. This upsurge of popular feeling may change the course of events. But it is still too early to say. The only answer is to keep on refusing.

In case any reader is confused, irradiated food does not mean it is radio-active but merely that it is dead. Wheat will normally germinate, but that which has been irradiated will not. Nothing will happen if it is moistened. So the arrival of these new technologies poses quite urgently the question whether any kind of life-energy exists in food, and how far the organic farming movement should be committed to such a belief? In using a lunar-gardening calendar, you are surely expressing an affirmative reply to this rather central issue.

In the past, organic farming has sometimes been defined ,rather negatively, as being free from the herbicides, pesticides and fungicides of the chemical industry and innocent of inorganic fertilizers (NPK). Organic growing appeared as mere romantic reaction by ageing hippies who were striving to recapture a lost rural idyll. Reality was that chemicals were needed to feed the world. All that has now changed, with huge food surpluses from over-production. Farmers are paid to set aside productive land. It is a positive advantage that the organic way involves a slower rate of growth and a lower final crop yield.

The bible of organic growers has been Nicolas Lampkin's *Organic Farming*.[60] The Soil Association's journal is called *The Living Earth*, which is for consumers, whereas growers might read *New Farmer and Grower*, Britain's journal for organic food production. There is also a wonderful new Euro-book, *Organic & Wholefoods, Naturally Delicious Cuisine* (expensive), which does have some quite positive comments upon Bio-Dynamics.[30]

Research in animal husbandry has made it plain that animals fed on organic diets are more fertile. One survey found that all fertility parameters for rabbits, such as litter size, were enhanced by an organic diet. Also, rabbits fed on chemically-produced foodstuffs were found to be more prone to disease. With human male fertility apparently continuing a long-established tendency to plummet this should be a matter of rather central importance.

Let's say it loud and clear: organic farms don't have BSE (Bovine Spongiform Encephalitis). To be more specific, cows born and bred on organic farms do not have BSE. Indeed, Bio-Dynamic farmers received quite a fillip when a a statement made in 1923 by Rudolf Steiner was unearthed: if cows were fed on meat produce, they would go mad.[81] And so they did.

A five-year study published by the US Department of Agriculture found that organic farms had yields roughly equal to, and costs considerably lower than, conventional farms.[95] The organic farms were found to use more labour per unit of produce but to consume less energy. With increasing shortages of energy the importance of this hardly needs stressing.

Panels of tasters tend to prefer organic food. Also, organics have longer shelf-life. The concept of quality is being refined by these and other investigations and should be of great relevance for future studies of lunar influence. We are moving towards a positive definition of what 'organic' means in terms of taste and other characteristics, not just the absence of chemical products.

There may be progress but still hedgerow removal continues; still only two per cent of the population works on the land; still the large-scale concepts of agribusiness and its awfully bogus concept of efficiency tend to prevail; and yet farmers continue to have the highest suicide rate of any profession, a full double the national average, due partly to social and work-induced isolation, partly to loneliness, partly to immense financial pressures and never helped by a lack of esteem amongst the predominantly town-dwelling public. But an organic farm may knit the community together, particularly when it endorses the concept of Community-Supported Agriculture. Young people hanging around the streets could be tossing bales of straw, collecting eggs from the chickens and making hedgerows.

Organic farming puts more people on the land, is more labour-intensive, *but* it gets more produce from the land per acre. Shops selling organic produce presently import 70 per cent of their vegetables from Europe, chiefly Holland. There, public subsidy contributes more to the equation than it does in Britain. Surveys show that over 50 per cent of the British public want more support for organic farming. Indeed, demand for organic food is increasing at over 20 per cent a year. With less than one per cent of UK farmers being organic there is a long way to go. The new official UK Register of Organic Farms keeps the facts and figures and will give helpful advice. For a farmer deciding to make the big transition, there is nothing more reassuring than having an expert turn up from Elm Farm.

Readers may well be interested in investing with a bank such as Triodos which supports organic agriculture and local community projects in return for a marginally lower interest rate. Originally this was a Dutch bank but is now based in Bristol. A next step for town-dwellers is to subscribe to a box-scheme, whereby organic vegetables are available or delivered to their door weekly. If one subscribes near the beginning of the year, the overall cost works out as little more than ordinary shop produce. Such a scheme gives one an experience of participating in the cycle of the year. Seriously, would you trust a tomato in January? A box scheme gives one vegetables as they come off the farm and you too may experience the country-person's 'hunger gap' when the fields are producing nothing more than a few roots before the flush of spring crops is ready.

A few stalwart readers will wish to spend a week or so on a Bio-Dynamic or organic farm – a chance to become totally exhausted, gaze at lovely countryside, converse with like-minded people, tune into Nature's rhythms, sleep like a log, work with appropriate-scale technology, taste more delicious food than one can remember, and ruminate on lunar cycles. There are about fifty Bio-Dynamic farms in Britain now.

As well as waterproof boots from Army Surplus, one should take a star map for the month, as this could be the only opportunity of the year to view the Milky Way, due to the creeping scourge of light pollution. Fewer and fewer townspeople ever get to gaze upon the glittering majesty of that starry wheel. Lie down on the grass at midnight GMT in the summertime and just gaze. Somewhere up there lies the Galactic Centre, with the Scorpion and the Archer on either side ...

One may notice two respects in which Bio-Dynamic farms differ from other organic farms.[11] Firstly, the cows have their horns on, reminding one of the line in Virgil's rustic poem:

> Glittering Taurus opens the year with his golden horns.

The horns express the dignity of the cow, as being that part of it which faces upwards. The highest concentration of gold in the cow is in the horns. In the human body, by comparison, the highest concentration of gold is around the heart. The cows have to be given enough space, so they are safe with their horns. There is something wonderfully mild about a cow, as if it had no idea of the harm which it could inflict with its horns. A farmer who leaves the horns on the cows is worthy of respect in the community.

The other difference lies in the use of a lunar calendar. 'We can't sow now, as the Moon isn't right,' I was first told in 1970 (at Tablehurst Farm in Forest Row near Ashdown Forest) and the question haunted me thereafter. Franz Rulni produced his first Bio-Dynamic calendar in 1948, followed later by the Thun calendars from 1963 which continued the difficult task of linking the cycles of Earth and Sky.

Nowadays, not only are cows fed with steroids, milked by machine and deprived of horns, but they don't even get sex. Semen, after being cryo-genically frozen in liquid nitrogen, is just injected. Farmers select the genes of the bull of their choice. What kind of view of Creation is this, to assume the dumb creatures can be so treated without repercussions on us?

The sidereal rhythms that I describe in this commentary and the calendar which follows are likely to work best for the gardener using organic methods. Research indicates that good organic soil produces crops healthy enough to respond well to these cycles, whereas that to which fertilizers are added may not, or at least not to the same extent. Such organic soil, ideally, is built up over the years with compost and is humus-rich, with well-rotted manure – its organic matter digested into a dark friable humus. If, on the other hand, inorganic fertilizers are relied upon, these will force the growth of plants, initially increasing quantity but not quality, and decreasing storage life, disease resistance and, eventually, soil quality.

Using the rhythms of Mother Earth is one aspect (but nonetheless a vital one) of organic gardening. In contrast to the high cost of agro-chemicals and their long-term effects on soil productivity, organic methods offer both a safer and more cost-effective alternative.

I take courage from a better gardener than myself, Jack Temple, who writes the organic gardening section for the magazine *Here's Health*. His columns were collected into a book, *Gardening without Chemicals*.[84] He would now and then assure readers that sowing by the correct Moon-element made a big difference, even, say, for cress grown indoors: it was worth waiting a few days until the leaf-days came round, he reckoned, even if it meant storing the cress in the fridge for a while.

Jack was keen on putting calcified seaweed into his compost preparations and also rock phosphate from Chile. This latter is an 'inorganic' chemical but one on the Soil Association's approved list because it is slow-release. Indeed, some gardeners don't like using it on the grounds that it is too insoluble.

After harvesting a vegetable plot Jack wouldn't dig. Organic kitchen waste was spread across, so were any vegetables the local shops were throwing out, then cut grass and nettles were added, with a dusting of calcified seaweed, and it was all covered with cardboard, empty cartons, and finally black plastic sheeting so that no weeds could grow. Worms and insects munched their way through beneath this until, in the spring, the soil was friable and ready for the next crop. The taste of his vegetables was an experience.

Once, a row of his beans was infested by blackfly. 'Needs some more compost,' Jack remarked. He was proud of his worm compost. What connec-tion compost application was supposed to have with blackfly infestation was far from clear to me but it was applied and the next week, lo! the blackfly were gone. There was an irrigation stream around his plot which provided enough frogs to control the slugs.

He seemed to have the right attitudes towards harnessing the forces of nature to the ends of man: ingenious, yet with proper respect.

Chapter 9

REMINDERS FOR THE VEGETABLE GARDEN

I: A Repertory of Plant Types

IT IS USEFUL TO HAVE a list to hand of which sort of plant belongs to which element or sign. The calendar itself is not filled with detailed instructions about which plants to tend at any particular time, but merely which *type* of plant. Every gardener will have their favourites and an infinity of space could be occupied with redundant suggestions.

WATER
LEAF PLANTS

Alexanders
Angelica
Asparagus
Basil
Bay
Brussels sprout
Cabbage
Cardoon
Celery
Chervil
Chicory
Chinese cabbage
Chive
Claytonia
Coriander
Cress, American
Dandelion
Dill
Endive

Fennel
Florence fennel
Good King Henry
Grass
Hyssop
Kale
Lamb's leaves
Lavender
Leaf beet
Lemon balm
Lettuce
Lovage
Marjoram
Mint
Mizuna
Mustard and cress
Orach
Oregano
Pak choi

Parsley
Pennyroyal
Purslain
Rhubarb
Rocket
Rosemary
Sage
Salad burnet
Saladings
Seakale
Sorrel
Spinach
Summer savory
Tansy
Tarragon
Thyme
Winter savory
Wormwood

EARTH
ROOT PLANTS

Asparagus
Beetroot
Carrot
Celeriac
Chinese artichoke
Garlic
Hamburg parsley
Horseradish

Jerusalem artichoke
Kohl rabi
Leek
Liquorice
Mushroom
Onion
Parsnip

Potato
Radish
Salsify
Scorzonera
Shallot
Spring onion
Swede
Turnip

AIR
FLOWERING PLANTS

Artichoke
Bergamot
Borage
Broccoli
Broom

Calabrese
Cauliflower
Chrysanthemum
Cowslip

Elderflower
Marigold
Nasturtium
The flower garden
Violet

FIRE
FRUIT & SEED PLANTS

Apple
Apricot
Asparagus pea
Aubergine
Blackberry
Blackcurrant
Broad bean
Cherry
Chilli pepper
Courgette
Cucumber
Damson
Fig
French bean

Gooseberry
Gourd
Grains
Greengage
Loganberry
Mange-tout pea
Marrow
Medlar
Mulberry
Nectarine
Pea
Peach
Pear
Plum

Pumpkin
Quince
Redcurrant
Runner bean
Squash
Strawberry
Sugar snap pea
Sweet corn
Sweet pepper
Tayberry
Tomato
Vine
White currant
Worcester berry

II: A Plan of Work

Ken Whyatt, who has spent many years using organic methods, has kindly provided this excellent and practical seasonal guide to organic vegetable gardening throughout the year. I hope it will prove useful to the reader, even though climates may not be quite the same as for Ken (51°N, south-west England).

January

Burn woody rubbish in a slow smother fire. The resultant ash, when sieved and mixed with leaf-mould in equal parts, will make a wonderful base for sowing seeds later on. Keep the ash in a dry place. If clods of earth are stacked round the bonfire, these will crumble and make a useful ingredient in a potting mixture for tomatoes later in the spring.

Spread compost on vacant land, to remain until the soil is suitable for making seed beds. Inspect all vegetables in store and safeguard against hard frosts by covering with straw, matting or other light, dry material.

Make a cropping plan for your plot, making sure that cabbages (and members of the cabbage family) and potatoes are rotated – planted in an area not occupied by these crops for at least two years previously.

Order seeds in good time. Early seed potatoes should be chitted – placed in trays in a light, frost-free place so that they may develop short green shoots – thus gaining several weeks' growth at planting time. If your soil is a sticky clay, do not walk on the garden unnecessarily unless it is frozen. Keep a supply of old planks to put down to walk on to pick sprouts and other winter crops in wet weather. This will ensure that your soil will be easier to dig in the spring.

If you have a sheltered area facing south and the soil is well-drained and crumbly, sowings may be made of early peas and broad beans (long-pod varieties). Cloches will give added protection. Shallots may also be planted, provided the soil is not sticky.

February

Lightly fork over the area intended for sowings of early carrots, lettuce, cabbage, beet and parsnips. Incorporate well-rotted compost or leaf-mould and sieved bonfire ash in the top two inches. If the soil is too sticky to rake to a fine tilth, keep it covered with cloches for a week or so. Small sowings may be made of early peas, short-horn carrots, lettuce, summer cabbage and Brussels sprouts.

Delay sowings of parsnips and beet (Boltardy is recommended) until late in the month. Even then, beet will require the protection of cloches. These seeds are large and can be spaced about two inches apart. A small sowing should provide salad beet in June if the spot chosen is a sheltered one.

Parsnips should be sown at intervals of about nine inches in rows eighteen inches apart. Seed must be fresh and it is advisable to sow in groups of three or four seeds to ensure even germination, the weaker plants being thinned out in April. To ensure the rows are well marked (parsnips are slow starters) sow radish about one inch apart in the same rows. These will be ready for pulling long before the parsnips have grown large.

Jerusalem artichokes may be planted about 12 inches apart. Remember they can attain a height of six feet so they can be used as a wind break, shade for late sowings of lettuce and as an excellent vegetable in their own right, provided they are properly prepared and cooked.

The main sowings of broad beans may be made now. It is worth planning to succeed broad beans by a crop that requires plenty of nitrogen such as cauliflower, autumn cabbage or broccoli. The beans' roots increase the soil's nitrogen content. When the crop has been picked, cut the haulm to ground level and leave the roots where they were.

March

A busy month if the weather is kind. It is better to wait until the end of the month before sowing than to sow on pasty soil. Broad beans are a worthwhile crop, but must be given plenty of room to develop. Pinch off the top six inches when they are in flower – the shoots make a delicious salad or cooked vegetable and the plants are less liable to attack from blackfly.

Sow main-crop Brussels sprouts, cabbages and short-horn carrots for summer use; celery or celeriac and leeks in seed boxes in garden frames or greenhouses. Plant out lettuces from February sowings, ensuring they have plenty of compost in drills directly under their roots. Further sowings of lettuce should be made from now throughout the spring and summer. A pinch of seed will sow a short row of about four feet and this will suffice if sowings are made fortnightly. The same rule applies to radish, which are large seeds and can be dropped in a drill singly about an inch apart.

Onions can be purchased as sets – normal onions whose growth has been arrested in the autumn. These are planted in fine soil manured for a previous crop. Just push them in the soil without bruising them and cover their necks. As they start to root they may push themselves out of the soil. Replant them with the tip of a trowel.

Parsnips may still be sown, but should be in by the end of the month if they are to attain maximum growth.

Peas may be sown in continuation. The taller kinds will need the support of twigs or netting and the rows should be far enough apart for ease in picking. Rows of lettuce or radish can be sown as catch crops between the peas at the same time, as these will mature before the peas are ready and will benefit from some shade.

Fine soil with plenty of compost is needed for a good yield of early potatoes. If these have two or three green shoots already formed (see January) they can be planted towards the end of March. Spinach, spinach-beet and Swiss chard can now be sown, the last being the most useful, its thick, fleshy midribs making a separate dish from the large spinach-like leaves.

Annual weeds, and even perennial ones, will wilt in the sun if the surface is hoed slightly. They may look unsightly for a while, but worms will assist in clearing them, and the dying material will act as mulch.

Continue to plant out Brussels sprouts, cabbages, savoys and broccoli. There is still time to plant marrows and cucumbers outdoors if plenty of humus is available to give them a good start.

Leeks may now be planted from seed beds. Trim about an inch off the leaf-tips and trim back straggly roots. They are then dropped in holes made by a dibber about eight inches apart and watered in without pressing back the soil.

Runner beans and tomatoes will require strong stakes, which are easier to push in if the ground is first soaked. Plant after the stakes are in position.

April

Tomatoes can be sown in late March, but plenty of light and an average temperature of 60°-65°F is necessary for a good start, so early April is soon enough. Minimum requirements are a warm window-sill not subject to draughts, a good seed compost in boxes of two-inch depth, and thin sowing. When the seedlings are about two inches high they should be planted in separate three-and-a-half-inch pots and grown until early May in a warm, light place before moving to a cold greenhouse. Do not plant outdoors until late May or early June.

A useful plant is land or American cress, similar in appearance, taste and food value to watercress. Sow in a damp spot such as the north side of a low wall, or close to a concrete path, where it is easy to keep them watered.

The main sowings of dwarf beans, beet, broccoli, spinach, autumn and winter cabbages, carrots and herbs of various kinds may be made this month (bearing in mind that dwarf beans are frost-tender, so these could be delayed to late April or even May). January King cabbage and the varieties of purple and white broccoli are useful winter vegetables which will withstand hard frosts when greens are so expensive to buy. Incidentally, broccoli and Brussels sprouts need an open situation and at least two feet between plants, with a good firm soil. Wind tends to rock them, so draw up some surrounding soil from time to time to hold their stems firm.

Early and maincrop potatoes should be planted before the end of the month, giving the maincrops a minimum gap of two feet in the rows and two feet six inches between the rows. If the early potatoes have come through the soil, earth them up slightly and cover with soil if frost threatens. Periodically, they should be earthed up leaving a curved rather than a sharp ridge.

May

Take the opportunity during dull, showery weather to plant out seedling cabbages, cauliflowers and Brussels sprouts. Plant to the base of the lowest leaf-stalks and make the soil really firm. Thinnings of lettuces may be planted out, but ensure the roots are not damaged. They must be thoroughly watered, unless the weather is showery, and prefer a spot with some daytime shade.

Runner beans, courgettes, marrows and ridge cucumber are all sown this month, but must have some protection from late frosts. Cloches are ideal for this and home-made polythene frames or tunnels ensure a good start. Close up the ends with a sheet of glass, as wind-tunnels are not appreciated by any plant.

Early May is the best time for sowing maincrop beetroot, the thinnings of earlier sowings being useful raw in salads. Pick them when they are the size of a golf ball.

Late broccoli, savoys and winter cabbage such as the excellent January King are sown this month. Swedes and turnips are useful as a winter crop and should be thinned to eight inches apart when one inch high.

Capiscums sown in the middle of May, given sufficient warmth, will provide green pods in the autumn. It is not too late to sow carrots; in fact, the later sowings are less prone to attack from carrot fly. Incidentally, when thinning carrots for salads, remove the tops to the compost heap and tread back the soil loosened in the rows. The fly is attracted by the smell of carrots and likes to lay its eggs in loose soil.

Keep cauliflowers well watered with diluted liquid manure. They are the hungriest and thirstiest of plants, although celery must run them very close. This vegetable is naturally a ditch plant and does well in a trench with soil banked on either side. These ridges are useful for catch crops of lettuce or radish; when they have been gathered, the soil is used for successive earthing up of the celery for obtaining well blanched stems.

Sweetcorn needs a sheltered, moist spot. Sow the seed to fill a square rather than in rows. This assists pollination.

Peas can still be sown, but it's a good plan to leave the finished seedbed, after raking it over, at least two inches below the surrounding soil. Water can then be given in plenty.

In the third week, tomato plants for outdoors should be hardened off. An improvised polythene-covered frame will suffice until the plants are put in their final quarters early in June.

June

Dwarf and runner beans may be sown for a continuation of supply or if previous sowings have failed.

Lettuces will bolt if planted out in sunny positions. It is far better to sow thinly, using any thinnings for salads. Afternoon shade provided by taller plants will lengthen the growing season.

Water will be required by most vegetables if rainfall is light: if it has been standing in tanks, so much the better. Always give a thorough watering; the effect of dribbles is to bring roots to the surface, only to be left high and dry. An all-night drenching from a sprinkler hose will do wonders to beans, lettuce, beet, celery and cauliflowers during a dry spell – if the state of the nation's water supply or the depth of your pocket, if on a water meter, permit. In fact, plants benefit from evening soakings far more than any in the morning; the morning is a good time to add a mulch of lawn mowings before the sun can bake the surface of the soil. Mowings will gradually disappear as earth worms take them down, thus helping to aerate the soil and increase its fertility.

July

Complete planting of cabbages, savoys, Brussels sprouts, broccoli and leeks. Swedes and hardy turnips can still be sown in the south of England. Spinach beet and Swiss chard can be sown for next spring cropping. Repeatedly pinch out side shoots from tomatoes, except bush varieties. Harvest shallots and onions as they ripen and keep runner and dwarf beans picked as soon as they are large enough. Beans must never be allowed to grow coarse or they'll become unproductive.

Sow winter radish and thin to six inches apart. A sowing of parsley in a sheltered spot should withstand the winter. Dig early potatoes if ready. Keep the soil moist, remembering that showery weather is usually a good time to give a crop a soaking.

As plots become vacant, for example after onions have been harvested, it is a good plan to dig the soil, incorporating leafy vegetable rubbish and compost in shallow trenches as the digging proceeds across the plot. Woody waste such as cabbage stems are best disposed of on a bonfire, the plant ash being collected and kept in a dry place.

A sowing of a suitable variety of spring cabbage may be made in northern districts during the last week of July. In the south, this is best deferred until the first week in August. Care in selection of a variety suitable to the district is advisable, this being one of the most valuable crops to be grown.

Cucumbers, marrows and beans will benefit from good soakings of rain-water warmed by the sun. An excellent liquid manure can be made by chopping nettles or comfrey into rain-storage tanks, allowing them to soak for a few days. Tomatoes, in particular, benefit from this liquid, supplemented by a dressing of wood ash round the roots and followed by a mulch of lawn mowings. The plants will make rapid growth and set their trusses of fruit early.

August

A problem with sowing seed at this time of year is the likelihood of the soil being too dry; it is not advisable to water seeds *after* they are sown. This may be overcome by drawing a drill rather deeper than normal, soaking this and sowing on top, finally covering the seeds with fine sifted soil mixed with leaf-mould or peat. The dry layer above the seeds will prevent rapid evaporation, keeping the seeds moist enough for quick germination. This method works well with seeds sown in August, such as onions, lettuce, winter radish and spring cabbage. If, however, drought conditions prevail, a soaking from a fine sprinkler or a can with a fine rose can be followed with a light covering of hedge trimmings. These will soon wilt, but will prevent caking of the surface, Alternatively, cloches may be used after the watering, the cloches being lightly covered with hay or prunings for a day.

From spring until autumn grass mowings not required for mulching should be rotted down on a compost heap. Layers of grass, not more than two or three inches thick, should be interspersed with garden and kitchen waste. Rotting will be faster if smaller quantities of animal manure are spread between layers and a dusting of lime is added from time to time. Good composting is an art in itself and there are many publications which deal fully with this subject. Suffice to say here that there is no finer material for plant feeding than a well-rotted compost. Spread as a mulch between crops or on vacant plots as a weed smother. Worms will be active in the autumn incorporating this material into the surface far more effectively than the gardener can ever do by digging it in.

Pick cobs of sweet corn while still green. Harvest onions as soon as the tops have died down. Continue to pick tomatoes as soon as ready. Surplus beans freeze well.

September

Sow varieties of lettuce that have been specially developed for over-wintering under cloches.

Continue to lift potatoes and maincrop carrots. Store sound roots for future use. Do not leave these vegetables in the ground when they have reached their maximum growth for slugs and other pests can do much damage.

September can be the worst month for weeds, many of which are hurrying to ripen their seeds for the autumn winds to scatter. Remove them to the compost heap where the warmth generated by lawn mowings should destroy them. Vacant plots can be utilized by filling (but not overcrowding) with cabbage, winter lettuce and spinach plants.

In dry spells, celery can be earthed up a few inches at a time. The stems will then be blanched. Plant out winter lettuce in land manured for a previous crop. On heavy soil it is advisable to plant on top of a slight ridge to avoid damping off. A further sowing of a winter-hardy variety may be made.

Use parsley as required from the seedling rows, leaving strong plants standing about six inches apart. Cover them with cloches if the plot is exposed to cold winds in the winter.

If your garden is exposed, or in a frost pocket, it is as well to prepare for a slight frost towards the end of the month. The risk is greatest during clear anti-cyclonic weather and the morning sun does the damage. Have polythene sheets or even newspaper handy to drape over tomatoes and peppers. They can be removed after an hour or so. Another way is to spray the plants with cold water. Gather ripened marrows for storage in a dry place.

Sow lamb's lettuce or corn salad. This is an invaluable salad which can be used during the early spring when lettuces are scarce and expensive. Cut like spinach.

October

Continue to pick tomatoes as they ripen and, if frosts are imminent, remove whole trusses of fruit to ripen in trays lined with newspaper. They will ripen in the dark providing they have warmth. The whole plants can be lifted, complete with roots, and hung in a cool greenhouse for the remaining fruits to ripen or they can be used green for chutney. With some care, it is possible to have ripened tomatoes until Christmas.

Dig the remainder of maincrop potatoes; they are liable to slug infestation if left in the soil. Ensure that the minute, undeveloped potatoes are removed, otherwise these can grow next year, possibly spreading disease to both tomatoes and potatoes. Parsnips may be dug as required but will improve if frosted and may remain in the soil until wanted. Beetroot and carrots will not withstand hard frosts and are better stored in dry sand or peat in a cool place.

Put annual weeds on the compost heap. Put tree leaves in a separate heap as they take much longer to rot. Keep the garden tidy, removing yellowing leaves of the cabbage family and other decaying matter which only harbours slugs and other pests in the garden and is far better on the compost heap. Heavy land should be rough dug during the autumn and given a good dressing of compost. Light soil is best composted in the spring.

Spring cabbages are planted this month. If two varieties have been sown, so much the better. They should be firmly planted, closer than other cabbages, say twelve inches apart in rows two feet apart. In spring, alternate cabbages may be cut, leaving the others to grow larger.

A final sowing of winter-hardy lettuce can be made early in the month, covering with cloches. Celery should be earthed up during dry spells and celeriac lifted as required, the remaining roots being covered with dry soil to protect from hard frosts.

November

Clear up fallen leaves and put in a heap. Chicken netting will prevent them blowing about and the resulting leaf-mould can be used at the bottom of next year's potato drills.

It is a good plan to turn semi-rotten compost, placing the outside to the middle and the middle to the outside of the new heap. When completed, give a sloping finish, dust with garden lime and cover with old matting to keep off excessive rain.

Woody waste, potato and tomato haulms and diseased plants should be burnt in a slow smother fire, if possible covered with clods. The ash and burnt soil can be sieved when cool, kept dry and used in sowing composts next spring.

Continue forking over vacant land and burning perennial weed roots. Leave the surface rough, or cover heavy land with rotted compost. A light forking is all that will then be necessary in the spring to prepare the soil for planting and sowing.

Jerusalem artichokes can be used as wanted and some stored in sand for use during hard frosts. Clear out all roots as they are dug. Even small pieces will grow next year and can become invasive. If horseradish is grown the same advice applies.

On dry soils, a sowing of broad beans will repay the effort by producing a finer crop than those sown in the spring. If land is in danger of becoming too wet the roots will rot. Cloches help prevent this.

Corn salad or lamb's lettuce thrives in a dry, sheltered spot and is most useful in early spring salads. Sown early this month under cloches it should provide plenty of tender green stuff in April.

December

It is better to dispose of soft vegetable waste in winter by digging it into trenches during the rough digging of vacant plots than to put it on the compost heap where vermin may be a problem.

Plan ahead for the coming year, making a list of crops which bear well on your soil and ensuring that they will be planted in proper rotation. Leaf vegetables do well on soil previously used for bean crops because of the latter's nitrogenous deposits created by bacteria from nitrogen in the air. Potatoes, if well manured, provide a well-dug soil suitable for beans and peas the following year. Roots can follow members of the cabbage family – give a scattering of lime prior to sowing; but keep lime away from land required for potatoes, otherwise scabby skins will result.

In a four-year crop rotation of this sort, lettuce, tomatoes, celery, leeks and onions can be fitted in where they are likely to do best; but it is advisable to move onions and leeks around from year to year.

III: THE EIGHTEENTH-CENTURY GARDENING YEAR

This is an edited extract from a grand cookery and household manual written by Mrs Martha Bradley and published in 1756 called *The British Housewife: or, the Cook, Housekeeper's, and Gardiner's Companion*. Martha Bradley arranged her work in twelve monthly instalments and at the end of each part she included a couple of chapters on the vegetable garden, flower garden and orchard. She was perhaps a more expert cook than gardener and most of her material seems to have been drawn directly from one of the most influential eighteenth-century manuals: Philip Miller's *Gardeners Kalendar*, first printed in 1731.

The reasons for printing this version here range from its intrinsic interest, to the fact that old gardening practices are often of current relevance, especially to people who are trying to give up sprays, chemicals and other toxins. Martha Bradley's ideas make a nice counterpoint to the more up-to-date suggestions of Ken Whyatt, above.

Martha Bradley did not include much about fruit bushes (gooseberries and currants) or soft fruit, nor did her idea of orchards extend far beyond beautifully espaliered stone fruits like peach and apricot.

Central to the internal economy of the Georgian vegetable garden was the dung-powered hot-bed. It fulfilled much the same role as the modern greenhouse for forcing early crops. I have omitted some of her instructions where they revolved around technicalities of dung selection and supply. For rather similar reasons, I have left out the paragraphs about raising melons and cucumbers. They were preoccupied mainly with hot-bed management: useful for maybe two or three people today.

In the instructions which follow, where she does refer to hot-beds, the modern gardener may think in terms of plastic or glass cloches or frames. Where there is doubt about a plant variety or name I have included a note in square brackets. Not everything she says or does will find favour today. She plants potatoes in February and harvests them in November; she sows crops very early. Some of her apparent anticipation of the spring and summer derives from the use of hot-beds, some from having well-protected walled gardens that had warmer or colder borders in them depending on orientation. These borders were played upon by the skilled gardener with an almost musical virtuosity.

These much-edited extracts do not include the recommendations about the flower garden made by Martha Bradley. The difficulties of relating old varieties and nomenclature to modern usage would make reproduction so burdened with notes and qualifications that it would constitute almost another book in itself.

January

This is a season at which very little is produced in the garden or orchard, and very little is done in them. What can be done this month will in a great measure depend upon the weather. If very hard frosts continue the ground will not bear working and all that can be done is to get things in readiness against its will. If it be a little milder, the beds are to be dug up for spring crops and you may sow radishes, carrots, lettuces, spinach and young salading, as well as Windsor beans.

Celery should be blanched, and the mushroom beds well covered to preserve them from the severity of the weather. Endive [*where she refers to endive she means the curly endive or chicory, not the Witloof chicory as is grown in Belgium*] may be transplanted and new asparagus beds earthed up if there be shoots. Cauliflower plants are also to be carefully watched [*against frost*].

A gentle hot-bed may also be made for raising mint, as also carrots and some other roots, to be transplanted out when the weather permits for early service. Some peas may also be sown in warm and sheltered places.

Where there are espaliers, this is the time to mend and repair them with new poles and good fastenings wherever they are loose. The earth is to be dug about old fruit trees and it will be very proper to dig in some old and perfectly rotted dung about them. At the same time, dig and prepare the borders for young fruit trees. Grafts for early fruits are to be cut at this time and laid in the earth in a warm, dry place.

If the weather prove moist, this is a good time for cleaning the old trees of moss and cutting off the dead branches, making the stumps smooth and even. Hardy fruit trees may also be pruned at this season. The roots of new planted trees are to be defended from the cold by mulch and the fig trees should be covered with a reed fence or with mats.

February

Most of the summer crops are to be sown this month, therefore let there be great care taken not to lose the opportunity. The mildest weather is best and is always to be seized upon. Sow leeks and onions, carrots and parsnips, cabbage lettuces and spinach. Begin now, and sow a small parcel again before the end of the month. Young salading is sown now in warm borders. Sow at the latter end of this month scorzonera, salsify, and skirrets [Sium sisarum, *a species of water parsnip, grown for its root, once widely eaten in England*]. Cauliflowers to be sown on moderate hot-beds; plant in open ground shallots, rocambole [*Spanish garlic or sand leek, used for flavouring dishes*], chives and garlic. Plant out some cabbage plants, particularly the sugar-loaf kind. Sow peas and beans twice this month so that the crops may follow [*to get succession*]. New beds should be made for asparagus. French beans should be sown at the end of the month on a moderate hot-bed. At the end of the month plant out cos lettuce where they are to stand; some cabbages and savoys are sown now for winter use. Celery should be sown now in a warm rich border; potatoes and Jerusalem artichokes should be planted. Finally, let the garden be well looked over for snails and other vermin and all killed that are to be found.

The hardier kind of fruit trees are now to be pruned and towards the end of the month some of the more tender kinds. All kinds of fruit trees are to be transplanted into the places where they are wanted; if the weather be favourable towards the end of the month, pears, plums and cherries may be grafted. Kernels of stone fruit may be sown, and in moist weather the moss should be pulled off from fruit trees and the greatest care is to be used to keeping off mischievous birds. Among these the principle and worst of all is the bullfinch. One week in the latter end of February, when the weather is mild and favourable, is often of more consequence than three at any other season.

March

It is a season in which much is to be done and he who would acquit himself to his own credit and his master's satisfaction must every day be busy. If there be any planting unfinished, it must be immediately undertaken; if apricot, peach and nectarine trees are left unpruned, let it be done without more loss of time. There will be some early blossoms in this month and the curious may shelter them to preserve them from the perpendicular fall of dews. By this means blossoms that would otherwise have been destroyed by these dews and frosts will set. Yew, holly, box, and the like may now be removed to where the gardener pleases, observing to open a hole large enough for them and to throw in well broken earth, and to see it well settled about their roots.

This is a very good season for grafting and inoculating. Towards the end of this month the fig trees are to be examined and all the old wood that can be spared is to be cut away as close to the stalk as possible for this does not bear. The bearing wood on the fig tree is principally the last year's shoot, these are therefore to be preserved. The beginning of the month is the best time for pruning cherry, plum and peach trees of one year's growth.

About the middle of this month look to your strawberry beds. Dress up the beds with a little fine manure, water them thoroughly. Clip away all the runners till they blossom. Plant out cauliflowers in a good warm bed. Uncover the asparagus, spread some loose mould about them and a little fresh manure. Plant out asparagus roots into new beds. Keep up a succession of salad plants by sowing fresh parcels once a week on warm borders. Sow cabbages and savoys for a winter crop, and celery for early blanching. Sow cardoons [*first cousin to globe artichokes, grown for their fleshy stalks or midribs, the plant is blanched before harvesting – see instructions below*] which are then transplanted towards the end of April. Globe artichokes must now be dressed so that you have three or four suckers on every strong root. The others should be slipped off carefully for transplanting. Sow lettuces, beets, fennel, chervil, spinach, dill, burnet and sorrel. Sow endive thinly. Divide tarragon roots and plant eight inches apart. Divide and plant out chives. Sow purslane and nasturtium on hot-beds. Continue sowing radishes, cabbage lettuces for soups and cos lettuce for salads. Continue sowing peas and beans for succession. Set out hardy sweet herbs such as mint, balm, penny-royal, savory, thyme, sage, and tansy. Parsnips and carrots should be sown, and onions, borage, bugloss. Sow Hamburg parsley in drills a foot apart in rich deep earth. When they are ready to be thinned leave them eight inches apart. Thin the early spinach beds: plants about four inches apart. Sow French beans in light and fine soil.

April

Put your last hand to the fruit trees to prepare them for the summer's service. The pruning and nailing, if any part be defective, must be supplied and finished with a very tender hand, for it is too far advanced for such operations. Look carefully for the last time and see if any dead wood escaped your eye. Cut it out with a sharp knife and a steady hand. Water those trees that have been planted this spring or autumn if the season be dry. Lay a heap of stones around the bottom of every new-planted tree. This answers two purposes: keeping the earth moist about the roots, and keeping the tree steady. Some content themselves with laying weeds or straw about the roots, but this answers only half the purpose. Watch the shoots of new-planted trees, rub off such as grow ill. Cherry trees that are in danger of being hidebound are now to be eased by slitting down the bark in such places with a knife. It is remarkable that the grain of cherry bark runs circularly, so that this method is sure to relieve them.[*This practice can be likened to that of whipping walnut tree trunks to release the tight grip of slow-growing bark and allow them to put on a spurt of growth.*] Let the vines be watched this month and all useless shoots removed; and the suckers be taken from the roots of fig trees.

Let the gardener now clean his alleys and lay all in order in his kitchen garden. Sow beets, sorrel, parsley, onions, and chibols [*spring onions*]. This is a very good time to sow French beans. Choose a dry soil and warm border and sow them in shallow trenches two feet apart, the seeds at four inch intervals. Rouncival peas [*a particularly large variety*] are to be sown as well as other peas and beans for late crops. Lettuce should be sown to succeed former crops. Purslane and nasturtium should be sown to take their chance in the naked ground. Water the strawberries every three days if the weather is dry: the fruit will come in such abundance as very well to repay the trouble. Cardoons to be sown directly where they are to grow: place four seeds in a hole made with a stick, make these holes at five feet distance. When the young plants come up keep the strongest and pull up the rest from each hole. Hoe the carrots and parsnips to destroy weeds and thin the plants. They should now be left about eight inches apart. Do the same to onions, leave four inches apart. Transplant young celery plants into beds of deep rich earth. Place about six inches apart. Water lightly until they take root. Hoe between the rows of beans and peas. Draw up the earth round the stems of cabbage and cauliflower plants.

This is the best season for propagating rosemary and lavender and the like by cuttings. Observe that cuttings of rosemary succeed in this way just as well as slips and do not hurt the mother plant in taking them off, whereas the slips tear and make wounds that do not easily heal. Many a fine shrub has died from this the next winter when the cause was forgot and the damage laid only to frosts.

There is no season at which the garden is so overrun with vermin.

May

This is a month when the sun has a great deal of power, and if there happen some rain, as there generally does, especially towards the beginning of it, a great deal of care must be taken in every quarter to keep down weeds. The useful crops will be at this time growing stoutly: but if they be not cleaned from weeds their progress will be checked and they will be backward and poor. Continue sowing all kinds of young saladings: they should be sown once a week or oftener, for they grow quickly too large for use. As to their situation, that should be now just the contrary to what it was to be early in the spring. Then they required a warm south aspect, now they should be set in a northern border, for the season favours them so much.

This is a very good season for endive: let it be sown for blanching. First it is to be thinned, for it will rise too thick; afterwards it must be kept very free from weeds. Purslane may now be sown upon a good warm south border in a sheltered place. This herb is too much neglected; it is wholesome as well as agreeable to the palate. If you intend to have late crops of beans, sow some in the third week in May upon the coldest and dampest border of the garden. Peas may be sown for the same purpose in the same manner. Choose a good, rich, moderately warm border for a second sowing of kidney beans. The cabbage and celery sown in April will now be of a height to plant out. Water them for the first three or four days. Prepare a bed for winter cauliflowers. Sow the seed carefully and defend it from birds. Lettuce of several kinds will now demand nice care in their management. Remember that, besides the present crop, there must be a succession. While continually drawing some for use, sow and transplant others. Where early cauliflowers begin to show the first signs of a head, break down two or three of the innermost leaves to cover the flower. This will preserve it white and make it grow thick and hard. Look over the early cabbages. They will begin to round. To assist this, tie the top leaves together with string. It makes for a better head which will be whiter and harder. Remove artichoke suckers. Sow turnips and broccoli. When turnips come up, thin them to stand a foot apart. At the end of the month, prepare gherkin cucumbers for pickling. Sow in the naked ground. Sow sweet marjoram and annual aromatic plants including sweet basil.

This is the season when the housekeeper begins to prepare for distilling. Plants are in their fullest perfection when they have grown to their height and are budding for flower. Some of them will be just in that condition at this season, particularly rosemary. Those that are cut now she uses to distil and any remaining bundles are preserved for drying. Hang them in small bundles in an airy garret on lines stretched from wall to wall. Other flowers to be gathered are borage and bugloss.

Look over the espaliers. Thin the wall-fruit. Apricots will hang in vast clusters and peaches grow together in lumps. They are carefully to be thinned. It is better to have a small number well ripened, large and truly flavoured, than a heap of ill-tasted and half-starved ones. The vines must be carefully looked after. Such shoots as have fruits above them must be stopped at the third joint above the bunch, and the others that are for next year's bearing are to be encouraged in the growth. Let the borders around the fruit trees be kept clear of weeds.

June

Sow a second crop of broccoli. If the weather be not too hot and dry, sow turnips in a shady place. They will very soon grow for the table. A crop of French beans and all kinds of lettuce should be sown also at this time. This is a good time for the planting out of those sweet herbs which have been sown for the use of the kitchen. Cabbage and savoy plants sown in the early months will now be fit for planting out. They can be planted between peas and beans and other early crops which will shade them till they have taken root. The early endive will also be ready for transplanting. They will be quickly fit for blanching. Plant out cardoons for the last time. It should stand in a bed of rich and light mould, each plant four foot from another. As it grows, the earth should be carefully hoed up to cover the stalks for blanching. When cardoons are not well blanched they look dirty and eat coarse.

Keep trees well weeded. Go over the fruit trees with a careful eye. Whenever the fruit stands too thick, thin it again. Where the fruit on the wall trees is too exposed to the sun, draw over some leaves by way of a covering. Whenever there happens a shower this month, be sure to visit the wall fruit and look carefully after snails; as also mornings and evenings. New planted trees must have some water at times and mulch should be laid about their roots. All side shoots and ill-placed branches of vines should be removed. Clear away the leaves from the bunches to give them all the advantages of ripening.

July

The products of the spring sowing are now many of them in their perfection, but the gardener should remember, while he is gathering one crop, to make preparation for another: there is the winter to come, in which the products of the kitchen garden are always very desirable and there is also a consideration to be had for the succeeding spring, for there is no time better than this for sowing many of the useful crops that are to come in very early.

Winter spinach is to be sown this month, and onions for the spring. Carrots sowed at this time and kept clear of weeds will also come in very well in spring: and coleworts [*kale*] and turnips may be sown now with great advantage. Late cauliflowers should now be planted out: and all of the cabbage kind intended for use early in spring. Endive is a herb so very useful by its continuance when others are gone that there always should be fresh sowings of it so long as the season calls for it. This is a very good season for sowing broccoli for the spring. At this time it will be proper to sow French beans and such as are sown now will bear till the very coming on of winter.

Celery and endive are now to be planted out for blanching. The celery is to be blanched by earthing up and the endive by tying it. The great care in drawing the earth up to the celery must be not to bury the head; and a proper time should be taken for tying up the endive; the middle of a dry day is the proper time, for if it be in wet weather, or even when there is a heavy dew, they will rot instead of blanching. Let it be a constant care to water those things which have been transplanted, for otherwise in these dry times they will come to little. Onions will show they now begin to be fit for pulling by the leaves fading. The same will be seen in the shallots and other plants of that kind. They must be laid in an airy room, spread at a distance upon the floor and upon shelves, that they may be thoroughly dried on the outside and may have a sufficient quantity of their juices gone from within to prepare them for keeping.

If asparagus beds have been made in the spring or young artichokes planted, this is the time for preparing and finishing them up. The asparagus beds must be carefully looked over and where any roots have failed the loss must be supplied by new ones. As to artichokes, great care must be taken that they be clear from weeds and the ground well dug about them. The lettuces sown last month will be fit for planting out and they must be watered for three or four evenings after. For these and for the repairing of the asparagus beds, there must be chosen a dripping day. We may assist the deficiencies of nature by artificial waterings: they do not answer like the real and proper drops from heaven: *Set Wet* is an everlasting good rule.

Many seeds will now be ripening, and they must be watched and gathered in due time. They must be gathered on a dry day and dried on a floor in an airy, shady place, after which they must be got out of the heads and pods, and put up for use.

The preceding month was a very favourable time for the budding of fruit trees but this will not be amiss, therefore let such as have omitted it entirely begin now. Cut suckers from the roots of young trees.

After every shower it will be proper to walk the rounds among the fruit trees to look after snails. They will now be seen crawling abroad and much good fruit may be saved by destroying them. Snails are not the only devourers of fine fruit, wasps will eat into it and even so contemptible an insect as the ant will be vastly mischievous. The way to guard against these is to tempt them from the fruit with something they like better; for this purpose let little gallipots of coarse sugar and water be stuck in the forks of trees and wide-mouthed bottles of the same syrup tied to the branches; they will be decoyed into these and the fruit will escape.

August

This is the time of providing for the winter and the following spring. Spinach must be sown and it will grow up for use in the season when most wanted. Onions may be sown also now, but they will be in danger if the winter proves hard. Cabbages that are to stand the winter should be sown about the second week in this month. Cauliflower should be sown a little later but they must be preserved with a great deal of care in winter in frames or under great shelter. Celery sown in preceding months will now be fit for transplanting in order to blanch; and endive will be in the same condition.

September

Few gardeners will have any great opinion of September sowings, yet there are some things to be done in that way very advantageous. Everyone concerned in providing for a table knows the value of spring carrots; the earlier they are brought in the greater is their value and this is one of those things that should be attempted by sowing in September. The chance of hard weather is against them but this is a risk the gardener must run who would take the advantage of the first season. For this purpose choose a well sheltered and warm bed. Sow beans and peas twice. If they escape the severity of winter they will yield very early crops. Taking the two opportunities a fortnight apart one of the two, if not both, may succeed. Sow also young salading and lettuce for the family. Cabbage lettuces are hardiest, but the cos the most valued. Sow mixed seed, let them take their chance together. Cover some with glass. Plant out the last sowing of broccoli and of cauliflower. The coleworts, lettuces and endive sown in July should also be transplanted. The cardoons that were planted out in June will be ready for earthing up in September. On a dry day tie up the leaves with string. Earth each plant up but take care not to bury the heart for then it will decay. Celery that was planted out early should also be earthed up at this time.

October

This is the time for transplanting many of those useful crops which are to stand through the winter and to preserve several others which the cold nights and frosts that are coming on will destroy. Look over your seedling lettuces and plant them out according to their coming in season. Some must be planted in the open ground and some under frames or on beds that may be sheltered from the frost. Dress your asparagus beds and plant cabbage and savoys in between the rows. The method to follow is this: cut down all the weeds on the beds and pile them up to one side. Dig a small trench between the rows of asparagus and bury the weeds at the bottom, replace the soil mixed with a little dung. Plant the cabbage and savoys on that. Earth up cardoons and finachia [*fennel bulbs*] and celery. Earth up the stalks of broccoli plants for it will defend them from frosts. Transplant cauliflower to sheltered spots where they can be covered with bell or hand glasses. Plant out the late-sown cabbage and coleworts. Cut down artichoke plants and trench the ground between the rows and throw the earth up from the trenches over the plants themselves. Put into the open trenches a mixture of two-thirds rotted dung and two-thirds coal ashes.

Prepare borders for new fruit trees. If the earth is too heavy, lighten it with sand and ashes. If it is too light, mix in some clay. Dig in compost. Prune apples, pears and plums. Gather in fruit that is to be kept for the winter. Winter pears should be laid up in heaps in a dry airy store room for a week. They will mellow and grow a little damp by lying together and this will prepare them for standing the rest of the season. They must be carefully wiped one by one; when this is done, they are to be laid upon shelves at such a distance as to be out of the reach of spoiling one another.

Plant gooseberries and currants. Prune currant bushes and work the soil around them. Harvest grapes on dry days. The best way of preserving the grapes is to cut off a joint of the vine with each bunch and to hang them up on strings or lines set a great distance from one another in a room where there is commonly a fire. They will thus keep very good a great part of the winter, and with right management may be preserved through the whole season. Towards the end of the month the vines may be pruned; there is no time fitter, because they will not lose their juices. Weed the strawberry beds, spread compost and rotted dung between the plants.

November

Frosts become severe and crack the earth about the stems of the plants; this lays the roots bare and a continuance of the same weather utterly destroys them. One method is universal against this disaster, which is the earthing up of their stalks.

The use of reed fences is very well known [*for protection against frost and wind*] and they never can be too much recommended. Where there are not a sufficient quantity of them, let others be procured and let them be well secured by tying to poles fast down into the ground. We have named also the use of furze bushes by way of defence against frost. The way of using these is by sticking them into the ground at different distances among the crop, and let them be of such a height as is sufficient for sheltering the growth and the more bushy the better.

Choose a warm border under a hedge or wall on a day when the earth is free from frost. Dig and work it well to a good depth to sow radishes and carrots to come in early. The chance of their succeeding or not depends entirely upon the weather [*but now we have plastic cloches*]. Sow young salading, peas and beans on hot-beds with a moderate degree of warmth. Take up potatoes and lay them by for the service of the kitchen. Where the quantity is considerable, choose a high, airy piece of ground where the soil is naturally dry. Dig a drench three foot deep and two foot and a half broad, and let the length be according to the quantity of potatoes to be preserved. Spread some dry, clean straw over the bottom of the trench and let it rise a little up the sides. Wipe the potatoes clean and lay them two days on the floor of an airy room, then fill the trench with them. Reserve a good quantity for the service of the family so long as they can be expected to keep good. Lay a covering of more clean straw upon the potatoes in the trench and pile over it a ridge of the earth that was dug out in the making of it. The ridge of earth is sufficient to defend them from frosts but may admit wet in a dripping winter. It should be covered with thatch.

Long and deep-rooting plants such as carrots, parsnips, beets, and Dutch parsley [*Hamburg parsley*] should be taken out of the ground, not only for their preservation, but because in continued hard frosts there will be no getting at them. The best method of preserving them is this: spread a large quantity of sand upon the floor that it may dry thoroughly. Take up these roots and wipe the earth clean from them. Lay them separate on a dry floor, from eleven to four o'clock some dry day and then taking them up, wipe them again and lay them separately upon a bed of dry sand. Cover them with more and thus have them for the winter. They will retain their true flavour at all times provided no wet be permitted to come at them.

Where there is an old and entirely useless tree in the orchard it should now be grubbed up without loss of time and a young one planted in its place. The business of pruning wall-trees may now be very well done, taking advantage of mild weather; and it is a work that should not be deferred much longer because the wounds do not heal well when weather is very severe. The several kinds of stone fruit, and the apples and pears, all admit the same time of pruning; but it is best to do the stone fruit first to be sure of a better season, their wounds not healing so easily as those of the others.

The winter pruning of the vine is a very peculiar article of the gardener's business. The hope of a good growth of fruit the succeeding year depends wholly upon this. Consider how quick a grower the vine is and keep that always in mind when pruning. Cut away with boldness and leave but few of the last year's branches. Those which are left must be the largest and the thickest. The smaller must all be taken away.

December

This is a dead season of the year for gardening; the winter crops are all in the ground and those to be sown in spring must not be put in for a considerable time. This would lead many to suppose there was nothing to be done in the garden at the present period and it is accordingly a custom with many who keep a gardener during the summer to discharge him at the approach of this season.

Look to the peas and beans sown late in autumn. Raise a couple of reed hedges at the ends of their bed and scatter some long, dry straw over them to protect against wind and frost. Get out the pods and plants of seeds and remove the seeds clean out of them, put up each in a paper with its proper name and lay them in readiness for sowing. Continue to blanch endives for following the last crop.

Mulch the newly planted fruit trees and stake any rocked by the wind. Cut away in a sloping manner, close to the trunk or stem, any irregular straggling branches, or dead wood, of older trees. Take care to leave the surface smooth otherwise the rains will get in and rot the tree. If you see any particular danger of this, lay over a coarse cloth with some wax and rosin, or a piece of sheet lead.

Cut any quickset hedges and mend any that are defective by cutting a good, stout shoot three parts through and laying it down a little sloping to thicken the bottom of the hedge, which is the most essential part.

Chapter 10

HOW TO USE THE CALENDAR IN FARM AND GARDEN

When you cut down elm, pine, walnut and all other timber, cut it when the moon
is waning, in the afternoon, and not under a south wind.

Cato, *On Farming*.

FROM ITS FIRST EDITION IN 1980, *Planting by the Moon* has claimed that the star-
zodiac was the framework that really worked. This claim grew out of the belief,
that two cycles, the sidereal four-element cycle and the waxing-waning phase
cycle of the Moon, were vitally relevant for growing crops and for the rearing
of farm animals. The calendar did not use the ascending-descending 'tropical'
cycle of the Moon. Readers who were also Bio-Dynamic farmers found this
different emphasis on lunar cycles at first difficult to support as they have long
been used to taking into account the ascending-descending tropical cycle. This
is indeed the underlying principle of all Bio-Dynamic lunar calendars, although
there appears little by way of published evidence that it works, and Rudolf
Steiner himself made no allusion to it in his original lectures on agriculture. On
the contrary, he strongly emphasized the Moon-phase cycle, though this latter
is hardly used in Bio-Dynamic calendars – a paradox.

A calendar should not be too complex. Bio-Dynamic calendars tend to
display at once five monthly cycles and planetary aspects, which is a lot for the
novice reader to absorb. However, we have seen how there exist only two
monthly cycles for which there is substantial evidence of important effects on
cultivating fruit and vegetables and rearing livestock. Others used in the present
calendar, for example the lunar node and perigee which we suggest as no-
planting days, have had comparatively little work done on them.

Originally, *Planting by the Moon* did not recommend sowing according to
lunar phase, despite the fact that in various parts of Britain and Europe beliefs
of this nature can be found which go back several hundred years. These folk-
beliefs may have become garbled over the centuries and a new start, a
rethinking of the situation, is necessary. It would be hard to find even sugges-
tive evidence that planting potatoes during the waning Moon, for example,
improves their growth. Would any of the popular almanacs which give this
advice to their gardening readers care to produce some evidence in support?

Readers may be inspired to try for themselves sowing one half of a crop at
a recommended optimal time and the other half at a negative time, to see

93

whether there is any difference. A proper experiment requires a dozen rows or more, as discussed in Chapter 4. Measured amounts of seed are sown equally in each row, on different days, then final yields per row are compared after each row has been grown for the same length of time, i.e. they are harvested in rotation. Then, over the years, one distinguishes astronomical-lunar rhythms present in the data from differences due to weather and so forth.

Putting together a lunar-gardening calendar and advocating that organic farmers and growers should adjust their work-schedules to fit into it is not done lightly. It does not mean that one is confident of knowing the answers, but more that one has an idea as to what are the right questions. Once in 18.6 years the lunar nodes revolve once round the zodiac and this period has gone by since the first edition of *Planting by the Moon* appeared: a node-cycle. Over this period the author has reached a clearer understanding of the fundamental principles involved ('the silver axioms') and of what evidence supports them. The millennium-synthesis edition you are now reading has one startling difference from the 1980s version: by advocating sowing crops at moonrise it is in effect using the waxing-Moon half of the cycle.

Organizing one's Schedule

The farmer is a busy man, especially in the growing season, and may have little choice when to do things. Beans have to be picked as they ripen, and corn may have to be harvested at the first dry spell. But even if he cannot in practice wait for the Moon it surely adds deeper interest and dignity to his craft to realise that these rhythms do exist and that, for example, the sensible and practical people of ancient Rome used them as a matter of course. Do apples keep better if picked at the New Moon and do tomatoes ripen quicker if picked at the Full? If a farmer can weave these cosmic rhythms into his programme then his productivity is sure to benefit.

So, in deciding when to sow, a farmer has to weigh, on the one hand, soil condition and prevailing weather and, on the other hand, the primary cosmic rhythms which affect his plants. For maximum yields he should sow at the peak times of the sidereal energy cycle involved. Yet there is no point in doing so if the ground is too wet, too dry or too cold. A balance or compromise has to be struck. Much of the farmer's craft involves such judgements.

As more people turn towards life-styles of ecological balance and self-sufficiency, so the demand must surely increase for natural methods of crop improvement which work in harmony with the universe of which we are a part. In this manual we have attempted to bring together the evidence so that the reader can make up his or her own mind upon this old, hardy perennial belief, that the Moon influences the growth and yield of crops.

The paragraphs which follow give some hints on how to use the calendar to best effect, and lay down certain broad principles which can be applied to each day or lunar circumstance.

The Calendar

The calendar of 2000 follows the same principles and layout as that published through the 1980s, plus one or two new features. One hopes the reader will appreciate these fairly novel features, as well as the sense of being linked with millennia of past tradition by using the star-zodiac of antiquity.

The Zodiac Rhythm

For sowing crops observe the four-element cycle. In the calendar these are shown as root, leaf, flower, and fruit or seed days. The table below gives some examples of what these include.

On Root-Days, sow carrots, onions, radishes & potato.

On Leaf-Days, sow cabbages, celery, spinach & lettuce.

On Flower-Days, sow cauliflower, artichoke, broccoli & all flowers.

On Fruit/Seed-Days, sow cucumber, corn, peas, beans & tomatoes.

If convenient, sowings are best made on the day nearest to the middle of any of the three Moon-signs of the appropriate element. Soil should be tilled on the day of such a sowing rather than before. Avoid sowing just before the Moon moves out of a sign. Such transition times are given to the nearest hour.

In Australia, one of the fathers of Bio-Dynamics, Alex Podolinsky (whose work is described in *Secrets of the Soil* by Bird & Tompkins) advocates sowing just as the Moon enters a new Moon-sign-element, so the seed has a full two days in that quality before it changes, on the grounds that it takes that long to germinate. That view may be important in drought-prone countries.

From a practical point of view it may be objected that, in the busy schedule of a farmer, it is very difficult to organize sowing activities so that resources are available every nine days or so to sow one particular type of crop. If this is the case, it is important and usually possible to note and avoid the worst days for sowing in any given lunar cycle, even if one cannot make use of the optimal time. By referring to Figure 19 which follows it can be seen that the cycle of four elements follows a regular wave pattern. For example, root crops should be sown during Earth-days for optimal yield. However, if this is impossible, one should at least avoid planting on days at the trough in the cycle when the Moon is in the opposite element, in this case Water-days. This inverse approach can be applied to each of the other elements; for example, Fire-days are the worst times to sow flower crops, which are related to Air-days. By checking the calendar in advance one can see which are the worst days as well as which are the best for planting a particular crop.

Bio-Dynamic farmers believe that any disturbance of the soil should be carried out in the same Moon-sign element in which the seed was sown. Lettuce, for example, is sown on a Leaf-day, so its soil preparation as well as subsequent thinning out, weeding and so forth should also be done on a Leaf-day to enhance the effect. This is something for the reader to mull over.

Potatoes, Carrots and Onions

For root crops to be stored over winter, harvest on a Root-day nearest to the New Moon. In previous editions, we have simply advised that it is best to harvest at New Moon if the crop is destined for storage. Since then, Maria Thun's investigations have found that harvesting as well as sowing can use the element-trigons, i.e. the four types of 'day', and Bio-Dynamic farmers seem to have confirmed this by experience.

For many gardening operations, at least in Britain, one just has to go ahead when weather permits. Once corn is ready, you can seldom wait a week to harvest it. This can undermine the practice of using a lunar calendar, but the harvesting of root-crops is an exception. There is no hurry in harvesting the carrots, so one has the option of selecting an optimal time.

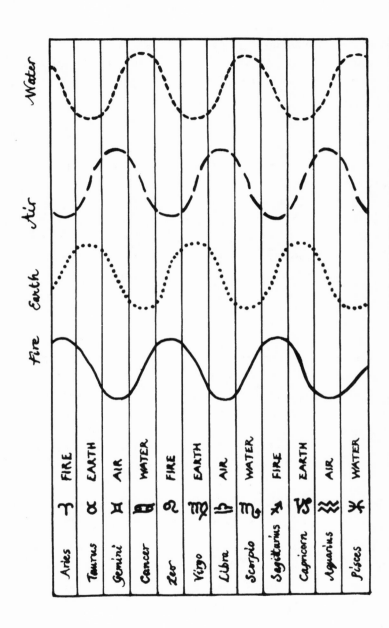

Figure 19. The four-element energy cycles.

Flowers and Venus

For Flower-days, the aspects between the Moon and Venus are given. A Moon-Venus energy is ideal for sowing or planting flowers, especially roses. Roses are ruled by Venus, that is to say, the rose *expresses the being* of Venus. The square aspects are also included, though some might view them as unsuitable, expressing difficulty and stress. Alternatively, they could be viewed as assisting the development of structure, so readers here have a choice.

Harmony of a Sun-Moon Trine

The calendar gives the trine (120°) angle between Sun and Moon, as happens twice monthly. This is a harmonious aspect free of stress or conflict, and its moment of linking the two luminaries is a good time for many things. Visualize it as a moment of harmony. Like the event of moonrise, it seems never before to have featured in a UK lunar gardening guide: the idea came from the American book *Gardening Success with Lunar Aspects* by Adele Barger (1976). She said that angels helped her with her book so perhaps they deserve the credit! This aspect is of particular interest for crops ruled by the Sun, for example oranges or vines.

Trees & Perennials

When working with plants that become woody or are veritable trees, seek a Saturn aspect for the most propitious time. The calendar gives three types of Moon-Saturn aspect each month: the opposition (180°), the trine (120°) and the sextile (60°). Growers should be mainly concerned with the Saturn aspects on fruit-days as most of their trees and bushes will be fruit-bearing. Because these plants are going to last for years there is all the more reason to identify the optimal date for planting. However, there are perennials that may be influenced by more than one factor. If you are planting a honeysuckle or clematis to grow up one's back wall seek a flower-day and then the calendar gives a choice: a Saturn aspect for durability or a Venus aspect for pretty flowers.

Moonrise

The calendar gives the daily event of moonrise, an hour either side being recommended as the best time of the day to undertake any planned planting, sowing or gardening that may be linked to the particular element-sign then in place. As a celestial aspect defines the optimal day, so does moonrise the hour.

In Britain, moonrise happens in the daytime during the waxing phase. The Calendar also gives night-time risings, not just for the benefit of insomniacs, but for persons in other time zones. The event of moonrise is given to within ten minutes. This event would be especially significant if some relevant aspect were being formed by the Moon that day, for example with the Sun or Saturn.

One may wish to sow at moonrise, i.e. in the waxing Moon phase, and just before Full Moon, that is in late afternoon. On the day of Full Moon, the Moon rises as the Sun sets, which might be rather late, so a day or two earlier could be preferable.

Moonrise times are given for zero longitude. For any other longitude, obtain the time of rising (GMT) by adding one hour per fifteen degrees of longitude due west. A user in Bristol, for example, which is three degrees due west, adds ten minutes to the times given in the calendar. There is also a latitude effect, whereby the Moon rises earlier due north, which readers in other latitudes can check by watching it rise and comparing the time of day to that given here.

Fish a-jumpin'

American almanacs give the best times for fishing each day as moonrise and the moment it culminates, that is it reaches its highest point in the sky. This last time can be obtained approximately from the calendar by adding six hours to your local moonrise. Some readers will recall the researches of the American biologist Frank Brown which demonstrated (in the laboratory) that the greatest metabolic rate in both plants and small animals was registered at the time of moonrise and culmination. The notion of fish being more active at these times is merely a practical illustration of his findings.

The Course of the Day

Gardeners are familiar with the idea that the time of day at which certain operations are performed is important. Planting-out of crops is in general best done in the evening so that they will have the night to settle in and rest. But pruning is best done in the morning so the Sun will dry up the cut surface, thereby inhibiting bleeding.

For effective lunar planting, seed should really begin to germinate as soon as it is sown by immediately beginning to absorb moisture from the soil. For this reason it is preferable, at least in warm weather, to sow seeds in the afternoons so the soil will remain moist for longer after sowing.

Traditionally, one harvested crops in the morning and sowed seeds in the afternoon. One would graft in spring and prune in late autumn and winter. It is likewise recommended that pruning should be done on the waning Moon, grafting on the waxing Moon. Planting-out should be done in the waxing Moon; if possible, in the same element in which the sowings were made.

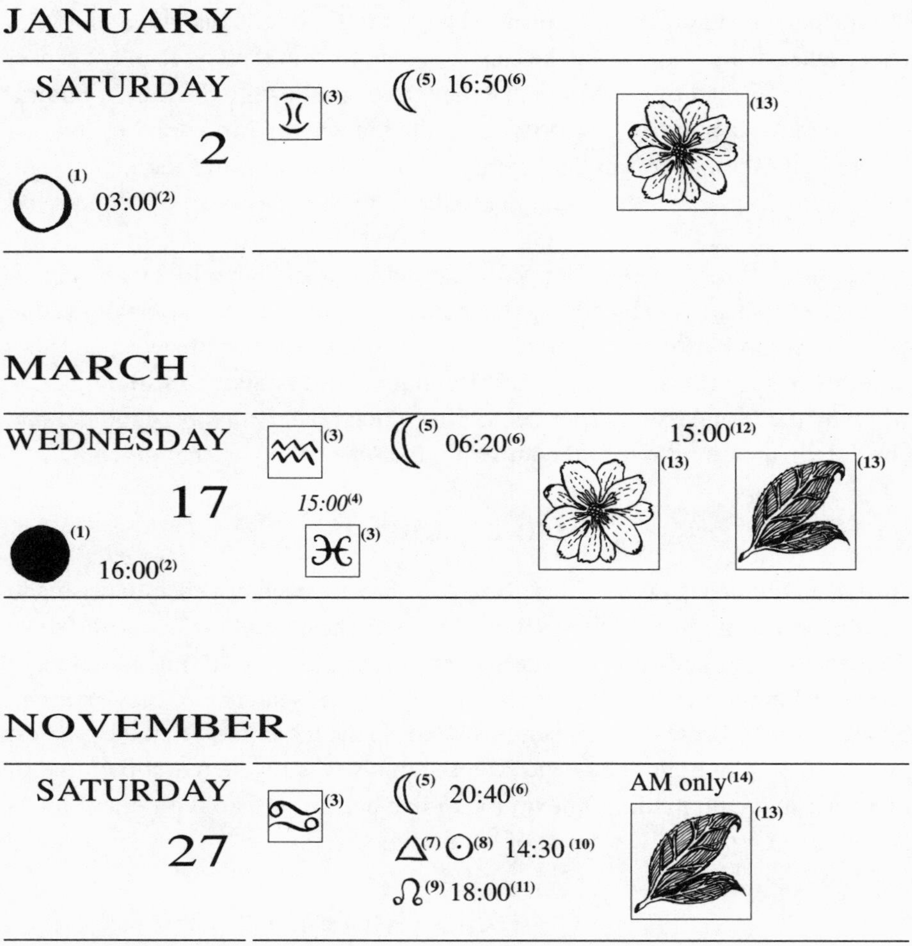

JANUARY

SATURDAY

2

$^{(1)}$ 03:00$^{(2)}$

$\mathfrak{X}$ $^{(3)}$ $^{(5)}$ 16:50$^{(6)}$

$^{(13)}$

MARCH

WEDNESDAY

17

●$^{(1)}$ 16:00$^{(2)}$

$\approx$ $^{(3)}$ *15:00*$^{(4)}$ $\mathcal{H}$ $^{(3)}$

$^{(5)}$ 06:20$^{(6)}$ 15:00$^{(12)}$

$^{(13)}$ $^{(13)}$

NOVEMBER

SATURDAY

27

$\mathcal{S}$ $^{(3)}$

$^{(5)}$ 20:40$^{(6)}$

$\triangle$$^{(7)}$ $\odot$$^{(8)}$ 14:30 $^{(10)}$

$\mathcal{S}$$^{(9)}$ 18:00$^{(11)}$

AM only$^{(14)}$ $^{(13)}$

Figure 20. Examples of calendar entries.

$^{(1)}$ Symbol of Moon phase.
$^{(2)}$ Time of New or Full Moon.
$^{(3)}$ Sidereal Moon sign.
$^{(4)}$ Hour of transition from one sign to another.
$^{(5)}$ Symbol indicating moonrise.
$^{(6)}$ Hour of moonrise.
$^{(7)}$ Trine symbol.
$^{(8)}$ Sun symbol (i.e. this is a Sun-Moon trine).
$^{(9)}$ Symbol for the Moon reaching its north node.
$^{(10)}$ Hour of the Sun-Moon trine.
$^{(11)}$ Hour of the Moon's crossing its north Node.
$^{(12)}$ Hour of transition from one element-sign to another.
$^{(13)}$ Symbols indicating which element-sign(s) is(are) in force that day.
$^{(14)}$ General advice about hours of work in a specific element-sign.

How to Read the Calendar

Opposite are some sample days from our calendar, showing what could then be happening in the sky. On the left is given the lunar cycle data and, on the right, the recommended type of plant best sown that day. All times are given in GMT and in the 24-hour form. Aspects and moonrise times are given to the nearest ten minutes, other times to the nearest hour.

JANUARY 2: this is a Flower-day, because the Moon is in Gemini, an Air-constellation. Each day, the ruling sign is denoted by the zodiacal glyph on the left of the entry. Each of the Moon's quarters is shown. This day is a Full Moon, its time to the nearest hour (GMT) is noted next to the sign. Moonrise times are always given next to the sign of a crescent moon at the top of each day's entry. Here it is 4.50 pm (correct to the nearest ten minutes).

MARCH 17: the 'ingress', that is the transition from one sign to another, occurs in the afternoon at 3pm. As the Moon progresses through the zodiac, so the ruling elements shift according to the same timetable. Hence, the morning was in Aquarius, an Air sign, which means working with flowering plants and the afternoon (after 3 pm) is in Pisces, a Water sign, which is the element which rules leaf plants. The transition from one sort of plant to another is recorded on the right of the entry. New Moon occurs at 4 pm.

NOVEMBER 27: this day, the Moon is in Cancer, a Water sign, which means that once more leafy plants are the subject of main attention. However, work is only recommended in the morning because the Moon reaches its north node at 6 pm, which means that the day is not recommended for sowing or planting crops. The calendar also records the occurrence of a Sun-Moon aspect of trine (120°) in the afternoon at 2.30 pm. All these aspects, mainly Moon-Saturn ones, but also some Sun-Moon and some aspects of the Moon with Venus, together with the crossing of the nodes, and the apogee and perigee of the Moon's circuit of the earth are recorded in this place in the calendar whenever they occur. Their significance or importance to the gardener and farmer has already been discussed in the preceding text and readers should refer to my comments in their proper place to draw any lessons from them. Generally, where it is felt that working in the garden is a bad idea, the fact is noted.

On the right-hand page of the calendar there is space for readers' notes and planting memoranda and there is a short commentary on the lunar and astronomical information expressed by symbols on the facing page. I hope that this may make the calendar easier to use for those who are unfamiliar with the whole concept. Notice, too, that the zodiacal glyphs are identified at the bottom of each calendar page.

Figure 21. Symbols and glyphs used in the calendar.

New Moon (and time)

Full Moon (and time)

Waxing Moon, first quarter

Waning Moon, third quarter

⊙ Sun

♈ Aries (Fire)

♀ Venus

♉ Taurus (Earth)

☾ Hour of moonrise

♊ Gemini (Air)

A Apogee

♋ Cancer (Water)

P Perigee

♌ Leo (Fire)

☊ North node

♍ Virgo (Earth)

☋ South node

♎ Libra (Air)

☌ Conjunction (aspect 0°)

♏ Scorpio (Water)

✳ Sextile (aspect 60°)

♐ Sagittarius (Fire)

□ Square (aspect 90°)

♑ Capricorn (Earth)

△ Trine (aspect (120°)

♒ Aquarius (Air)

☍ Opposition (aspect 180°)

♓ Pisces (Water)

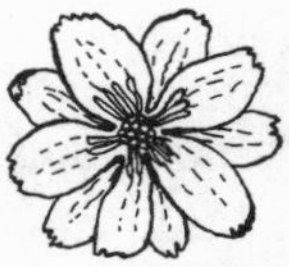

Flower (Air) element sign

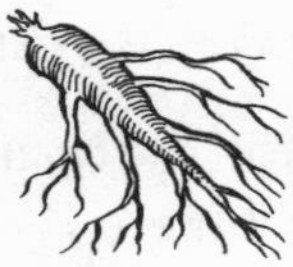

Root (Earth) element sign

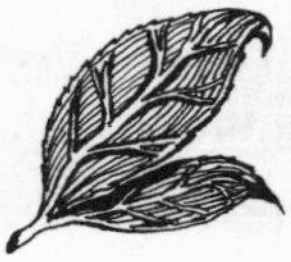

Leaf (Water) element sign

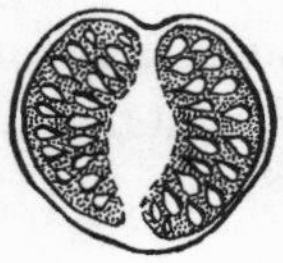

Fruit/seed (Fire) element sign

The attentive reader needs to have absorbed some of the earlier comments on the possible significance of various astronomical combinations but a bare summary of recommendations would go along the following lines:

Annual crops: follow the four-element rhythms, sowing as near to the centre of the relevant sign as is convenient to you. The same element-sign (Leaf, Root, Fruit, Flower) reappears every nine days, so if you miss the appropriate period the next may still be convenient.

Perennial crops, shrubs or trees: try to take advantage of a Saturn-Moon aspect when planting – these are the most common aspects noted in the calendar; aspects of the Moon and the Sun and the Moon and Venus are less frequently recorded and are always distinguished by their identifying glyphs. If a tree or bush is fruit-bearing try also to plant or graft it on a fruit-day.

The waxing and waning Moon is relevant to diverse gardening and farming activities from grafting and transplanting during a waxing Moon to pruning and gelding livestock during its wane.

The hour of moonrise: this is an important moment in the gardening day, particularly with a view to obtaining maximum yields. Try to sow and plant as close to the hour noted on each day (with adjustments to your longitude and latitude) whenever convenient.

The nodes and perigee: avoid critical times in these cycles. Maria Thun claims to have found that seed quality is impaired in crops sown near the nodes. Bio-Dynamic farmers also avoid sowing at perigee. Our limited experience with these cycles supports the view that planting at such times – including **eclipses** – is best avoided. At the two nodes there may be forces involved which are not beneficial to crops and, in general, sowing at least several hours either side of the Moon's nodes is not recommended.

The ascending/descending Moon: referred to in US almanacs as the Moon riding high or riding low is sometimes considered important. Bio-Dynamic farmers use the concept but we remain unconvinced that it has any relevance.

Pruning: the lunar water-uptake cycle is here relevant and near Full Moon is not recommended for pruning. As Pliny wrote, 'All cutting, gathering and trimming is done with less injury to the trees and plants when the Moon is waning than when it is waxing.'

Harvesting: here the old rule recorded by Pliny applies. Fruits to be preserved are best picked at New Moon since these will store better whereas fruits to be eaten fresh are best picked at Full Moon. Crops should be harvested in the same Moon-sign element in which they were sown if the requirement is to obtain seeds for next year's crop.

Full Moon: where drought is a problem, the tendency of seeds to absorb the greatest amount of water on the days prior to the Full Moon should be noted. In dry regions, sowing at this time could well lead to optimal germination. Many people swear by sowing crops just before the Full of the Moon but one should not rely on this improving crop yield.

APPENDIX
Calculating Times

All times given in this book are Greenwich Mean Time. As far as British Summer Time is concerned, between the relevant dates in March and October, British users will have to add one hour to the given times. Users in other parts of the world will need to adjust the times according to the time zone their country adopts with respect to GMT. Such time-zone differences for North America and Australasia are given below.

Time Zone Adjustments for North America

Atlantic	-4 hours
Eastern	-5 hours
Central	-6 hours
Mountain	-7 hours
Pacific	-8 hours
Yukon	-9 hours
Alaska-Hawaii	-10 hours
Bering	-11 hours

Time Zone Adjustments for Australasia

Western Australia	+8 hours
South Australia	+9 $\frac{1}{2}$ hours
Northern Territory	+9 $\frac{1}{2}$ hours
New South Wales	+10 hours
Victoria	+10 hours
Queensland	+10 hours
Tasmania	+10 hours
New Zealand	+12 hours

REFERENCES AND FURTHER READING

1. Abele, U., PhD thesis, U. of Giessen, Germany, 1973.
2. ——, 'Saatzeitversuche mit Radies', *Lebendige Erde* 6 223–5, 1975.
3. Abrami, G., 'Correlations between Lunar Phases and Rhythmicities in Plant Growth under Field Conditions', *Canadian Journal of Botany*, 1972, No. 50, 2157–2166.
4. Andrews, E., 'Moon Talk, the Cyclic Periodicity of Postoperative Hemorrhage', *Journal of Florida Medical Assocn.*, May 1960, 1362–66.
5. Baker, M., *Gardener's Magic and Folklore*, Universe, New York, 1978.
6. Barger, A., *Gardening Success with Lunar Aspects*, 1977, AFA US.
7. Beeson, C., 'The Moon and Plant Growth', *Nature*, 1946, 158, 572–3.
8. Bell, B. & Defouw, R., 'Concerning a Lunar modulation of Geomagnetic Activity' *Journal Geophysical Research* 1964, 69, 3169–3174.
9. ——, 'Dependence of the Lunar Modulation of Geomagnetic Activity on the Celestial Latitude of the Moon', *Journal Geophysical Research*, 1966, 71, 3, 951–957.
10. Best, S., 'Lunar Influence in Plant Growth: A Review of the Evidence', *Phenomena*, 2.3–2.4, August 1978.
11. *Biodynamics: New Directions for Farming and Gardening in New Zealand*, Random Century N.Z., 1989.
12. Bishop, C., 'Moon Influences in Lettuce Growth', *Astrological Journal*, 10, No. 1, Winter 77/78.
13. Bose, J. C., *Plant Response as a Means of Physiological Investigation*, Longmans, London, 1906.
14. Bradley, D., Woodbury, M., and Brier, G., 'Lunar Synodical Period and Widespread Precipitation', *Science*, 137, 1962, 748–9 (also Adderley, E. & Bowen, E., Ibid, 749–50).
15. Brier, G. & Bradley, D., 'Lunar Synodic Precipitation in the United States', *Journal Atmos. Sci.*, 1964, 21, 386–395.
16. Brown, F., 'The Rhythmic Nature of Animals and Plants', *Cycles*, April, 1960, 81–92.
17. ——, & Chow, C., 'Lunar-correlated Variations in Water Uptake by Bean Seeds', *Biological Bulletin*, Oct., 1973, 145, 265–278.
18. Burns, J.T., *Cosmic Influences on Humans, Animals and Plants, An Annotated Bibliography*, Magill (US), 1997.
19. Burr, H. S., 'Diurnal Potentials in the Maple Tree', *Yale Journal of Biology & Medicine*, 1945, 17, 727–734.
20. ——, *The Fields of Life: Our Links with the Universe*, NY, 1973.
21. Carpenter, T. *et al.*, 'Observed Relationship between lunar tidal cycles and formation of hurricanes and tropical storms', *Monthly Weather Review*, 1972, 100, 451–6.
22. Culpeper, N., *Complete Herbal*, Foulsham, London.
23. Currie, R. 'Evidence for 18.6-year signal in Temperature and Drought conditions in North America since AD 1800', *Journal of Geophysical Research*, 1981, 86, 11055.
24. ——, 'Examples & Implications of 18.6- and 11-yr Terms in World Weather Records', in *Climate*, Ed. Rampino *et al.*, NY, 1987.
25. Cutler, W., 'Lunar and Menstrual Phase Locking', *American Journal of Obstetric Gynecology*, 1980, 137, 834.
26. ——, *et al.*, 'Lunar influences on the reproductive cycle in women', *Human Biology*, 1987, 59, 959–72.
27. *Dariotus Redivivus, or a brief introduction to the judgement of the stars*, 1653 (agricultural section by Nathaniel Spark).

28. Dewey, E. & Mandino, O., *Cycles–the mysterious forces that trigger events*, New York, 1973.
29. Dixon, B., 'Plant Sensations', *Omni,* Dec., 1978, 24.
30. Domin, A., ed., *Organic Wholefoods, Naturally Delicious Cuisine,* Konemann, 1997.
31. Dubrov, A., *The Geomagnetic Field and Life* (trans. from Russian), 1978.
32. ——, *Human Biorhythms and the Moon*, Nova Science, NY, 1996, 117.
33. Elliott, J., *Plants & Planets*, Astrological Gardening, 1996.
34. *Elm Farm Research Centre Bulletin*, April 1995 (Info. on Organic Farming)
35. Estienne, C., & Liebault, J., *La Maison Rustique*, trans. Surfleet, 1616.
36. Fagan, C., *Zodiacs Old and New,* Anscombe and Co., London, 1951.
37. Farbridge K. & Leatherland, J., 'Lunar Periodicity of Growth Cycles in Rainbow Trout', *Journal of Interdisciplinary Cycles Research*, 1987, 18, 169–177.
38. Farrar, J., 'Sunspot Weather', *Farmers Weekly,* Feb. 28, 1975.
39. Field, J., 'A Lutheran Astrologer: Johannes Kepler', *Arch. Hist. Exact Sci.* 1984, 31, 190–268 (has his calendar predictions for 1602).
40. Graf, U., PhD thesis. Zurich E.T.H., 1977.
41. Grau, G. *et al.*, 'Lunar Phasing of the Thyroxine Surge', *Science,* 1981, 211, 607–9.
42. Graviou, E., 'Analogies between Rhythms in Plant Material in Atmospheric Pressure and Solar-Lunar Periodicities', *International Journal of Biometeorology*, 1978, Vol. 22, No. 2.
43. Hesiod, *The Homeric Hymns and Homerica,* trans. H.G. Evelyn-White, 1977.
44. Hill, T., *The Gardener's Labyrinth*, 1577, OUP, 1987.
45. Joly, N., *Le Vin du Ciel à la Terre*, Paris, 1997.
46. Kerr, A. & Marshall,C., 'Planting by the Moon', *Harvests* [Journal of N.Z. Bio-Dynamic Assoc.], Summer 1997.
47. Kerr, R. A, 'Fickle Sun could be altering Earth's Climate after all', *Science*, 269, Aug. 1995, 633.
48. King, J., 'Solar Radiation Changes and the Weather', *Nature,* 245, Oct., 1973, 443–446.
49. ——, *et al.,* 'Agriculture and Sunspots', *Nature,* 252, Nov 1, 1974, 2–3.
50. Kokus, M., 'The 18.6-year Cycle in Drought and Flood: A Review of the Climate Research of Robert Currie', *Cycles,* Aug 1988,189–191,
51. Kolisko, L., *The Moon and the Growth of Plants,* Anthroposophical Press, London, 1938, 1975 (1933, in German).
52. ——, *Agriculture of Tomorrow*, 1939, 1982.
53. Kollerstrom, N., 'Zodiac Rhythms in Plant Growth – Potatoes', *Mercury Star Journal*, Summer 1977.
54. ——, 'Plant Response to the Synodic Lunar Cycle: A Review', *Cycles,* 31, 1980, 61–63.
55. ——, 'A Lunar Sidereal Rhythm in Crop Yield', *Correlation,* Jun 81, 1, 44–53.
56. ——, 'Testing the Lunar Calendar' *Biodynamics* 185 (US), Winter 1993, 44–48.
57. ——, 'The Star-Zodiac of Antiquity', *Culture and Cosmos,* Winter 1997, 5–22.
58. Knight, J. 'Moon Up – Moon Down: the story of the Solunar Theory', *Biodynamics* (US), 1972.
59. Lai, T. M., 'Phosphorus and Potassium Uptake by Plants Relating to Moon Phases', *Biodynamics* (US), Summer, 1976.
60. Lampkin, N. *Organic Farming,* 1990.
61. Lethbridge, M., 'Relationship between thunderstorm frequency and lunar phase', *Journal of Geophysical Research,* 1970, 75, 5153.
62. Lieber, A. L., *The Lunar Effect,* Corgi, 1979.
63. Lücke, J., *Untersuchungen...* PhD, U. of Giessen 1982, 71, 74.
64. Mather, M., 'The Effect of Temperature and the Moon on Seedling Growth', *Journal of the Royal Horticultural Society,* 1942, 67, 264–270.
65. Markham, G., *The Whole Art of Husbandry,* 1631 (trans. of a continental work, originally published in the 1570s).

66. Maw, M. G., 'Periodicities in the Influences of Air Ions on the Growth of Garden Cress, *Lepidium Sativum* L.', *Canadian Journal of Plant Science,* 1967, 47, 499–505.
67 Messegu , M., *Of Men and Plants,* NY, 1972, 9.
68. McClintock, M., 'Menstrual Synchrony and Suppression', *Nature,* 1971, 229, 244–5.
69. Oehmke, M.G., 'Lunar Periodicity in Flight Activity of Honey Bees', *Journal of Interdisciplinary Cycles Research,* 1973, 4, 319–335.
70. Panzer, J. J., 'Lunar Correlated Variations in Water Uptake and Germination in 3 Species of Seeds', PhD, U. of Tulane, 1976.
71. Playfair, G. & Hill, S., *The Cycles of Heaven,* Pan Books, 1979.
72. Pliny, *History of Nature,* Vol. 18, Section 75 (Loeb Classics, 1961).
73. Podolinsky, A. *Bio-Dynamic Agriculture Introductory Lectures,* Vol. 1, Australia 1990.
74. Powell, R. and Treadgold, P., *The Sidereal Zodiac,* Anthroposophical Publications, 1979.
75. Rossignol M. *et al.*, 'Lunar Cycle and Nuclear DNA variations in Potato callus', *Geocosmic Relations* (Ed Tomassen, Pudoc, Netherlands 1990), 116–126.
76. Rounds, H. D., 'A semi-lunar periodicity of neurotransmitter-like substances from plants', *Physiologia Plantarium,* 1982.
77. Sattler, F. & Wistinghausen E., *Bio-Dynamic Farming Practice*, CUP 1989.
78 Spiess, H., 'Chronobiological Investigations...', *BAH,* 1990, 7, 165–89.
79. ——, *Biologische Rhythmen im Landbau,* 3 vols., Darmstadt 1994.
80. Steiner, R. *Agriculture,* 1938, 1993 (US).
81. ——, *Health & Illness,* Anthropological Press NY, 1983 edition.
82. Stolov, H. & Cameron A., 'Variation of Geomagnetic Activity with Lunar Phase'm, *Journal Geophysical Research,* 1964, 69, 4975–4982.
83. Taverner, E., 'The Roman Farmer and the Moon', *Transactions & Proceedings of the American Philological Association,* 1918, 49, 67–82.
84. Temple, J., *Gardening Without Chemicals,* 1986.
85. ——, 'Checking the value of planting by the zodiac', *Here's Health,* November 1982, 144–5.
86. Theroux, M., 'Lunar Influence on ... Colloidal Silver', *Borderlands, A Quarterly Journal of Borderlands Research* (US), 1997, 3, 52–4.
87. Thompson, L., 'The 18.6-year and 9.3-year Lunar cycles Their Possible Relation to Agriculture', *Cycles,* Dec. 1988, 286–7.
88. ——, 'The 18.6-year Lunar cycle: Its possible Relation to Agriculture', *Cycles*, March 1989, 65–9.
89. Thun, M., 'Nine Years Observation of Cosmic Influences on Annual Plants', *Star and Furrow*, 22, Spring 1964.
90. ——, & Heinze, H., *Mondrhythmen im Siderischen Umlauf und Pflanzenwachstum,* Darmstadt, 1979.
91. ——, *Work on the Land & the Constellations*, Lanthorn Press, East Grinstead, 1991.
92. ——, *Milch und Milchverarbeitung,* 1992.
93. Timmins, C., *Planting by the Moon,* Aries Press, Chicago, 1939.
94. Treloar A., *et al.*, 'Variations of the Human Menstrual Cycle through Reproductive Life', *International Journal of Fertility,* 1967, 12, 77–126.
95. *New Scientist,* 19 March, 1981, 740, 'US Study shows that back to Nature Farming makes sense'.
96. Vines, R. G., 'Possible Relationships between Rainfall, Crop Yields and the Sunspot Cycle', *Journal of the Australian Institute of Agricultural Science,* March/June, 1977, 3–13.
97. Vollman, F., 'The Menstrual Cycle', *Major Problems in Obstetrics & Gynecology,* Philadelphia, Vol 7, 1977, 54–56.
98 Walker, C., ed., *Astronomy Before the Telescope* , 1996, Ch. 3: 'Astronomy & Astrology in Mesopotamia'.

PLANTING BY THE MOON

2000

JANUARY

SATURDAY

1

☽ 02:40

⚭ 06:10

SUNDAY

2

☽ 03:40

10:00

_10:00_

JANUARY

The Moon is in opposition to Saturn early in the morning. Often this is thought a stressful period, although Bio-Dynamic gardeners maintain the contrary.

SATURDAY

1

The shift from Libra to Scorpio (Air to Water) happens quite early in the day giving a chance to shift attention from flowering to leaf plants.

SUNDAY

2

 Libra
Air

 Scorpio
Water

 Sagittarius
Fire

  Capricorn
Earth

 Aquarius
Air

 Pisces
Water

JANUARY

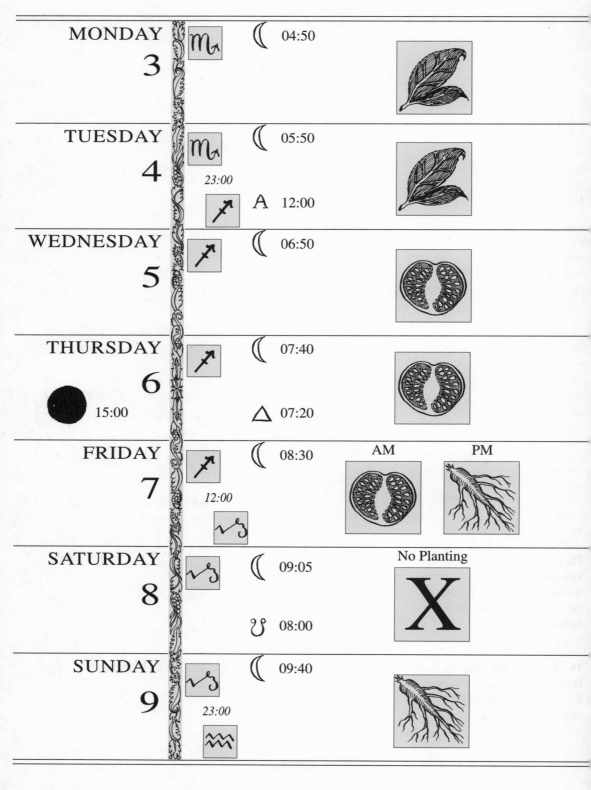

MONDAY
3

♏   ☾ 04:50

TUESDAY
4

♏   ☾ 05:50

23:00

♐   A 12:00

WEDNESDAY
5

♐   ☾ 06:50

THURSDAY
6

♐   ☾ 07:40

● *15:00*

△ 07:20

FRIDAY
7

♐   ☾ 08:30

12:00

♑

AM   PM

SATURDAY
8

♑   ☾ 09:05

☋ 08:00

No Planting

X

SUNDAY
9

♑   ☾ 09:40

23:00

♒

 Aries *Fire*   Taurus *Earth*   Gemini *Air*    Cancer *Water*    Leo *Fire*   Virgo *Earth*

JANUARY

If you have glass or plastic cloches, think about sowing some early salad crops.	**MONDAY** **3**
At the end of the evening, the sign changes from Water to Fire (leaf to fruit or seed). The Moon's apogee, i.e. furthest point from the Earth, is at midday.	**TUESDAY** **4**
Remember that the hour after moonrise is the most propitious time to work with the designated plant type. That may mean an early start today.	**WEDNESDAY** **5**
Because the Moon has only just passed its apogee, its passage through the various signs is at its slowest.	**THURSDAY** **6**
A shift of signs from Fire (fruit or seed) to Earth (root) element occurs at midday.	**FRIDAY** **7**
The passing of the Moon through its south node is the reason for advising against any form of planting activity. The south is reckoned even less favourable than the north node.	**SATURDAY** **8**
The change in ruling signs happens right at the end of the evening, leaving the whole day free for roots.	**SUNDAY** **9**

 Libra *Air*   Scorpio *Water*   Sagittarius *Fire*  Capricorn *Earth*   Aquarius *Air*   Pisces *Water*

JANUARY

MONDAY 10 ♒ ☾ 10:10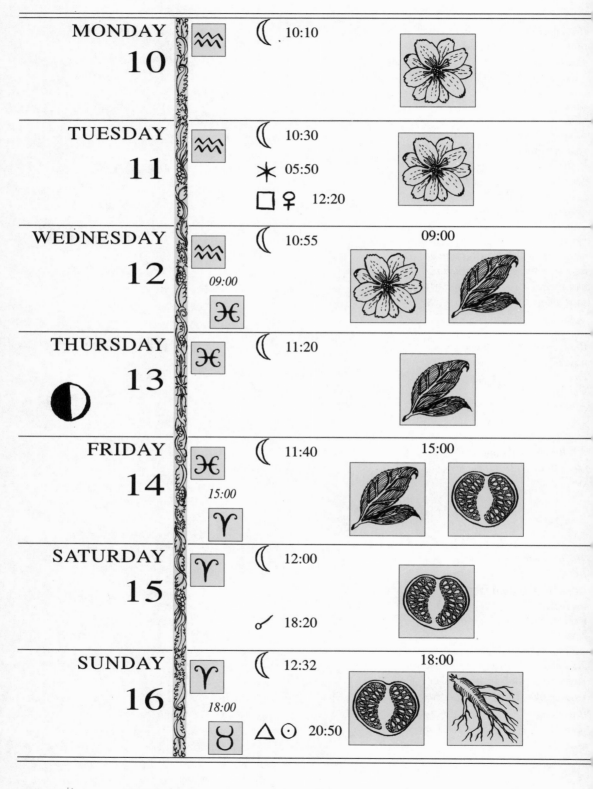

TUESDAY 11 ♒ ☾ 10:30   ✳ 05:50   □ ♀ 12:20

WEDNESDAY 12 ♒ ☾ 10:55   09:00   *09:00* ♓

THURSDAY 13 ♓ ☾ 11:20

FRIDAY 14 ♓ ☾ 11:40   15:00   *15:00* ♈

SATURDAY 15 ♈ ☾ 12:00   ⚸ 18:20

SUNDAY 16 ♈ ☾ 12:32   18:00   *18:00* ♉   △ ☉ 20:50

 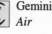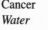

JANUARY

MONDAY
10

Moon and Saturn form a propitious sextile (60°) aspect. The square of the Moon and Venus, at around midday, is more ambiguous. The square is not generally thought a helpful aspect.

TUESDAY
11

The element signs change from Aquarius (Air) to Pisces (Water) – flower to leaf plants – at the outset of the working day. The hour after moonrise is the best time to select for sensitive operations.

WEDNESDAY
12

THURSDAY
13

The change from leaf to fruit occurs at teatime.

FRIDAY
14

The conjunction of the Moon and Saturn at the end of the day is not a brilliant aspect, so pruning vines, fruit trees and bushes, or treating them with any winter washes should be done towards midday.

SATURDAY
15

The trine of the Moon and Sun is a very good governing aspect, especially for work with fruit trees and things like vines. The shift from fruiting plants to roots comes at the end of the day.

SUNDAY
16

 Libra *Air*

 Scorpio *Water*

 Sagittarius *Fire*

 Capricorn *Earth*

 Aquarius *Air*

 Pisces *Water*

JANUARY

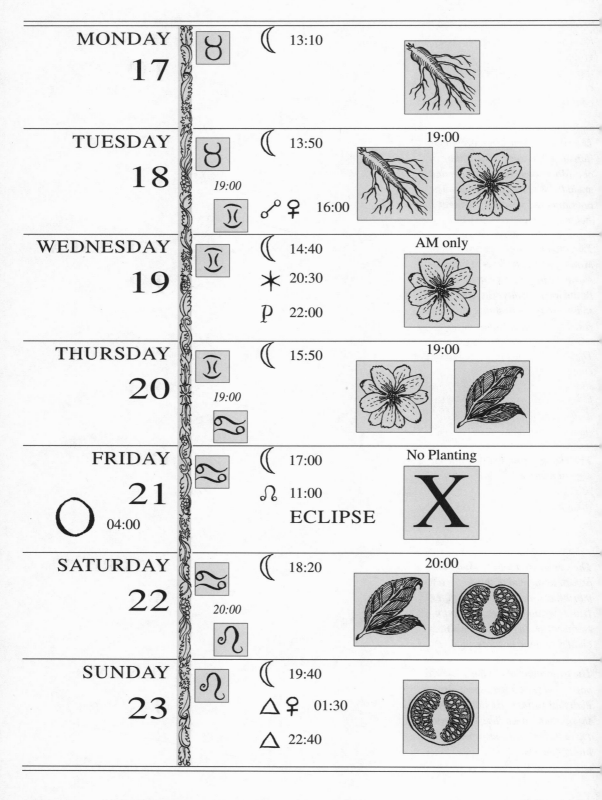

MONDAY 17 — Taurus — ☽ 13:10

TUESDAY 18 — Taurus — ☽ 13:50 — *19:00* Gemini — ☌ ♀ 16:00 — 19:00

WEDNESDAY 19 — Gemini — ☽ 14:40 — ✳ 20:30 — ♇ 22:00 — AM only

THURSDAY 20 — Gemini — ☽ 15:50 — *19:00* Cancer — 19:00

FRIDAY 21 — Cancer — ☽ 17:00 — ☊ 11:00 ECLIPSE — ○ 04:00 — No Planting **X**

SATURDAY 22 — Cancer — ☽ 18:20 — *20:00* Leo — 20:00

SUNDAY 23 — Leo — ☽ 19:40 — △ ♀ 01:30 — △ 22:40

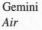

JANUARY

Remember that for best results the ground should be worked during the element-sign of its intended crop. If the soil is right, shallots could be planted today.

MONDAY

17

The shift in ruling signs does not influence the day's work, but the opposition of the Moon and Venus noted for 4 o'clock in the afternoon is a moment of stress.

TUESDAY

18

The beneficent effects of the sextile Moon-Saturn aspect is overshadowed by the passage of the Moon through its perigee (nearest point to the Earth). Hence the advice to restrict work to the morning.

WEDNESDAY

19

The change from flower to leaf element is late in the evening so should not affect the day's plans, however, planting or sowing is best done in the middle of each period shown for the appropriate element.

THURSDAY

20

The lunar eclipse is the significant event, as it passes through its north node. No work on plants today: do some burning, clearing, or building.

FRIDAY

21

The elements change from leaf plants to fruit/seed plants during the evening.

SATURDAY

22

There are two trine aspects at opposite ends of the day: of the Moon with Saturn and with Venus. The trine is a harmonious moment. Think of sowing early peas and broad beans in a warm spot.

SUNDAY

23

 Libra
Air

 Scorpio
Water

 Sagittarius
Fire

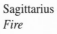 Capricorn
Earth

 Aquarius
Air

 Pisces
Water

JANUARY

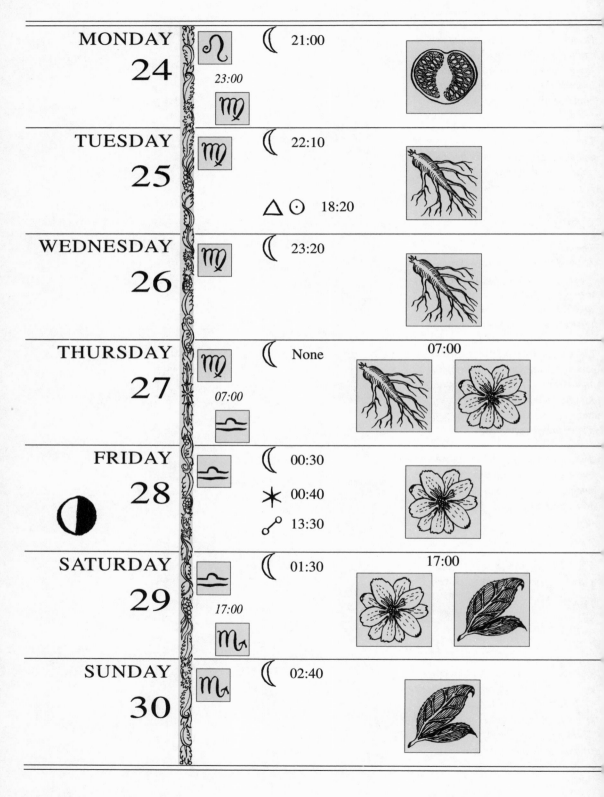

MONDAY 24
♌
23:00
♍
☽ 21:00

TUESDAY 25
♍
☽ 22:10
△ ☉ 18:20

WEDNESDAY 26
♍
☽ 23:20

THURSDAY 27
♍
07:00
♎
☽ None
07:00

FRIDAY 28
♎
☽ 00:30
✳ 00:40
☍ 13:30

SATURDAY 29
♎
17:00
♏
☽ 01:30
17:00

SUNDAY 30
♏
☽ 02:40

 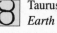
 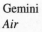

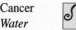

JANUARY

The change in the element sign happens late in the evening.	**MONDAY** **24**
The Moon forms a trine aspect with the Sun: generally a good thing.	**TUESDAY** **25**
Think of chitting early potatoes.	**WEDNESDAY** **26**
The shift from roots to flowering plants leaves the whole day free for the latter.	**THURSDAY** **27**
The sextile Moon/Saturn aspect is somewhat counteracted by the less harmonious opposition formed in the afternoon.	**FRIDAY** **28**
A change of elements towards the end of the afternoon. The Moon being on the wane, it is a good time to think of pruning shrubs and trees.	**SATURDAY** **29**
This may be time to think of blanching celery and curly endive.	**SUNDAY** **30**

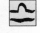 Libra
Air

 Scorpio
Water

 Sagittarius
Fire

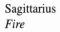 Capricorn
Earth

 Aquarius
Air

 Pisces
Water

JANUARY/FEBRUARY

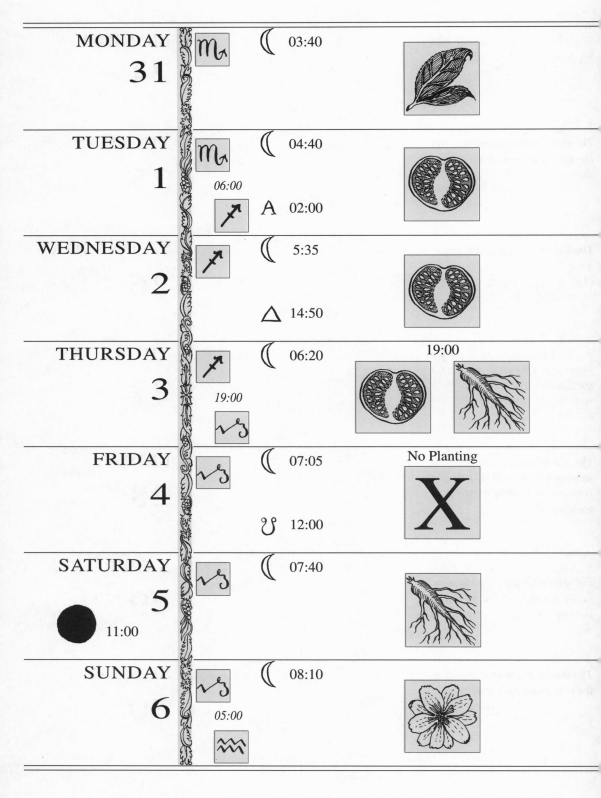

MONDAY
31

♏   ☽ 03:40

TUESDAY
1

♏   ☽ 04:40

06:00

♐   A 02:00

WEDNESDAY
2

♐   ☽ 5:35

△ 14:50

THURSDAY
3

♐   ☽ 06:20   19:00

19:00

♑

FRIDAY
4

♑   ☽ 07:05   No Planting

☋ 12:00   **X**

SATURDAY
5

♑   ☽ 07:40

● 11:00

SUNDAY
6

♑   ☽ 08:10

05:00

♒

 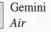

JANUARY/FEBRUARY

MONDAY

31

The apogee of the Moon's orbit (furthest from the Earth) happens during the night.

TUESDAY

1

The Saturn/Moon aspect this afternoon is the harmonious trine (120°). Work ground for sowings of peas and beans.

WEDNESDAY

2

There is a change in governing signs at the end of the day. Work up ground for carrots, radishes and parsnips.

THURSDAY

3

The moon's crossing through its south node in the middle of the day is reason enough to suspend any planting.

FRIDAY

4

Plant Jerusalem artichokes.

SATURDAY

5

The change in element-signs is in the earliest part of the day, before sunrise. Start some early cauliflowers (protected).

SUNDAY

6

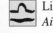 Libra
Air

 Scorpio
Water

 Sagittarius
Fire

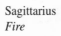 Capricorn
Earth

 Aquarius
Air

 Pisces
Water

FEBRUARY

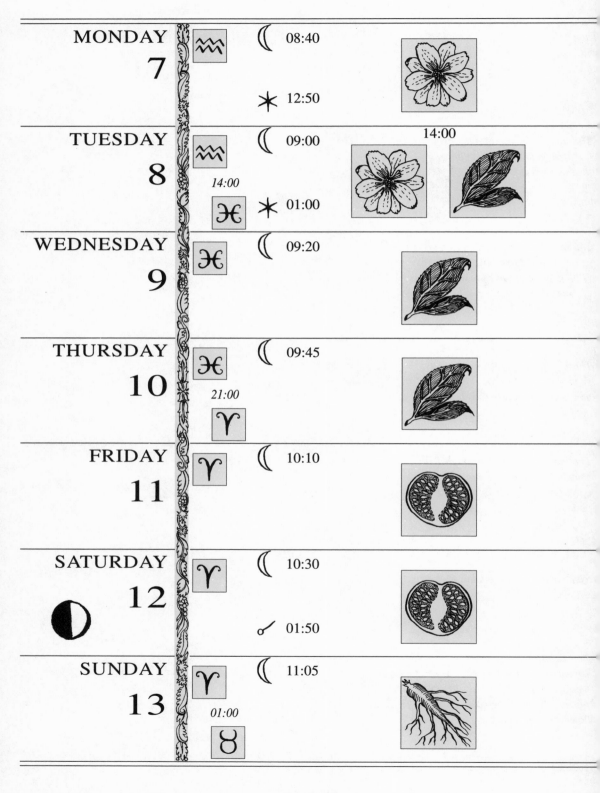

MONDAY 7 ♒ ☽ 08:40 ✳ 12:50

TUESDAY 8 ♒ ☽ 09:00 — 14:00 — ♓ ✳ 01:00 — 14:00

WEDNESDAY 9 ♓ ☽ 09:20

THURSDAY 10 ♓ ☽ 09:45 — 21:00 — ♈

FRIDAY 11 ♈ ☽ 10:10

SATURDAY 12 ♈ ☽ 10:30 — 01:50

SUNDAY 13 ♈ ☽ 11:05 — 01:00 — ♉

 ♈ Aries *Fire*
 ♉ Taurus *Earth*
 ♊ Gemini *Air*
 ♋ Cancer *Water*
 ♌ Leo *Fire*
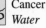 ♍ Virgo *Earth*

FEBRUARY

The sextile is good: act on it. Work within an hour of moonrise for best effect.

MONDAY

7

The good vibes continue: catch up on things left undone. Start sowing saladings and spinach; and some early cabbage and Brussels sprouts.

TUESDAY

8

WEDNESDAY

9

There is a shift in element-signs from leaf to fruit in the night.

THURSDAY

10

A day, perhaps, for sowing peas and beans.

FRIDAY

11

The fire element, governing fruit or seed crops, continues to rule the working day, a shift to the earth element (roots) occurring in the night. The Moon-Saturn conjunction is a moment of slight stress.

SATURDAY

12

SUNDAY

13

 Libra
Air

 Scorpio
Water

 Sagittarius
Fire

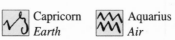 Capricorn
Earth

 Aquarius
Air

 Pisces
Water

FEBRUARY

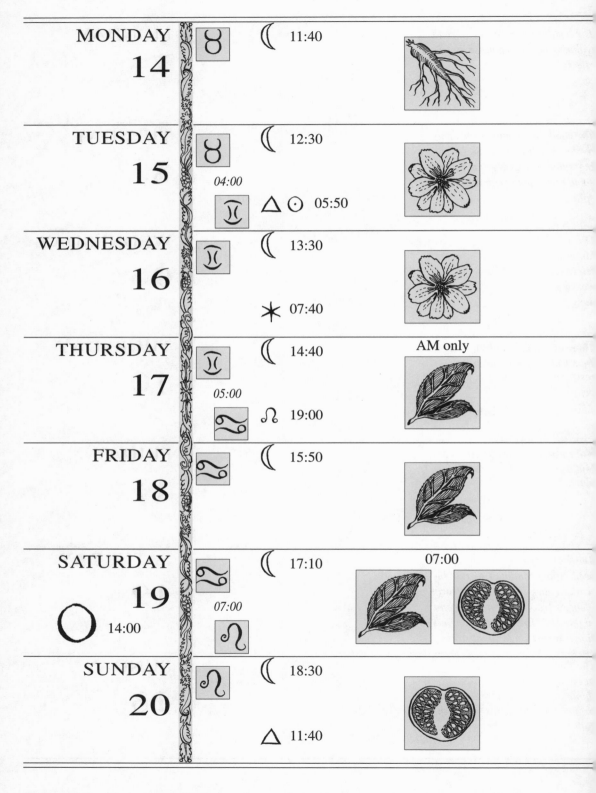

| MONDAY 14 | ♉ | ☾ 11:40 | |

| TUESDAY 15 | ♉ | ☾ 12:30 | |
| | *04:00* ♊ | △ ☉ 05:50 | |

| WEDNESDAY 16 | ♊ | ☾ 13:30 | |
| | | ✳ 07:40 | |

| THURSDAY 17 | ♊ | ☾ 14:40 | AM only |
| | *05:00* ♋ | ♌ 19:00 | |

| FRIDAY 18 | ♋ | ☾ 15:50 | |

| SATURDAY 19 | ♋ | ☾ 17:10 | 07:00 |
| ◯ 14:00 | *07:00* ♌ | | |

| SUNDAY 20 | ♌ | ☾ 18:30 | |
| | | △ 11:40 | |

 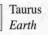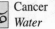

FEBRUARY

MONDAY

14

There is a Moon-Sun trine aspect (120°). Taurus (Earth) gives way to Gemini (Air) – roots to flowering plants – before the Sun is up.

TUESDAY

15

The sextile aspect (60°) of the Moon and Saturn has particular relevance to trees and perennials: work with fruit trees on fruit/seed days.

WEDNESDAY

16

The crossing of the north node in the evening is the reason for the restriction of work to the hours before midday.

THURSDAY

17

Many people think just before Full Moon is the ideal time to sow or plant.

FRIDAY

18

Full Moon.

SATURDAY

19

There is a Moon-Saturn trine aspect: altogether a good thing, though not an ideal moment for pruning, given the proximity of the Full Moon.

SUNDAY

20

 Libra
Air

 Scorpio
Water

 Sagittarius
Fire

 Capricorn
Earth

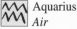 Aquarius
Air

 Pisces
Water

FEBRUARY

MONDAY 21

♌︎
10:00
♍︎
☾ 19:45

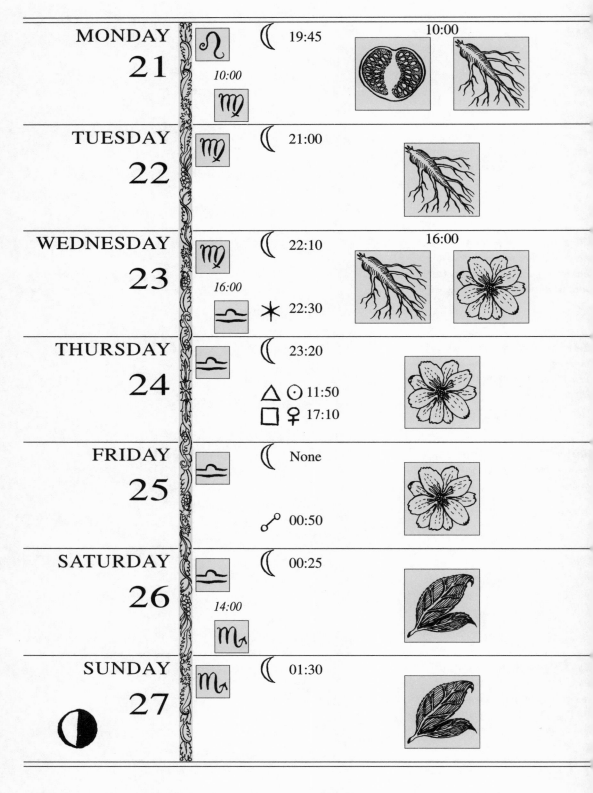

10:00

TUESDAY 22

♍︎
☾ 21:00

WEDNESDAY 23

♍︎
16:00
♎︎ ✳ 22:30
☾ 22:10

16:00

THURSDAY 24

♎︎
☾ 23:20

△ ☉ 11:50
□ ♀ 17:10

FRIDAY 25

♎︎
☾ None

⚯ 00:50

SATURDAY 26

♎︎
14:00
♏︎
☾ 00:25

SUNDAY 27

♏︎
☾ 01:30

 ♈ Aries *Fire*   ♉ Taurus *Earth*   ♊ Gemini *Air*   ♋ Cancer *Water*    ♌ Leo *Fire*   ♍ Virgo *Earth*

FEBRUARY

The change from fruit or seed to root element happens at mid-morning.	**MONDAY** **21**
Parsnips, garlic, carrots and radishes might be sown.	**TUESDAY** **22**
Divide the day between root and flower elements. The Moon and Saturn form a sextile aspect late in the evening.	**WEDNESDAY** **23**
The Moon-Sun aspect is trine in the morning, whereas the less beneficent square aspect between the Moon and Venus is formed at the end of the day.	**THURSDAY** **24**
There is a Moon-Saturn opposition just after midnight.	**FRIDAY** **25**
The shift from flower to leaf element happens in the middle of the night, leaving the whole day for the latter.	**SATURDAY** **26**
Chives and other leaf plants for early crops could be sown today.	**SUNDAY** **27**

 Libra *Air*   Scorpio *Water*   Sagittarius *Fire*  Capricorn *Earth*   Aquarius *Air*   Pisces *Water*

FEBRUARY/MARCH

MONDAY 28

♏︎↗︎ 14:00 ↗︎

☾ 02:30

A 20:00

AM   PM

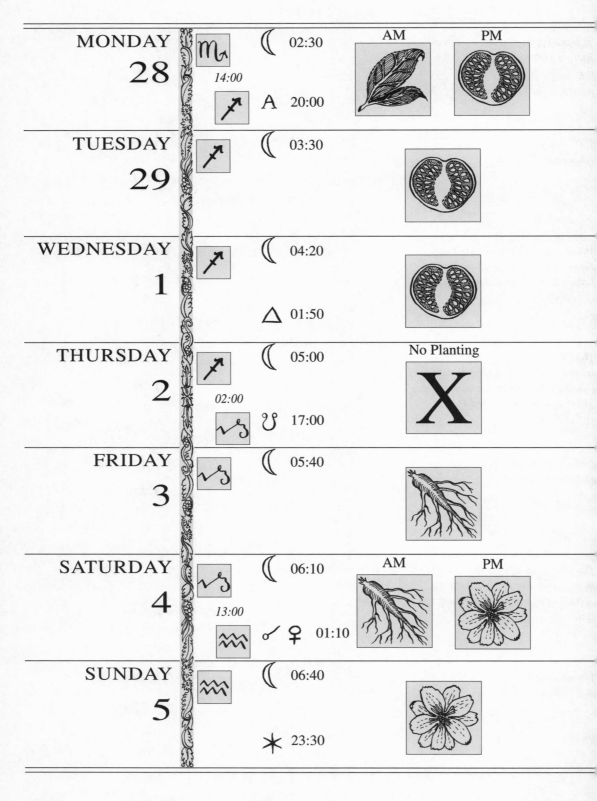

TUESDAY 29

↗︎

☾ 03:30

WEDNESDAY 1

↗︎

☾ 04:20

△ 01:50

THURSDAY 2

↗︎ 02:00 ♑︎

☾ 05:00

☊ 17:00

No Planting

X

FRIDAY 3

♑︎

☾ 05:40

SATURDAY 4

♑︎ 13:00 ♒︎

☾ 06:10

☌ ♀ 01:10

AM   PM

SUNDAY 5

♒︎

☾ 06:40

✳ 23:30

♈ Aries *Fire*   ♉ Taurus *Earth*   ♊ Gemini *Air*   ♋ Cancer *Water*   ♌ Leo *Fire*   ♍ Virgo *Earth*

FEBRUARY/MARCH

MONDAY
28

The elements divide the day between them, but the Moon's apogee later in the evening is a slight disturbance that should be noted.

TUESDAY
29

WEDNESDAY
1

There is a Moon-Saturn trine aspect during the night: its influence is benign. This may be a good time to graft any fruit trees.

THURSDAY
2

The passage of the Moon through the south node is the reason for advising against planting on this day.

FRIDAY
3

Onions and celeriac are two root crops that could be planted or sown now.

SATURDAY
4

The Moon-Venus aspect is in conjunction (0°) at the beginning of the morning. Think of working particularly with perennials.

SUNDAY
5

The Moon forms a sextile aspect with Saturn.

 Libra
Air

 Scorpio
Water

 Sagittarius
Fire

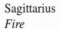 Capricorn
Earth

 Aquarius
Air

 Pisces
Water

MARCH

MONDAY 6

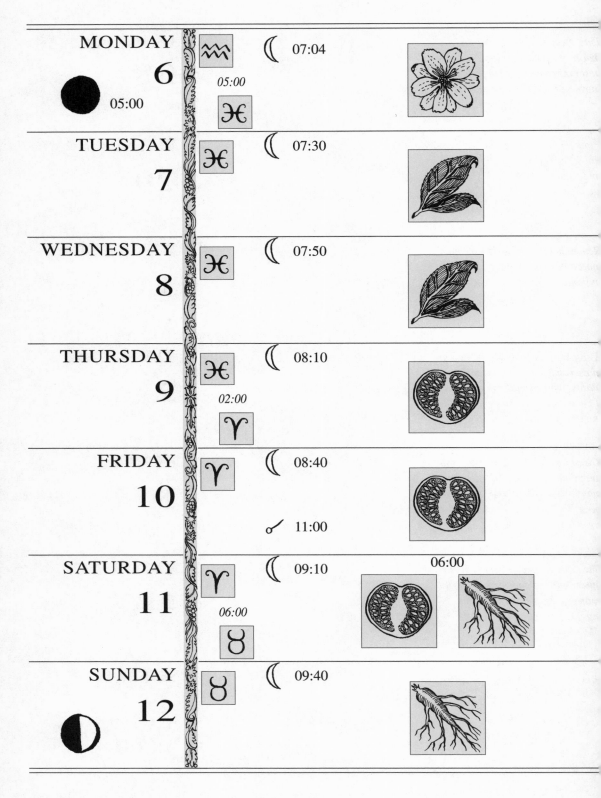

● 05:00

♒ *05:00*
♓

☽ 07:04

TUESDAY 7

♓

☽ 07:30

WEDNESDAY 8

♓

☽ 07:50

THURSDAY 9

♓
02:00
♈

☽ 08:10

FRIDAY 10

♈

☽ 08:40

⚸ 11:00

SATURDAY 11

♈
06:00
♉

☽ 09:10

06:00

SUNDAY 12

◐

♉

☽ 09:40

MARCH

There is a shift in element-signs before breakfast. New Moon: the best time for tree felling and pruning – and for surgical operations!	**MONDAY** **6**
Plant out lettuce seedlings, continue sowings of leaf vegetables and salads.	**TUESDAY** **7**
Remember that one hour round moonrise is the best time for sowing and planting.	**WEDNESDAY** **8**
At the outset of the day there is a move from leaf plants to fruit/seed plants. With the moon waxing, it is a good time to consider any grafting or transplanting of trees.	**THURSDAY** **9**
The Moon-Saturn aspect is in conjunction: slightly stressful in some people's eyes, but still a Saturn aspect that will influence work with trees and perennials.	**FRIDAY** **10**
The move from one element to another – from fruit/seed plants to roots – happens early in the morning.	**SATURDAY** **11**
	SUNDAY **12**

 Libra
Air

 Scorpio
Water

 Sagittarius
Fire

 Capricorn
Earth

 Aquarius
Air

Pisces
Water

MARCH

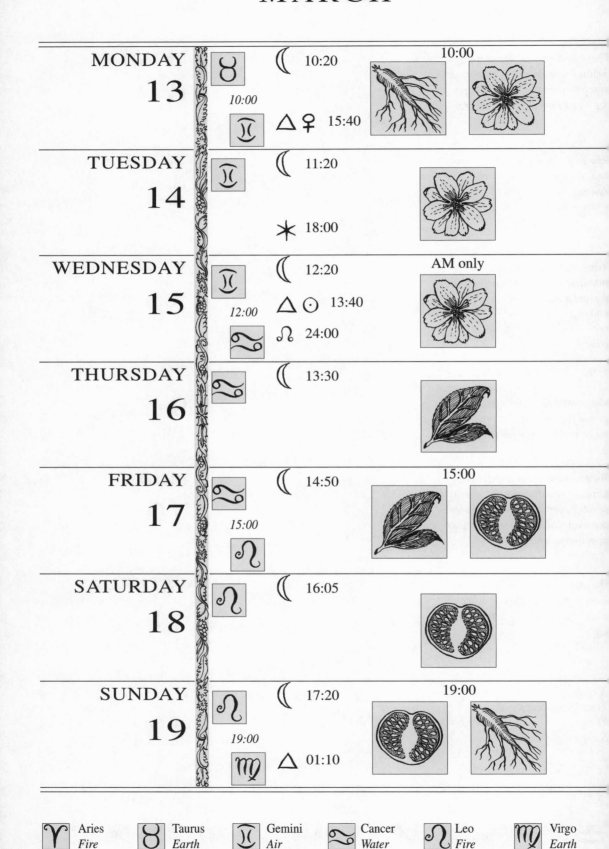

MONDAY **13**	♉	☽ 10:20		10:00
	10:00 ♊	△ ♀ 15:40		
TUESDAY **14**	♊	☽ 11:20		
		✳ 18:00		
WEDNESDAY **15**	♊	☽ 12:20	AM only	
	12:00 ♋	△ ☉ 13:40		
		♌ 24:00		
THURSDAY **16**	♋	☽ 13:30		
FRIDAY **17**	♋	☽ 14:50		15:00
	15:00 ♌			
SATURDAY **18**	♌	☽ 16:05		
SUNDAY **19**	♌	☽ 17:20		19:00
	19:00 ♍	△ 01:10		

♈ Aries *Fire*	♉ Taurus *Earth*	♊ Gemini *Air*	♋ Cancer *Water*	♌ Leo *Fire*	♍ Virgo *Earth*

MARCH

The trine aspect of the Moon with Venus is a good moment for working with flowers.

MONDAY
13

The Moon forms a sextile aspect to Saturn during the evening. Think of working especially with perennials.

TUESDAY
14

There is a shift in element-signs at midday, but the passage of the Moon through its north node at the end of the day casts a blight on afternoon working. The Sun-Moon trine is a good thing.

WEDNESDAY
15

THURSDAY
16

A change from Water (leaf) to Fire (fruit and seed) element at the end of the afternoon. Try to time planting or sowing to the middle of the appropriate sign period.

FRIDAY
17

SATURDAY
18

A change from fruit or seed to an Earth sign occurs in the evening. The trine aspect of the Moon and Saturn is generally benevolent.

SUNDAY
19

 Libra
Air

 Scorpio
Water

 Sagittarius
Fire

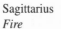 Capricorn
Earth

 Aquarius
Air

 Pisces
Water

MARCH

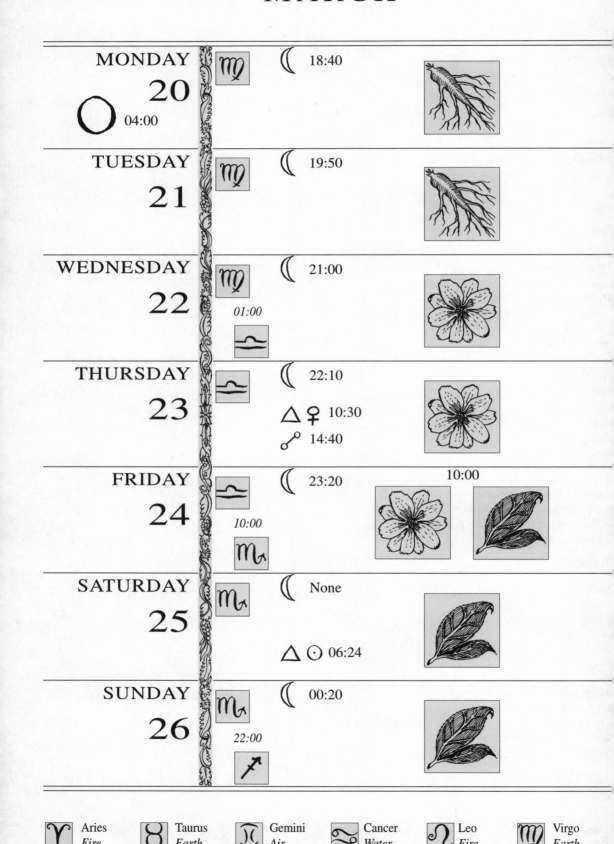

MONDAY **20** ⭘ 04:00	♍	☽ 18:40		
TUESDAY **21**	♍	☽ 19:50		
WEDNESDAY **22** *01:00* ♎	♍	☽ 21:00		
THURSDAY **23**	♎	☽ 22:10 △ ♀ 10:30 ⚹ 14:40		
FRIDAY **24** *10:00* ♏	♎	☽ 23:20	10:00	
SATURDAY **25**	♏	☽ None △ ☉ 06:24		
SUNDAY **26** *22:00* ♐	♏	☽ 00:20		

MARCH

Full Moon and spring tides. The time just before Full Moon is the ideal moment to sow seeds.

MONDAY

20

TUESDAY

21

The shift from roots to flower element-signs happens during the night.

WEDNESDAY

22

The Moon forms a trine aspect to Venus in the morning. This is a particularly good day to wait for if work with flowering plants is on the agenda though the Moon-Saturn opposition should be avoided.

THURSDAY

23

FRIDAY

24

The Moon-Sun aspect is trine early in the morning. This is a good things, especially for work with vines.

SATURDAY

25

The change in ruling signs happens in the evening, so the whole day is free for work with leaf plants.

SUNDAY

26

 Libra
Air

 Scorpio
Water

 Sagittarius
Fire

 Capricorn
Earth

 Aquarius
Air

 Pisces
Water

MARCH/APRIL

MONDAY **27**	↗	☾ 01:20 A 18:00	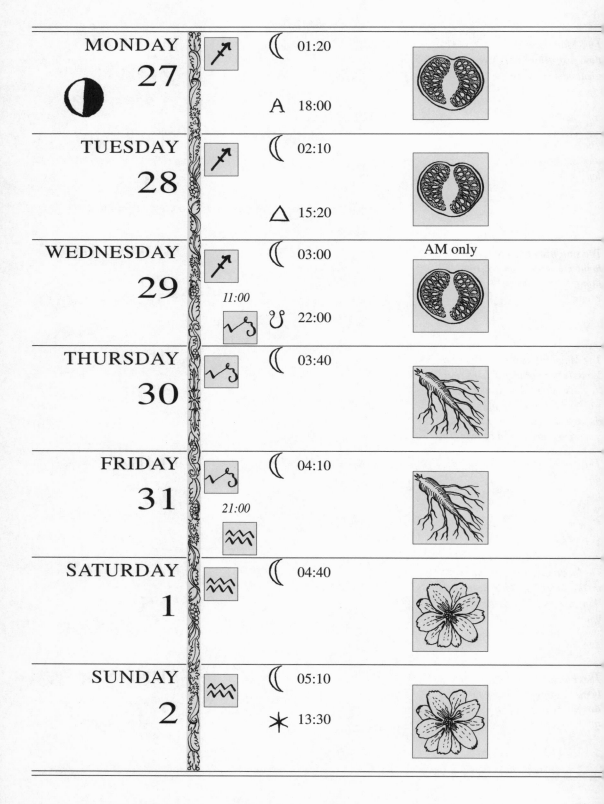
TUESDAY **28**	↗	☾ 02:10 △ 15:20	
WEDNESDAY **29**	↗ *11:00* ♑	☾ 03:00 ☋ 22:00	AM only
THURSDAY **30**	♑	☾ 03:40	
FRIDAY **31**	♑ *21:00* ♒	☾ 04:10	
SATURDAY **1**	♒	☾ 04:40	
SUNDAY **2**	♒	☾ 05:10 ✳ 13:30	

MARCH/APRIL

The Moon is at its apogee at the end of the day.

MONDAY

27

The trine aspect (120°) of the Moon and Saturn is especially benevolent.

TUESDAY

28

Work in the morning only, because of the baleful influence of the Moon crossing its south node during the evening.

WEDNESDAY

29

THURSDAY

30

The change in element-signs does not occur until the evening, leaving the whole day to fiddle with your roots.

FRIDAY

31

SATURDAY

1

The Moon-Saturn sextile aspect (60°) is another good one for gardeners. It is best to plant as soon after moonrise as possible.

SUNDAY

2

 Libra
Air

  Scorpio
Water

 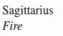 Sagittarius
Fire

 Capricorn
Earth

 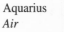 Aquarius
Air

 Pisces
Water

APRIL

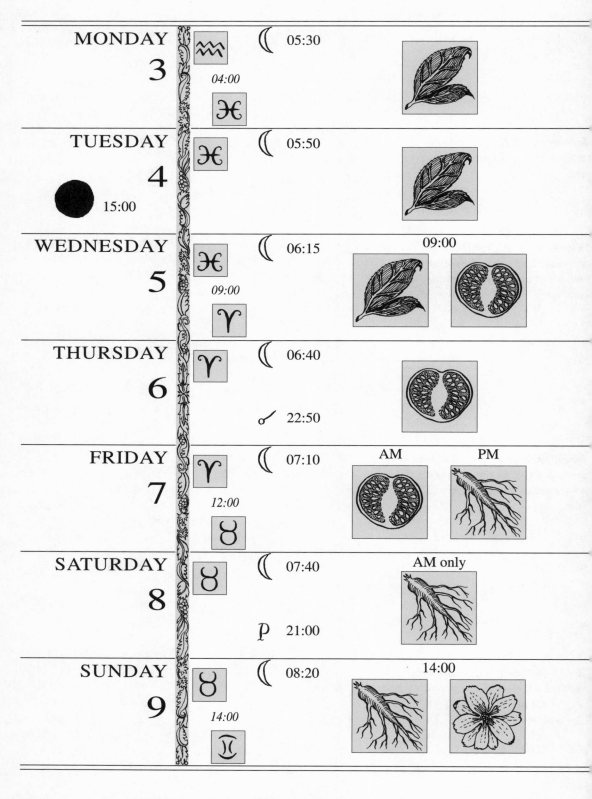

MONDAY 3
♒
04:00
♓
☾ 05:30

TUESDAY 4
♓
15:00
☾ 05:50

WEDNESDAY 5
♓
09:00
♈
☾ 06:15
09:00

THURSDAY 6
♈
☾ 06:40
♂ 22:50

FRIDAY 7
♈
12:00
♉
☾ 07:10
AM   PM

SATURDAY 8
♉
♇ 21:00
☾ 07:40
AM only

SUNDAY 9
♉
14:00
♊
☾ 08:20
14:00

APRIL

	MONDAY 3
New Moon, a moment of enhanced plant activity.	**TUESDAY** 4
The change in element means that effectively the whole day may be devoted to fruit-bearing plants.	**WEDNESDAY** 5
The conjunction as an aspect is not so bad as opposition or square. Seventeenth-century British writers thought it as benign as the sextile and trine aspects.	**THURSDAY** 6
Divide the day between fruit and seed plants on the one hand, and root plants on the other.	**FRIDAY** 7
The perigee of the lunar orbit is the reason for recommending work during the morning only.	**SATURDAY** 8
The element-signs change after lunch.	**SUNDAY** 9

 Libra *Air*   Scorpio *Water*   Sagittarius *Fire*   Capricorn *Earth*   Aquarius *Air*   Pisces *Water*

APRIL

MONDAY **10**	♊	☽ 09:10	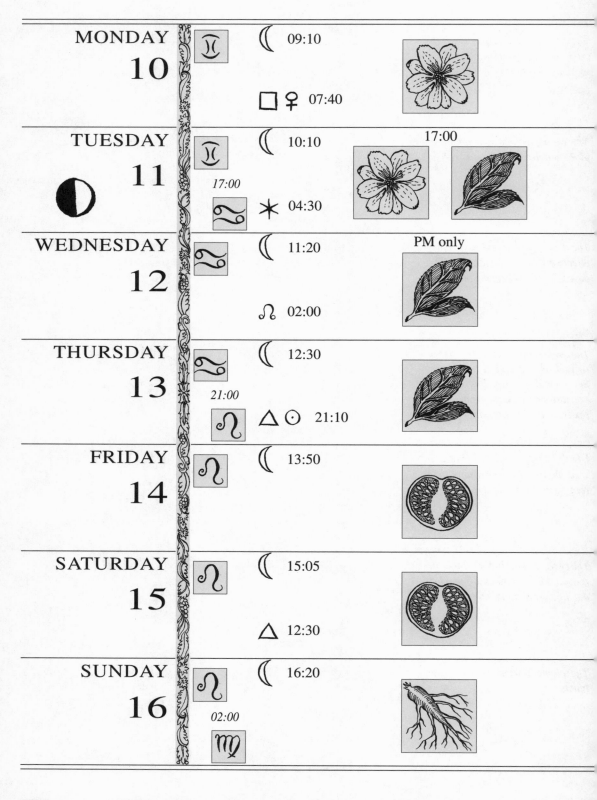
		□ ♀ 07:40	

TUESDAY 11

◗ ♊ ☽ 10:10

17:00 ♋ ✳ 04:30 17:00

WEDNESDAY 12 ♋ ☽ 11:20 PM only

♌ 02:00

THURSDAY 13 ♋ ☽ 12:30

21:00 ♌ △ ☉ 21:10

FRIDAY 14 ♌ ☽ 13:50

SATURDAY 15 ♌ ☽ 15:05

△ 12:30

SUNDAY 16 ♌ ☽ 16:20

02:00 ♍

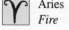 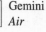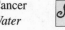

APRIL

<table>
<tr><td>*The Moon's square aspect to Venus early in the morning may affect working with flowering plants.*</td><td>MONDAY
10</td></tr>
<tr><td>*The sextile aspect to Saturn suggests emphasis on perennials.*</td><td>TUESDAY
11</td></tr>
<tr><td>*The Moon crosses its north node in the early hours; hence the advice to restrict work to the afternoon.*</td><td>WEDNESDAY
12</td></tr>
<tr><td>*The change of element-sign is in the evening so the whole day can be given over to leaf plants. The Sun-Moon trine is harmonious. Oranges and vines are two types of plant especially affected.*</td><td>THURSDAY
13</td></tr>
<tr><td></td><td>FRIDAY
14</td></tr>
<tr><td>*The Saturn-Moon trine impacts especially on perennials and trees. Planting should be concentrated on the hour of moonrise.*</td><td>SATURDAY
15</td></tr>
<tr><td>*The change of element-signs occurs in the early hours: the day therefore belongs to roots.*</td><td>SUNDAY
16</td></tr>
</table>

 Libra
Air

 Scorpio
Water

 Sagittarius
Fire

 Capricorn
Earth

 Aquarius
Air

 Pisces
Water

APRIL

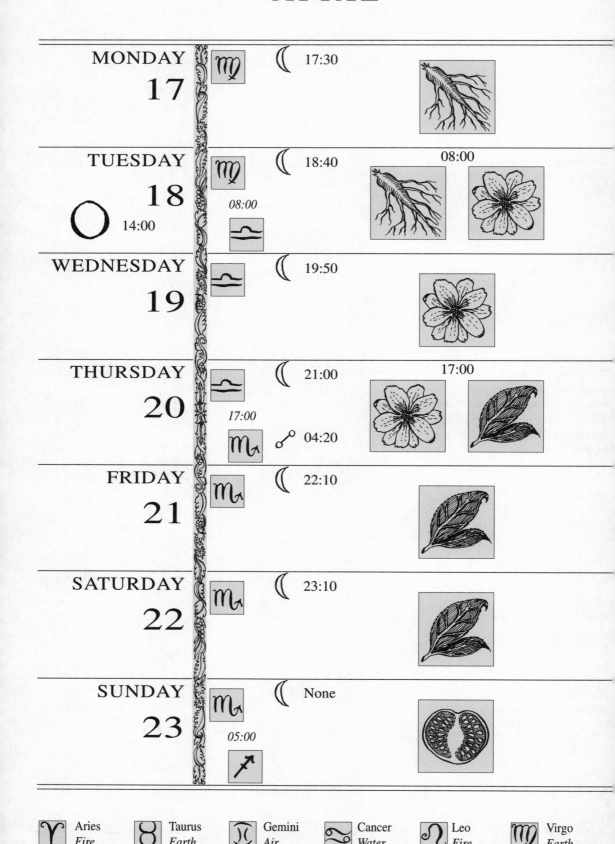

MONDAY 17 — ♍ — ☽ 17:30

TUESDAY 18 — ♍ — ☽ 18:40 — ○ 14:00 — ♎ 08:00 — 08:00

WEDNESDAY 19 — ♎ — ☽ 19:50

THURSDAY 20 — ♎ — ☽ 21:00 — ♏ 17:00 — ☍ 04:20 — 17:00

FRIDAY 21 — ♏ — ☽ 22:10

SATURDAY 22 — ♏ — ☽ 23:10

SUNDAY 23 — ♏ — ☽ None — ♐ 05:00

♈ Aries *Fire*   ♉ Taurus *Earth*   ♊ Gemini *Air*   ♋ Cancer *Water*   ♌ Leo *Fire*   ♍ Virgo *Earth*

APRIL

MONDAY 17

TUESDAY 18

Full Moon in the afternoon. The optimum time for sowing and planting.

WEDNESDAY 19

THURSDAY 20

The Moon and Saturn are in opposition (180°): thought stressful by some, although Bio-Dynamic farmers think it a very suitable moment to sow or plant.

FRIDAY 21

SATURDAY 22

SUNDAY 23

The element-signs change just before breakfast.

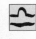 Libra *Air*   Scorpio *Water*   Sagittarius *Fire*  Capricorn *Earth*   Aquarius *Air*   Pisces *Water*

APRIL

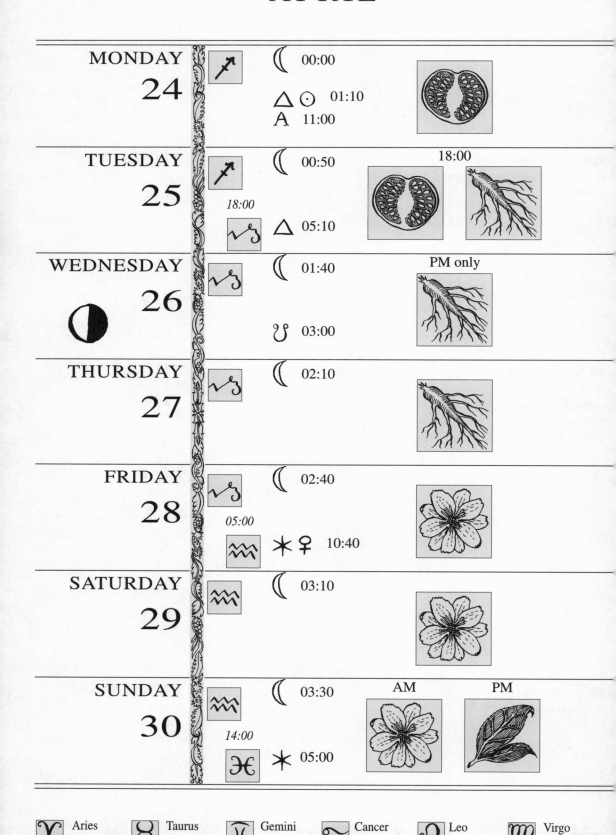

MONDAY 24
- ☾ 00:00
- △ ☉ 01:10
- A 11:00

TUESDAY 25
- ☾ 00:50
- *18:00*
- △ 05:10
- 18:00

WEDNESDAY 26
- ☾ 01:40
- ☋ 03:00

THURSDAY 27
- ☾ 02:10

FRIDAY 28
- ☾ 02:40
- *05:00*
- ✳ ♀ 10:40

SATURDAY 29
- ☾ 03:10

SUNDAY 30
- ☾ 03:30
- *14:00*
- ✳ 05:00
- AM
- PM

PM only

♈ Aries *Fire*	♉ Taurus *Earth*	♊ Gemini *Air*	♋ Cancer *Water*	♌ Leo *Fire*	♍ Virgo *Earth*

APRIL

MONDAY 24

The Sun-Moon trine in the early hours is a good omen for working with fruit trees; the apogee is never so menacing as the perigee.

TUESDAY 25

The Moon-Saturn trine continues the good omens for working with perennials.

WEDNESDAY 26

As the Moon crosses the South node in the early hours, restrict work to the afternoon.

THURSDAY 27

FRIDAY 28

The Moon-Venus aspect is sextile (60°): good for work with flowers. The element-sign has already changed by the start of the working day.

SATURDAY 29

SUNDAY 30

The element-signs change again, splitting the day into two. The sextile aspect is harmonious.

 Libra
Air

 Scorpio
Water

 Sagittarius
Fire

  Capricorn
Earth

 Aquarius
Air

 Pisces
Water

MAY

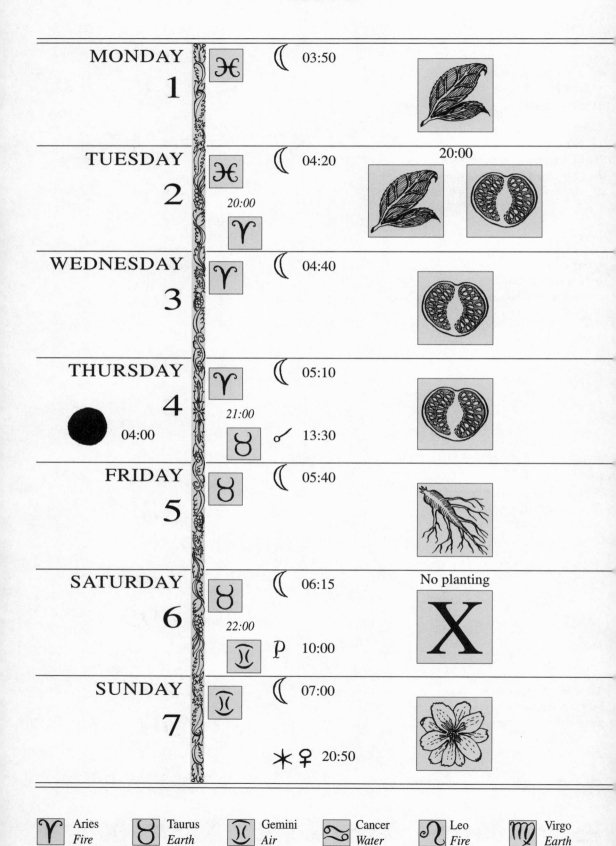

MONDAY **1**	♓	☽ 03:50	
TUESDAY **2**	♓ *20:00* ♈	☽ 04:20	20:00
WEDNESDAY **3**	♈	☽ 04:40	
THURSDAY **4** ● 04:00	♈ *21:00* ♉	☽ 05:10 ♂ 13:30	
FRIDAY **5**	♉	☽ 05:40	
SATURDAY **6**	♉ *22:00* ♊	☽ 06:15 ℞ 10:00	No planting **X**
SUNDAY **7**	♊	☽ 07:00 ⚹ ♀ 20:50	

♈ Aries *Fire*	♉ Taurus *Earth*	♊ Gemini *Air*	♋ Cancer *Water*	♌ Leo *Fire*	♍ Virgo *Earth*

MAY

	MONDAY 1
The change in element happens at the end of the working day.	TUESDAY 2
	WEDNESDAY 3
New Moon. The Moon-Saturn aspect is conjunction (0°): not brilliant but not a villain in everyone's eyes.	THURSDAY 4
	FRIDAY 5
The perigee is the reason for advising against planting or sowing on this day.	SATURDAY 6
There is a Moon-Venus sextile aspect at the end of the day: good for flowering plants. Some recommend working up to six hours before the exactitude, but not after it.	SUNDAY 7

 Libra *Air*   Scorpio *Water*   Sagittarius *Fire*    Capricorn *Earth*   Aquarius *Air*   Pisces *Water*

MAY

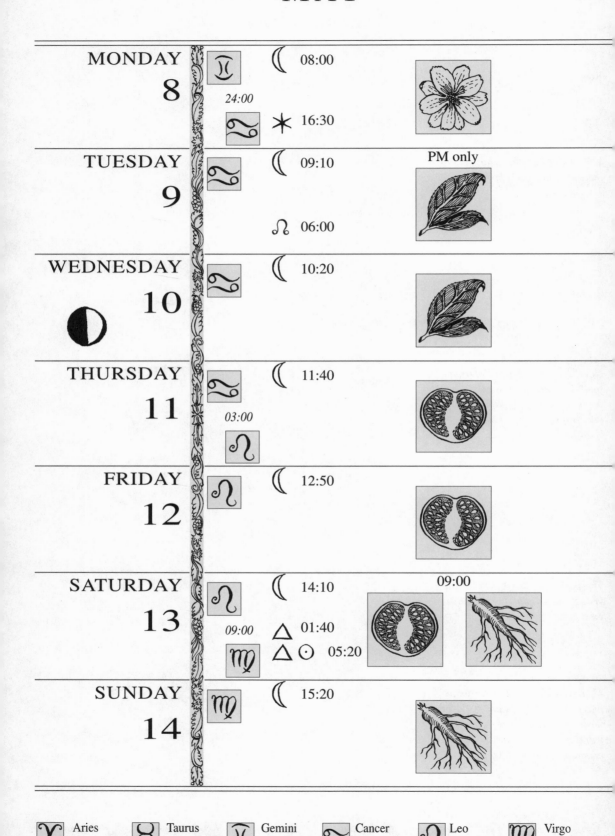

MONDAY **8**	Gemini ♊	☾ 08:00	
	24:00 Cancer ♋	✳ 16:30	
TUESDAY **9**	Cancer ♋	☾ 09:10	*PM only*
		♌ 06:00	
WEDNESDAY **10**	Cancer ♋	☾ 10:20	
THURSDAY **11**	Cancer ♋ *03:00* Leo ♌	☾ 11:40	
FRIDAY **12**	Leo ♌	☾ 12:50	
SATURDAY **13**	Leo ♌ *09:00* Virgo ♍	☾ 14:10 △ 01:40 △ ☉ 05:20	*09:00*
SUNDAY **14**	Virgo ♍	☾ 15:20	

♈ Aries *Fire*   ♉ Taurus *Earth*   ♊ Gemini *Air*   ♋ Cancer *Water*   ♌ Leo *Fire*   ♍ Virgo *Earth*

MAY

The Moon-Saturn aspect is sextile in the afternoon. The element-signs change at midnight, leaving the whole day for flowering plants.

MONDAY
8

As the Moon crosses its north node, so work is confined to the afternoon.

TUESDAY
9

WEDNESDAY
10

Again, the change of element occurs conveniently in night hours.

THURSDAY
11

FRIDAY
12

There are two trines today: one Moon-Saturn, the other Moon and the Sun.

SATURDAY
13

SUNDAY
14

 Libra *Air*   Scorpio *Water*   Sagittarius *Fire*   Capricorn *Earth*   Aquarius *Air*   Pisces *Water*

MAY

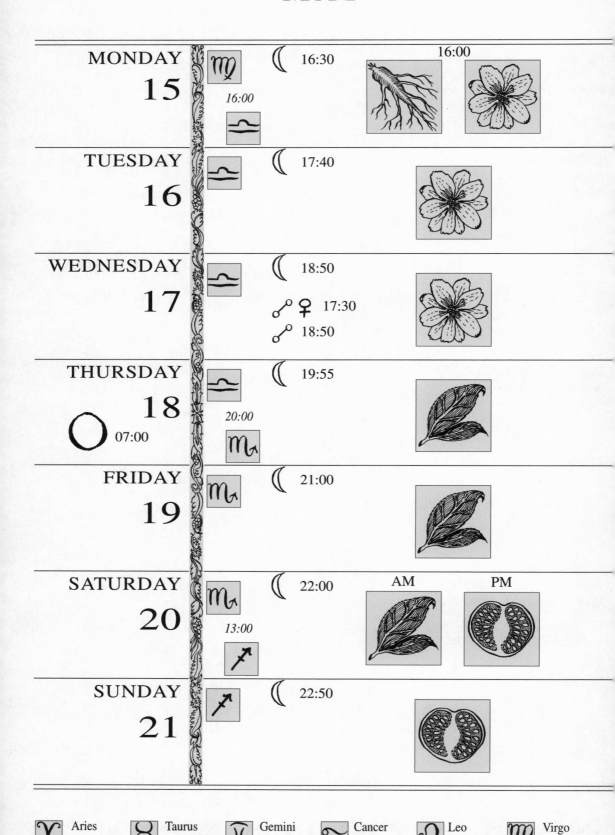

MONDAY **15**	♍ *16:00* ♎	☾ 16:30	16:00
TUESDAY **16**	♎	☾ 17:40	
WEDNESDAY **17**	♎	☾ 18:50 ☌ ♀ 17:30 ☌ 18:50	
THURSDAY **18** ◯ 07:00	♎ *20:00* ♏	☾ 19:55	
FRIDAY **19**	♏	☾ 21:00	
SATURDAY **20**	♏ *13:00* ♐	☾ 22:00	AM PM
SUNDAY **21**	♐	☾ 22:50	

♈ Aries *Fire*   ♉ Taurus *Earth*   ♊ Gemini *Air*   ♋ Cancer *Water*   ♌ Leo *Fire*   ♍ Virgo *Earth*

MAY

There is a shift from root (Earth) to flower (Air) element at the end of the afternoon.

MONDAY
15

TUESDAY
16

Two oppositions: Moon-Saturn and Moon-Venus. Opposition is thought a good thing by Bio-Dynamic growers.

WEDNESDAY
17

The element changes from Air (flower) to Water (leaf) during the night. There is a Full Moon at the beginning of the day.

THURSDAY
18

FRIDAY
19

SATURDAY
20

SUNDAY
21

 Libra *Air*   Scorpio *Water*   Sagittarius *Fire*   Capricorn *Earth*   Aquarius *Air*   Pisces *Water*

MAY

MONDAY 22
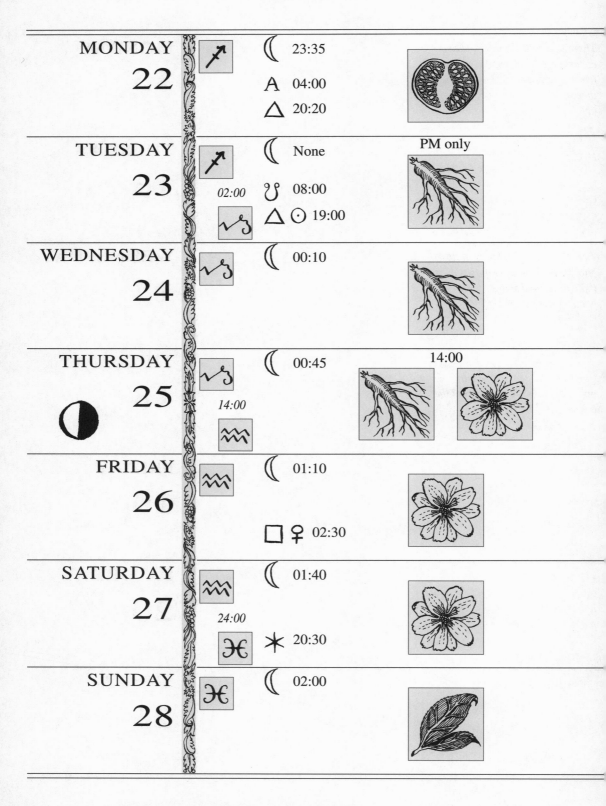

☽ 23:35
Λ 04:00
△ 20:20

TUESDAY 23

02:00

☽ None
☊ 08:00
△ ☉ 19:00

PM only

WEDNESDAY 24

☽ 00:10

THURSDAY 25

14:00

☽ 00:45

14:00

FRIDAY 26

☽ 01:10

□ ♀ 02:30

SATURDAY 27

24:00

☽ 01:40

✳ 20:30

SUNDAY 28

☽ 02:00

 Aries *Fire*   Taurus *Earth*   Gemini *Air*    Cancer *Water*   Leo *Fire*   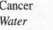 Virgo *Earth*

MAY

MONDAY 22

The Moon touches its apogee in the early hours (when it is furthest from the Earth). Come evening, there is a trine aspect of the Moon and Saturn.

TUESDAY 23

The element change is at night. The crossing of the south node at breakfast-time means afternoon working is best. The Sun-Moon trine in the evening is more benevolent.

WEDNESDAY 24

THURSDAY 25

FRIDAY 26

There is a Moon-Venus square aspect. A moment of stress when working with flowering plants.

SATURDAY 27

The Moon-Saturn aspect is sextile (60°). The move out of flowers into leaf plants is not until the hours of night.

SUNDAY 28

 Libra
Air

 Scorpio
Water

 Sagittarius
Fire

 Capricorn
Earth

 Aquarius
Air

 Pisces
Water

MAY/JUNE

MONDAY **29**	♓	☾ 02:20	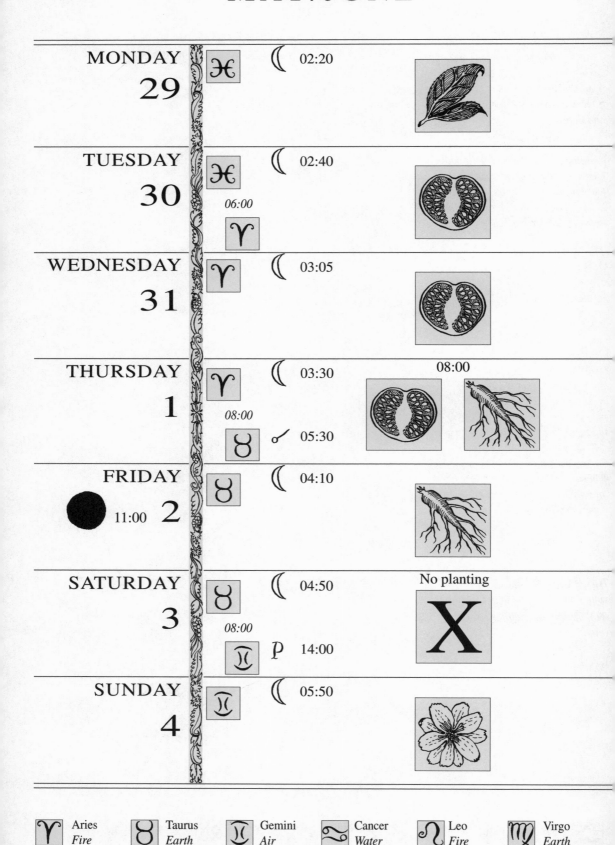
TUESDAY **30**	♓ *06:00* ♈	☾ 02:40	
WEDNESDAY **31**	♈	☾ 03:05	
THURSDAY **1**	♈ *08:00* ♉	☾ 03:30 ☌ 05:30	*08:00*
FRIDAY ● 11:00 **2**	♉	☾ 04:10	
SATURDAY **3**	♉ *08:00* ♊	☾ 04:50 ☊ 14:00	No planting **X**
SUNDAY **4**	♊	☾ 05:50	

♈ Aries *Fire*	♉ Taurus *Earth*	♊ Gemini *Air*	♋ Cancer *Water*	♌ Leo *Fire*	♍ Virgo *Earth*

	MONDAY
	29

	TUESDAY
A change from leaf to fruit/seed plants happens in the early morning.	**30**

	WEDNESDAY
	31

	THURSDAY
The shift of elements is early in the day so that most should be devoted to root crops. The stressful influence of the conjunction is also safely confined to hours of sleep.	**1**

	FRIDAY
New Moon at 11:00.	**2**

	SATURDAY
The perigee is the reason for advising against planting or sowing on this day.	**3**

	SUNDAY
	4

 Libra
Air

 Scorpio
Water

 Sagittarius
Fire

 Capricorn
Earth

 Aquarius
Air

 Pisces
Water

JUNE

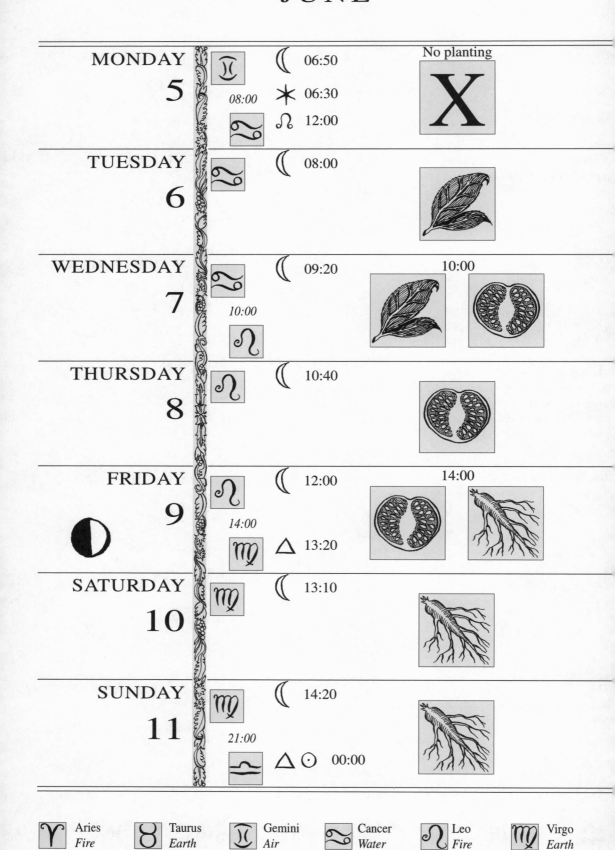

MONDAY **5**	♊ 08:00 ♋	☾ 06:50 ✳ 06:30 ♌ 12:00	No planting **X**
TUESDAY **6**	♋	☾ 08:00	
WEDNESDAY **7**	♋ 10:00 ♌	☾ 09:20	10:00
THURSDAY **8**	♌	☾ 10:40	
FRIDAY **9**	♌ 14:00 ♍	☾ 12:00 △ 13:20	14:00
SATURDAY **10**	♍	☾ 13:10	
SUNDAY **11**	♍ 21:00 ♎	☾ 14:20 △ ☉ 00:00	

♈ Aries *Fire*	♉ Taurus *Earth*	♊ Gemini *Air*	♋ Cancer *Water*	♌ Leo *Fire*	♍ Virgo *Earth*

JUNE

The passage through the North node at midday is the cause of the day's advice, notwithstanding the harmony of the sextile aspect of the Moon and Saturn.

MONDAY
5

TUESDAY
6

Move from leaf plants to fruit/seed plants at the end of the morning.

WEDNESDAY
7

THURSDAY
8

The Moon-Saturn aspect is trine, a good day to work on perennials and trees.

FRIDAY
9

SATURDAY
10

There is a trine aspect again to-day, this time of the Moon and the Sun.

SUNDAY
11

 Libra
Air

 Scorpio
Water

 Sagittarius
Fire

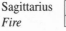 Capricorn
Earth

 Aquarius
Air

 Pisces
Water

JUNE

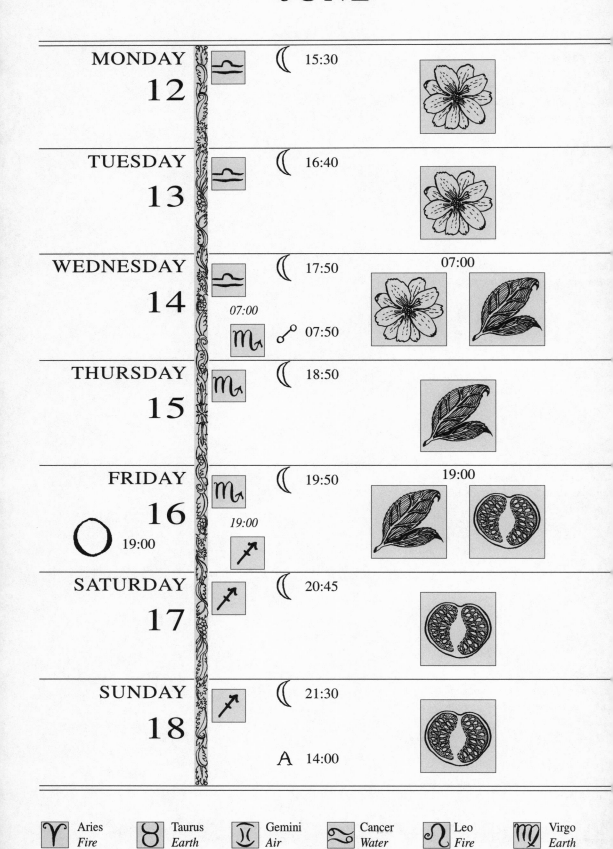

MONDAY 12 ☊ ☾ 15:30

TUESDAY 13 ☊ ☾ 16:40

WEDNESDAY 14 ☊ ☾ 17:50
07:00 ♏ ☍ 07:50
07:00

THURSDAY 15 ♏ ☾ 18:50

FRIDAY 16 ♏ ☾ 19:50
○ 19:00
19:00 ♐
19:00

SATURDAY 17 ♐ ☾ 20:45

SUNDAY 18 ♐ ☾ 21:30
A 14:00

| ♈ Aries *Fire* | ♉ Taurus *Earth* | ♊ Gemini *Air* | ♋ Cancer *Water* | ♌ Leo *Fire* | ♍ Virgo *Earth* |

JUNE

MONDAY
12

TUESDAY
13

The Moon-Saturn aspect is opposition, not brilliant. The afternoon might be the better time to work.

WEDNESDAY
14

The day before a Full Moon is optimal for sowing seeds (water absorption is at its highest).

THURSDAY
15

The change from leaf (Water) to fruit/seed (Fire) in the evening, leaves the day for fruiting and seed-bearing plants. Full Moon coincides.

FRIDAY
16

SATURDAY
17

The Moon reaches its apogee (less stressful than its perigee) in the middle of the day.

SUNDAY
18

 Libra
Air

 Scorpio
Water

 Sagittarius
Fire

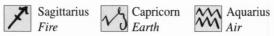 Capricorn
Earth

 Aquarius
Air

 Pisces
Water

JUNE

MONDAY 19

♐ ☽ 22:10
08:00
♑ △ 09:50
☊ 11:00

No planting
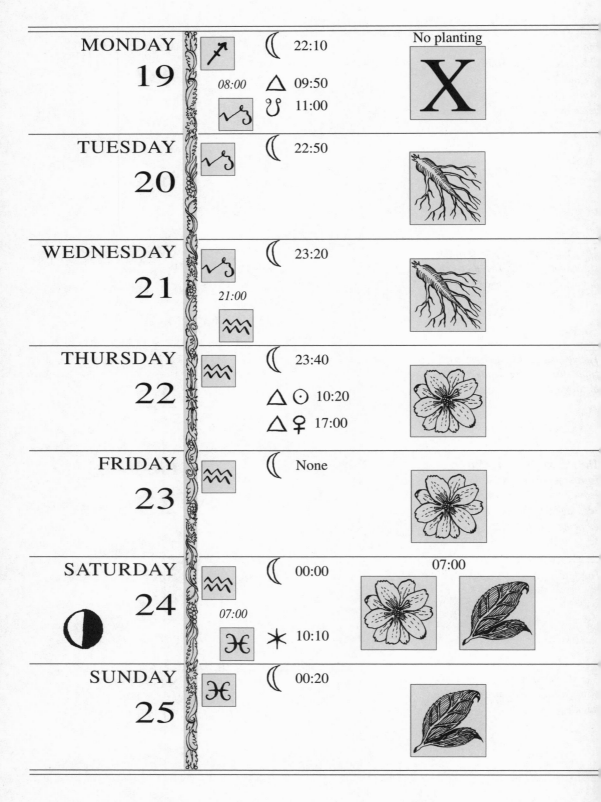
X

TUESDAY 20

♑ ☽ 22:50

WEDNESDAY 21

♑ ☽ 23:20
21:00
♒

THURSDAY 22

♒ ☽ 23:40
△ ☉ 10:20
△ ♀ 17:00

FRIDAY 23

♒ ☽ None

SATURDAY 24

♒ ☽ 00:00
07:00
♓ ✳ 10:10

07:00

SUNDAY 25

♓ ☽ 00:20

JUNE

Moon-Saturn form a trine aspect (120°). But its benevolent influence is cancelled by the passage of the Moon through its south node, hence the advice to avoid planting.

MONDAY
19

TUESDAY
20

Midsummer, the longest day.

WEDNESDAY
21

The Moon forms two trines, first with the Sun, then with Venus: a good day for flowering plants.

THURSDAY
22

FRIDAY
23

The sextile aspect is harmonious.

SATURDAY
24

SUNDAY
25

 Libra *Air*

 Scorpio *Water*

 Sagittarius *Fire*

 Capricorn *Earth*

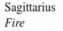 Aquarius *Air*

 Pisces *Water*

JUNE/JULY

MONDAY 26
♓
15:00
♈
☾ 00:40
15:00
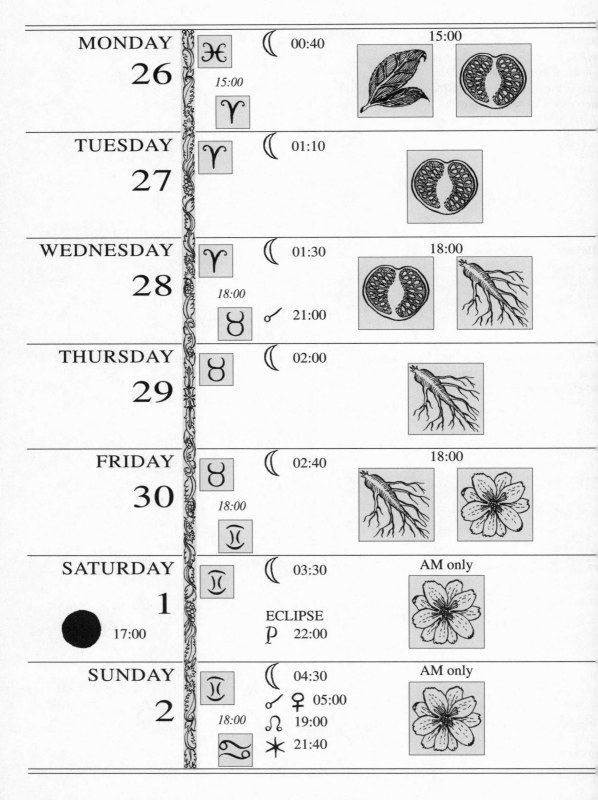

TUESDAY 27
♈
☾ 01:10

WEDNESDAY 28
♈
18:00
♉ ☌ 21:00
☾ 01:30
18:00

THURSDAY 29
♉
☾ 02:00

FRIDAY 30
♉
18:00
♊
☾ 02:40
18:00

SATURDAY 1
● 17:00
♊
☾ 03:30
ECLIPSE
♇ 22:00
AM only

SUNDAY 2
♊
18:00
♋
☾ 04:30
☌ ♀ 05:00
☊ 19:00
✳ 21:40
AM only

 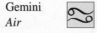

JUNE/JULY

A change in element-signs from leaf to fruit or seed plants in the afternoon. The most propitious time to work is in the middle of a sign's spell of dominance, when that is possible.

MONDAY

26

TUESDAY

27

There is a Moon-Saturn conjunction (aspect 0°), which is thought harmonious by some observers.

WEDNESDAY

28

The Moon crosses its south node at midnight, hence the recommendation to work only during the morning.

THURSDAY

29

The change in elements happens at the end of the working day.

FRIDAY

30

There is a solar eclipse, a time of disturbance, at about the same time as the New Moon. The Moon is also at its perigee. Work is advised in the morning only.

SATURDAY

1

Work in the morning once more. The Moon crosses its north node in the early evening; there is a Moon-Venus conjunction in the early morning; and a Moon-Saturn sextile aspect later on.

SUNDAY

2

 Libra
Air

 Scorpio
Water

 Sagittarius
Fire

 Capricorn
Earth

 Aquarius
Air

 Pisces
Water

JULY

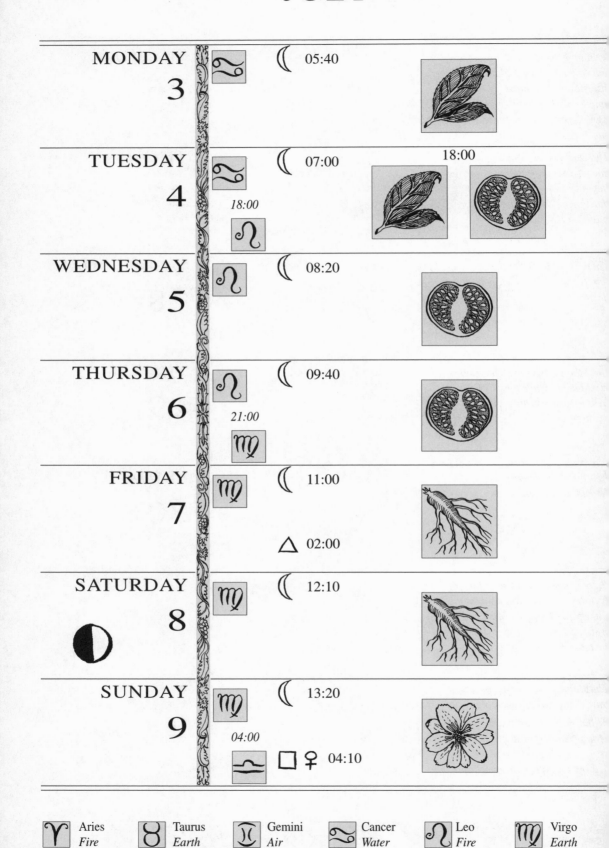

MONDAY 3 ♋ ☾ 05:40

TUESDAY 4 ♋ ☾ 07:00 · 18:00
18:00 ♋

WEDNESDAY 5 ♌ ☾ 08:20

THURSDAY 6 ♌ ☾ 09:40
21:00 ♍

FRIDAY 7 ♍ ☾ 11:00
△ 02:00

SATURDAY 8 ♍ ☾ 12:10

SUNDAY 9 ♍ ☾ 13:20
04:00
♎ □ ♀ 04:10

| ♈ Aries *Fire* | ♉ Taurus *Earth* | ♊ Gemini *Air* | ♋ Cancer *Water* | ♌ Leo *Fire* | ♍ Virgo *Earth* |

JULY

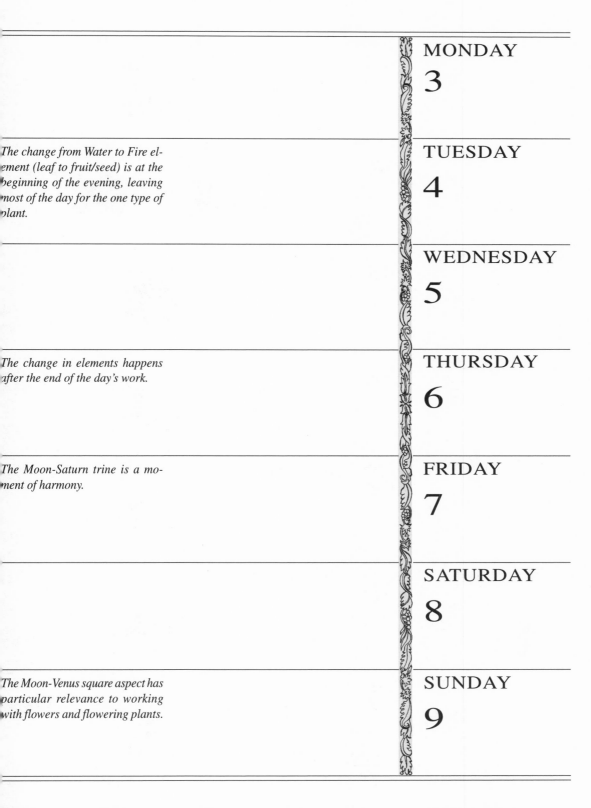

MONDAY

3

TUESDAY

4

The change from Water to Fire element (leaf to fruit/seed) is at the beginning of the evening, leaving most of the day for the one type of plant.

WEDNESDAY

5

THURSDAY

6

The change in elements happens after the end of the day's work.

FRIDAY

7

The Moon-Saturn trine is a moment of harmony.

SATURDAY

8

SUNDAY

9

The Moon-Venus square aspect has particular relevance to working with flowers and flowering plants.

 Libra
Air

 Scorpio
Water

 Sagittarius
Fire

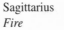 Capricorn
Earth

 Aquarius
Air

 Pisces
Water

JULY

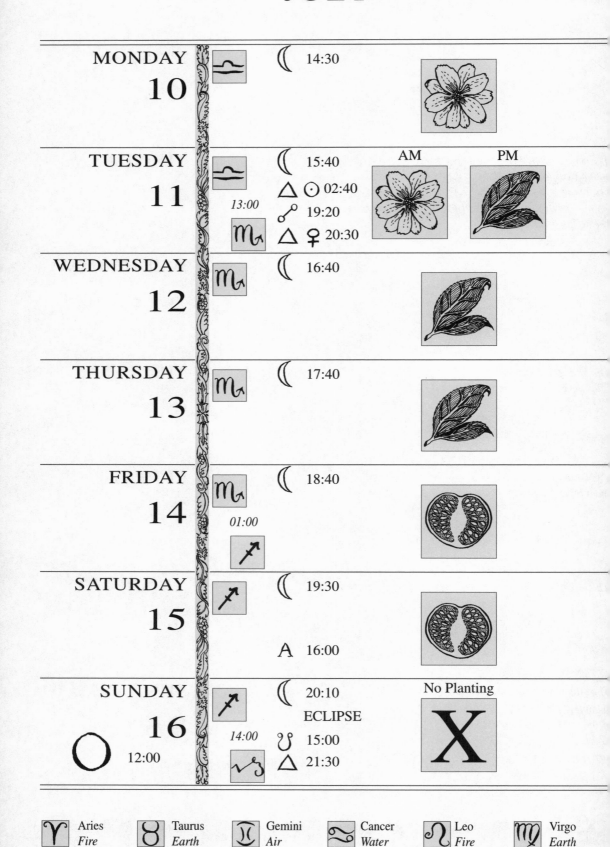

MONDAY **10**	♎	☾ 14:30	*flower illustration*

TUESDAY
11

♎
13:00
♏

☾ 15:40
△ ☉ 02:40
☍ 19:20
△ ♀ 20:30

AM PM

WEDNESDAY
12

♏

☾ 16:40

THURSDAY
13

♏

☾ 17:40

FRIDAY
14

♏
01:00
♐

☾ 18:40

SATURDAY
15

♐

☾ 19:30

A 16:00

SUNDAY
16

○ 12:00

♐
14:00
♑

☾ 20:10
ECLIPSE
☊ 15:00
△ 21:30

No Planting

X

| ♈ Aries
Fire | ♉ Taurus
Earth | ♊ Gemini
Air | ♋ Cancer
Water | ♌ Leo
Fire | ♍ Virgo
Earth |

JULY

	MONDAY
	10

The Moon has a trine aspect to both Venus and the Sun at opposite ends of the day and is in opposition to Saturn as well. It is the time before, not after, these events that matters to plants.

TUESDAY
11

WEDNESDAY
12

THURSDAY
13

FRIDAY
14

The Moon is at its apogee.

SATURDAY
15

Not a good day for work. There is a lunar eclipse when the Full Moon occurs; it also passes through its south node. Finally, the Moon-Saturn aspect is trine.

SUNDAY
16

 Libra
Air

 Scorpio
Water

 Sagittarius
Fire

 Capricorn
Earth

 Aquarius
Air

 Pisces
Water

JULY

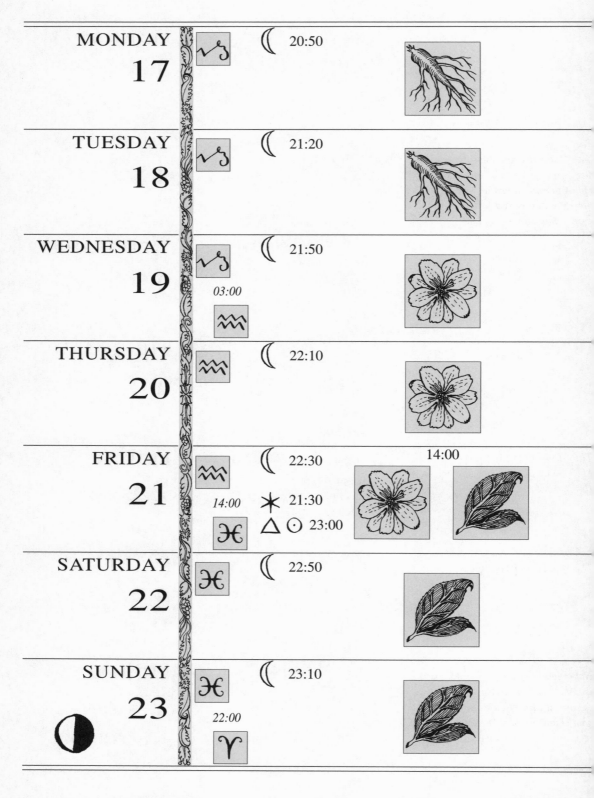

MONDAY 17 ♑ ☾ 20:50

TUESDAY 18 ♑ ☾ 21:20

WEDNESDAY 19 ♑ ☾ 21:50
03:00 ♒

THURSDAY 20 ♒ ☾ 22:10

FRIDAY 21 ♒ ☾ 22:30
14:00 ♓ ✳ 21:30 △ ☉ 23:00
14:00

SATURDAY 22 ♓ ☾ 22:50

SUNDAY 23 ♓ ☾ 23:10
22:00 ♈

JULY

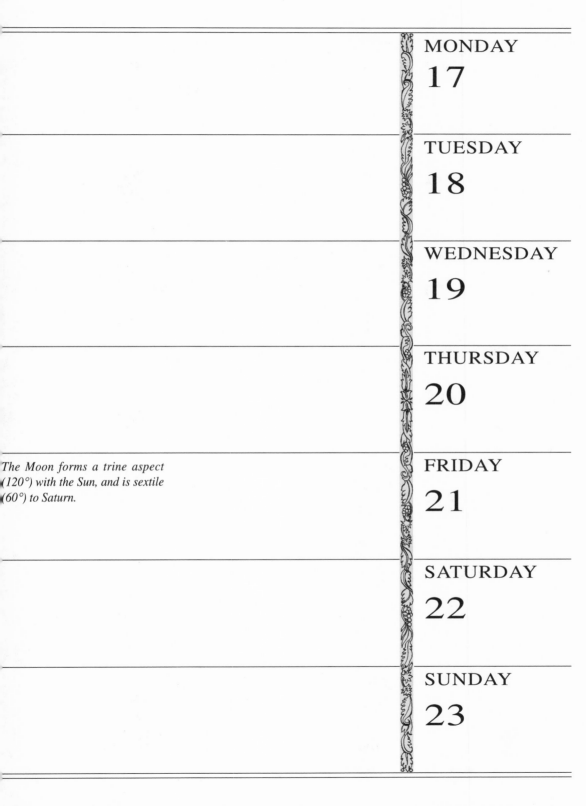

MONDAY
17

TUESDAY
18

WEDNESDAY
19

THURSDAY
20

The Moon forms a trine aspect (120°) with the Sun, and is sextile (60°) to Saturn.

FRIDAY
21

SATURDAY
22

SUNDAY
23

 Libra
Air

 Scorpio
Water

 Sagittarius
Fire

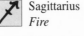 Capricorn
Earth

 Aquarius
Air

 Pisces
Water

JULY

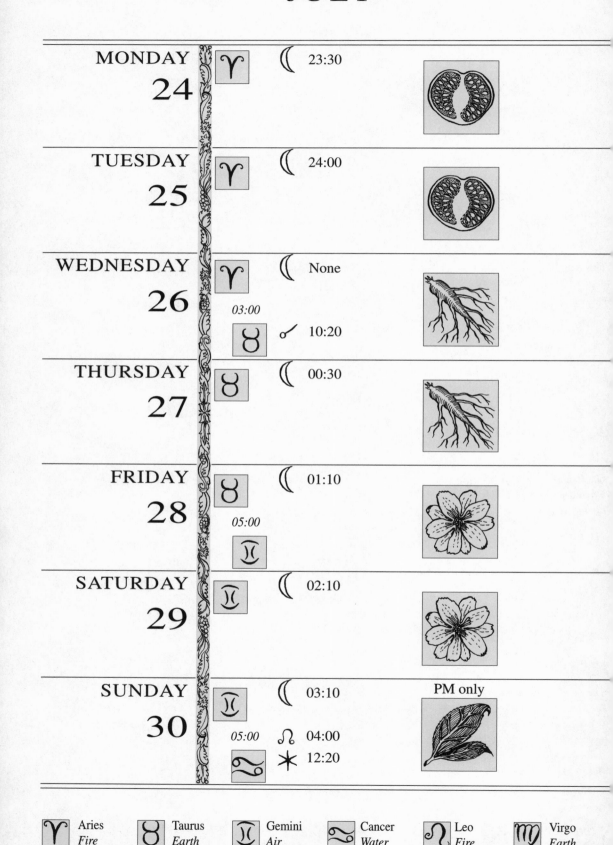

MONDAY **24**	♈	☽ 23:30
TUESDAY **25**	♈	☽ 24:00
WEDNESDAY **26**	♈ *03:00* ♉	☽ None ☌ 10:20
THURSDAY **27**	♉	☽ 00:30
FRIDAY **28**	♉ *05:00* ♊	☽ 01:10
SATURDAY **29**	♊	☽ 02:10
SUNDAY **30**	♊ *05:00* ♋	☽ 03:10 ♌ 04:00 ✳ 12:20 — PM only

♈ Aries *Fire*   ♉ Taurus *Earth*   ♊ Gemini *Air*   ♋ Cancer *Water*   ♌ Leo *Fire*   ♍ Virgo *Earth*

JULY

MONDAY
24

TUESDAY
25

The elements change during the night. The Moon-Saturn aspect is conjunction (0°).

WEDNESDAY
26

THURSDAY
27

The change in elements happens at the outset of the day.

FRIDAY
28

SATURDAY
29

The crossing of the north node by the Moon is the reason for limiting work to the afternoon. The benign sextile (60°) aspect of the Moon and Saturn may be seen as a settler to earlier disturbance.

SUNDAY
30

 Libra
Air

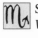 Scorpio
Water

 Sagittarius
Fire

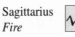 Capricorn
Earth

 Aquarius
Air

  Pisces
Water

JULY/AUGUST

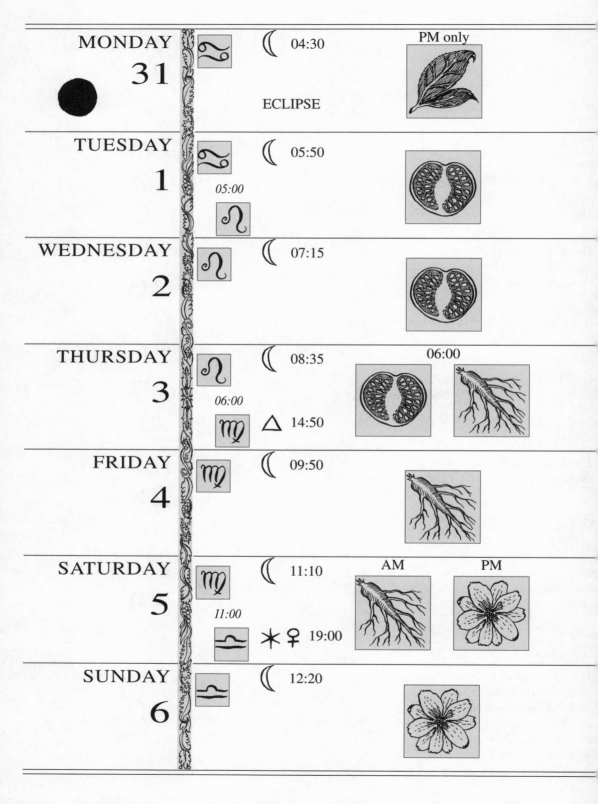

MONDAY 31
♋ ☾ 04:30

ECLIPSE

PM only

TUESDAY 1
♋ ☾ 05:50

05:00
♌

WEDNESDAY 2
♌ ☾ 07:15

THURSDAY 3
♌ ☾ 08:35

06:00
♍ △ 14:50

06:00

FRIDAY 4
♍ ☾ 09:50

SATURDAY 5
♍ ☾ 11:10

11:00
♎ ✳ ♀ 19:00

AM   PM

SUNDAY 6
♎ ☾ 12:20

 Aries
Fire

 Taurus
Earth

 Gemini
Air

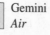 Cancer
Water

 Leo
Fire

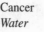 Virgo
Earth

JULY/AUGUST

There is a solar eclipse at the time of the New Moon. Work only in the afternoon.

MONDAY
31

There is a change from Water to Fire element (leaf to fruit/seed) before work starts for the day.

TUESDAY
1

WEDNESDAY
2

The Moon/Saturn aspect is trine (120°). There is also a progression through the elements from fruit/seed to roots.

THURSDAY
3

FRIDAY
4

There is a change from root to flowering plants. The sextile aspect of the Moon to Venus relates especially to flowering plants.

SATURDAY
5

SUNDAY
6

 Libra *Air*

 Scorpio *Water*

 Sagittarius *Fire*

 Capricorn *Earth*

 Aquarius *Air*

Pisces *Water*

AUGUST

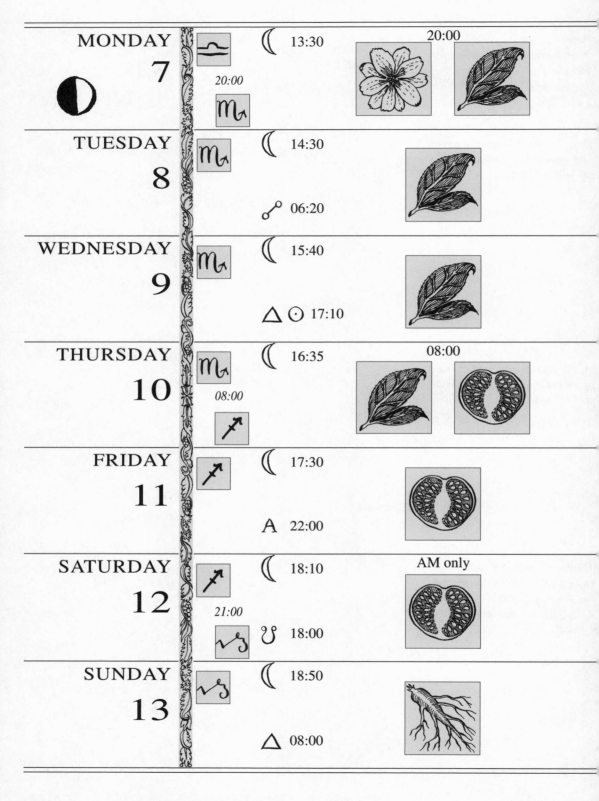

MONDAY 7

◑

♎ 13:30
♏ 20:00

🌙 13:30
20:00

TUESDAY 8

♏

🌙 14:30
⚷ 06:20

WEDNESDAY 9

♏

🌙 15:40
△ ☉ 17:10

THURSDAY 10

♏
08:00
♐

🌙 16:35
08:00

FRIDAY 11

♐

🌙 17:30
A 22:00

SATURDAY 12

♐
21:00
♑

🌙 18:10
☊ 18:00
AM only

SUNDAY 13

♑

🌙 18:50
△ 08:00

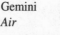

AUGUST

MONDAY
7

At the end of the day the elements change from those favouring flowering plants to those promoting leaf plants.

TUESDAY
8

The Moon-Saturn opposition is generally thought stressful.

WEDNESDAY
9

The Moon-Sun trine aspect has a particular bearing on vines and the vineyard.

THURSDAY
10

FRIDAY
11

The Moon reaches its apogee.

SATURDAY
12

The crossing of the Moon's south node is the reason for restricting work to the morning.

SUNDAY
13

The Moon-Saturn trine restores harmony in the garden.

 Libra
Air

 Scorpio
Water

 Sagittarius
Fire

 Capricorn
Earth

 Aquarius
Air

 Pisces
Water

AUGUST

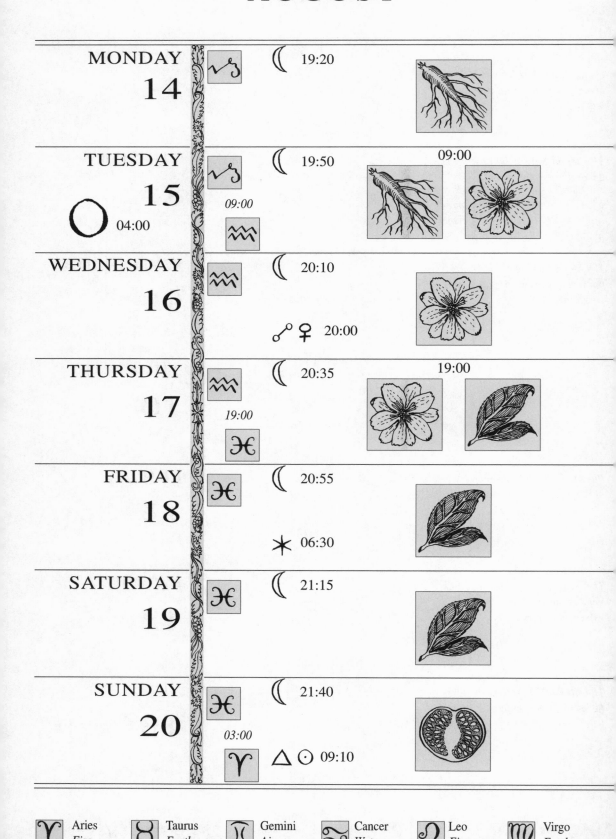

MONDAY 14

♑ ☽ 19:20

TUESDAY 15

♑ ☽ 19:50
09:00
♒
○ 04:00
09:00

WEDNESDAY 16

♒ ☽ 20:10
☌ ♀ 20:00

THURSDAY 17

♒ ☽ 20:35
19:00
♓
19:00

FRIDAY 18

♓ ☽ 20:55
⚹ 06:30

SATURDAY 19

♓ ☽ 21:15

SUNDAY 20

♓ ☽ 21:40
03:00
♈ △ ☉ 09:10

♈ Aries *Fire*   ♉ Taurus *Earth*   ♊ Gemini *Air*   ♋ Cancer *Water*   ♌ Leo *Fire*   ♍ Virgo *Earth*

AUGUST

	MONDAY **14**
Full Moon: a good time to harvest, especially things that are not to be stored. There is a change in elements in the morning, leaving most of the day to deal with flowering plants.	**TUESDAY** **15**
The Moon forms an oppositional aspect with Venus.	**WEDNESDAY** **16**
	THURSDAY **17**
In the early morning, the Moon and Saturn have a sextile (60°) aspect.	**FRIDAY** **28**
	SATURDAY **19**
The elements change in the hours of night; there is a Moon-Sun trine aspect as work begins.	**SUNDAY** **20**

 Libra
Air
 Scorpio
Water
 Sagittarius
Fire
 Capricorn
Earth
 Aquarius
Air
 Pisces
Water

AUGUST

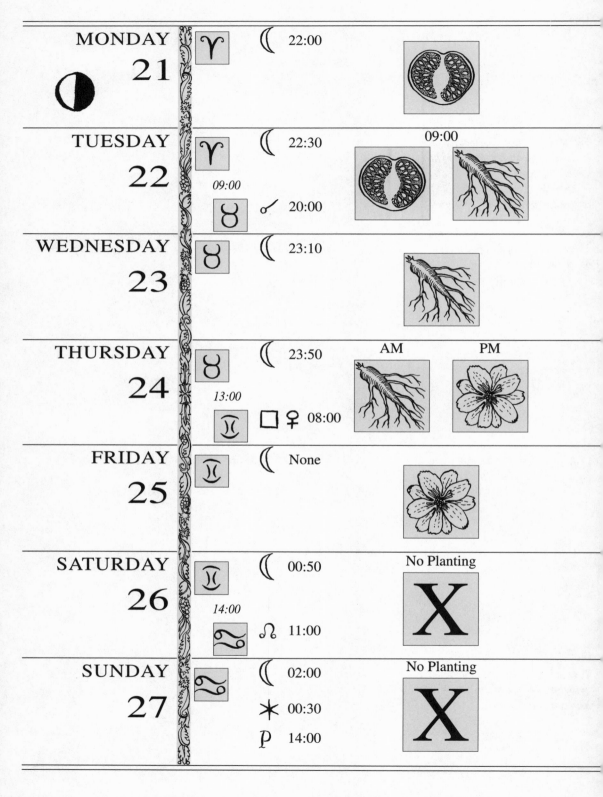

MONDAY **21** (first quarter moon)	♈	☽ 22:00	

| **TUESDAY** **22** | ♈ *09:00* ♉ | ☽ 22:30 ☌ 20:00 | 09:00 |

| **WEDNESDAY** **23** | ♉ | ☽ 23:10 | |

| **THURSDAY** **24** | ♉ *13:00* ♊ | ☽ 23:50 □ ♀ 08:00 | AM   PM |

| **FRIDAY** **25** | ♊ | ☽ None | |

| **SATURDAY** **26** | ♊ *14:00* ♋ | ☽ 00:50 ♌ 11:00 | No Planting **X** |

| **SUNDAY** **27** | ♋ | ☽ 02:00 ✳ 00:30 ♇ 14:00 | No Planting **X** |

 Aries *Fire*    Taurus *Earth*   Gemini *Air*   Cancer *Water*   Leo *Fire*   Virgo *Earth*

AUGUST

MONDAY
21

The Moon-Saturn conjunction is a mild stress point.

TUESDAY
22

WEDNESDAY
23

The change in elements happens in the middle of the day. The Moon is square to Venus at the outset.

THURSDAY
24

FRIDAY
25

Suspend planting today as the Moon passes through its north node.

SATURDAY
26

Another day of inactivity is proposed due to the perigee some time after lunch.

SUNDAY
27

 Libra
Air

 Scorpio
Water

 Sagittarius
Fire

  Capricorn
Earth

 Aquarius
Air

 Pisces
Water

AUGUST/SEPTEMBER

MONDAY 28
♋ ☽ 03:20
15:00
♌
15:00
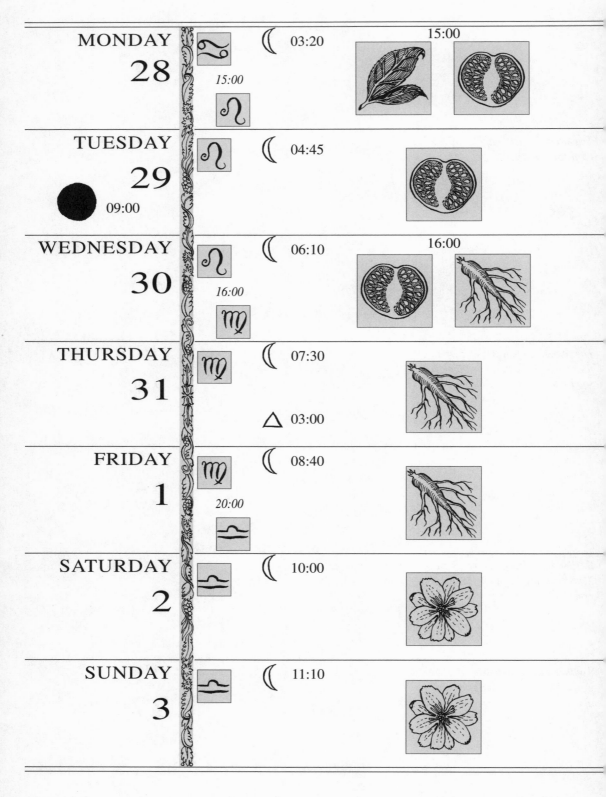

TUESDAY 29
♌ ☽ 04:45
● 09:00

WEDNESDAY 30
♌ ☽ 06:10
16:00
♍
16:00

THURSDAY 31
♍ ☽ 07:30
△ 03:00

FRIDAY 1
♍ ☽ 08:40
20:00
♎

SATURDAY 2
♎ ☽ 10:00

SUNDAY 3
♎ ☽ 11:10

AUGUST/SEPTEMBER

There is a change from Water to Fire element (leaf to fruit/seed).

MONDAY

28

New Moon: a good time to harvest those things that are to be stored for eating later, or used for seed during the next season.

TUESDAY

29

There is a progression through the elements from fruit/seed to root plants.

WEDNESDAY

30

The Moon-Saturn aspect is trine.

THURSDAY

31

FRIDAY

1

SATURDAY

2

SUNDAY

3

 Libra
Air

 Scorpio
Water

 Sagittarius
Fire

 Capricorn
Earth

 Aquarius
Air

 Pisces
Water

SEPTEMBER

MONDAY 4

☾ 12:20

04:00

♐ ☍ 16:00

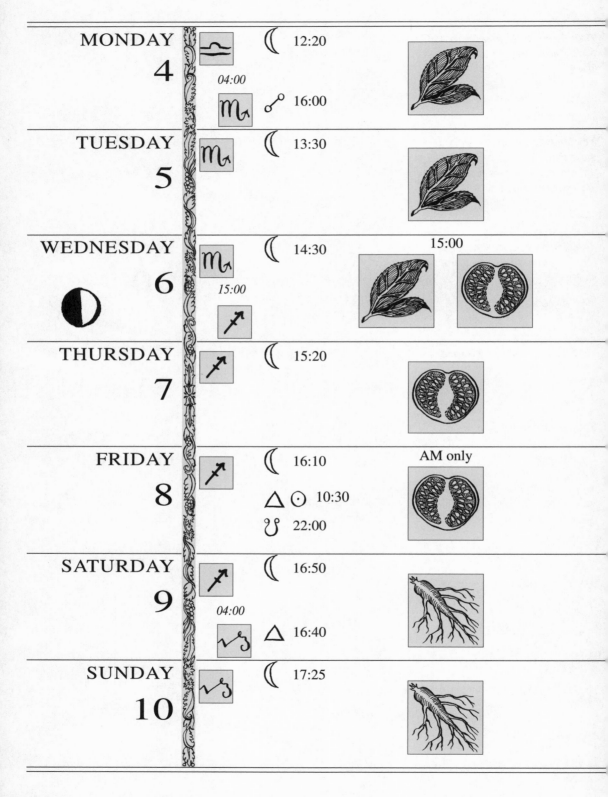

TUESDAY 5

☾ 13:30

WEDNESDAY 6

☾ 14:30

15:00

15:00

♐

THURSDAY 7

☾ 15:20

FRIDAY 8

☾ 16:10

△ ☉ 10:30

☋ 22:00

AM only

SATURDAY 9

☾ 16:50

04:00

△ 16:40

SUNDAY 10

☾ 17:25

SEPTEMBER

Moon and Saturn are in opposition. Moonrise is conveniently timed in daylight hours, take advantage of it for sowing and planting autumn crops.

MONDAY

4

TUESDAY

5

Progression through the ruling signs, from leaf to fruit or seed plants.

WEDNESDAY

6

THURSDAY

7

The crossing of the south node is the cause of restriction to morning working. There is also a trine aspect of the Moon and the Sun during that time.

FRIDAY

8

A Moon-Saturn trine.

SATURDAY

9

SUNDAY

10

 Libra
Air

 Scorpio
Water

 Sagittarius
Fire

 Capricorn
Earth

 Aquarius
Air

 Pisces
Water

SEPTEMBER

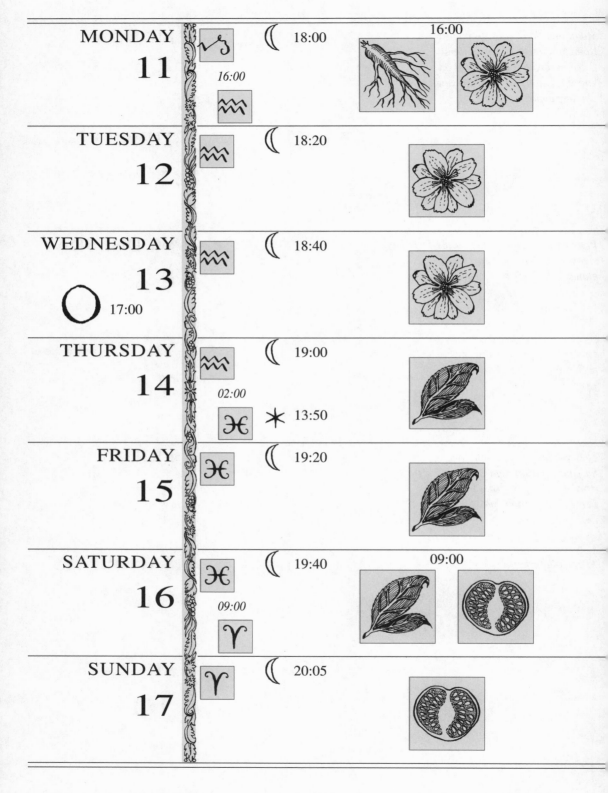

MONDAY 11 ♑ ☾ 18:00 — 16:00 / ♒ 16:00

TUESDAY 12 ♒ ☾ 18:20

WEDNESDAY 13 ♒ ☾ 18:40 — ○ 17:00

THURSDAY 14 ♒ ☾ 19:00 — 02:00 / ♓ ✳ 13:50

FRIDAY 15 ♓ ☾ 19:20

SATURDAY 16 ♓ ☾ 19:40 — 09:00 / ♈ — 09:00

SUNDAY 17 ♈ ☾ 20:05

 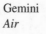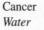

SEPTEMBER

MONDAY
11

TUESDAY
12

Full Moon.

WEDNESDAY
13

There is a Moon-Saturn sextile aspect: a time free from stress.

THURSDAY
14

FRIDAY
15

SATURDAY
16

SUNDAY
17

 Libra *Air*   Scorpio *Water*   Sagittarius *Fire*    Capricorn *Earth*   Aquarius *Air*   Pisces *Water*

SEPTEMBER

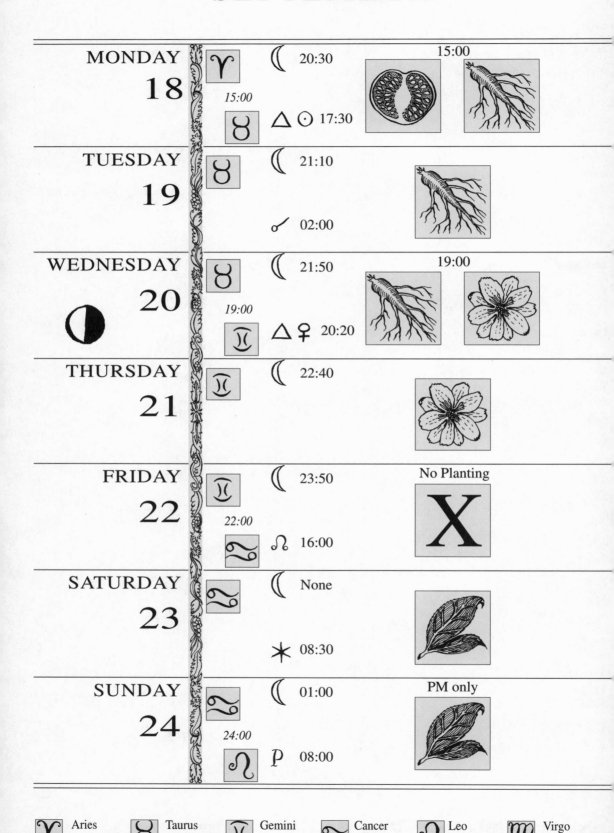

MONDAY **18**	♈ *15:00* ♉	☾ 20:30 △ ☉ 17:30	15:00
TUESDAY **19**	♉	☾ 21:10 ♂ 02:00	
WEDNESDAY **20**	♉ *19:00* ♊	☾ 21:50 △ ♀ 20:20	19:00
THURSDAY **21**	♊	☾ 22:40	
FRIDAY **22**	♊ *22:00* ♋	☾ 23:50 ♌ 16:00	No Planting **X**
SATURDAY **23**	♋	☾ None ✳ 08:30	
SUNDAY **24**	♋ *24:00* ♌	☾ 01:00 ℞ 08:00	PM only

♈ Aries *Fire*	♉ Taurus *Earth*	♊ Gemini *Air*	♋ Cancer *Water*	♌ Leo *Fire*	♍ Virgo *Earth*

SEPTEMBER

The Moon and Sun form a trine. While the previous week was quiet, this week is more interesting.	**MONDAY** **18**
The Moon and Saturn are in conjunction (0°).	**TUESDAY** **19**
The change in elements happens at the end of the working day. There is a trine aspect beetween the Moon and Venus.	**WEDNESDAY** **20**
	THURSDAY **21**
No planting: because of the crossing of the north node.	**FRIDAY** **22**
There is a Moon-Saturn sextile aspect.	**SATURDAY** **23**
The perigee of the Moon's orbit is a time of imbalance, thus the advice to work only in the afternoon.	**SUNDAY** **24**

 Libra
Air

 Scorpio
Water

 Sagittarius
Fire

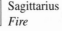 Capricorn
Earth

 Aquarius
Air

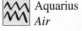 Aquarius
Air

 Pisces
Water

SEPTEMBER/OCTOBER

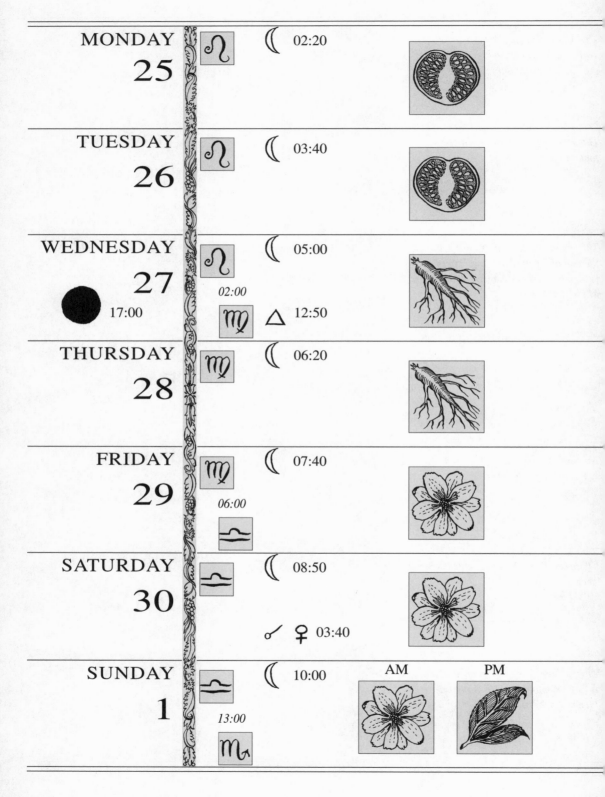

MONDAY 25
☊ ☽ 02:20

TUESDAY 26
☊ ☽ 03:40

WEDNESDAY 27
● 17:00
☊ ☽ 05:00
02:00
♍ △ 12:50

THURSDAY 28
♍ ☽ 06:20

FRIDAY 29
♍ ☽ 07:40
06:00
♎

SATURDAY 30
♎ ☽ 08:50
☌ ♀ 03:40

SUNDAY 1
♎ ☽ 10:00
13:00
♏
AM   PM

   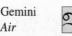

SEPTEMBER/OCTOBER

MONDAY
25

TUESDAY
26

New Moon. The change in element-signs is in the middle of the night. There is a Moon-Saturn trine at midday. The afternoon is a good time to work with perennials.

WEDNESDAY
27

THURSDAY
28

FRIDAY
29

There is a Moon-Venus conjunction (0°): of special relevance to flowering plants.

SATURDAY
30

Divide the day between the two types of plant.

SUNDAY
1

 Libra
Air

 Scorpio
Water

 Sagittarius
Fire

 Capricorn
Earth

 Aquarius
Air

 Pisces
Water

OCTOBER

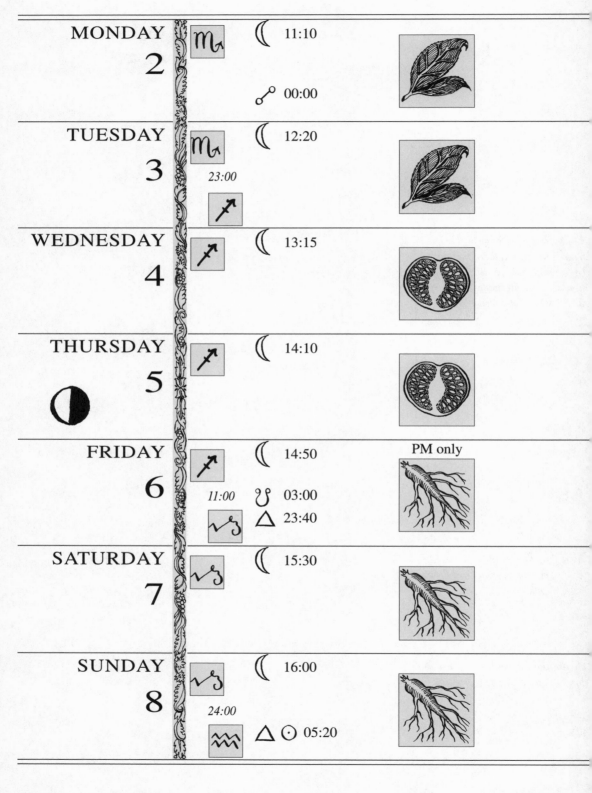

MONDAY 2
♏ ☾ 11:10
☊ 00:00

TUESDAY 3
♏ ☾ 12:20
23:00
♐

WEDNESDAY 4
♐ ☾ 13:15

THURSDAY 5
♐ ☾ 14:10

FRIDAY 6
♐ ☾ 14:50
PM only
11:00
♉ 03:00
♑ △ 23:40

SATURDAY 7
♑ ☾ 15:30

SUNDAY 8
♑ ☾ 16:00
24:00
♒ △ ☉ 05:20

 Aries *Fire*   Taurus *Earth*  Gemini *Air*   Cancer *Water*  Leo *Fire*   Virgo *Earth*

OCTOBER

The Moon-Saturn aspect is opposition (180°).

MONDAY

2

TUESDAY

3

WEDNESDAY

4

THURSDAY

5

Work only in the afternoon; the traverse of the south node is stressful. The trine aspect of the Moon and Saturn come later in the evening.

FRIDAY

6

SATURDAY

7

There is a trine aspect of the Moon and the Sun. The shift in element-signs happens tidily at the end of the day.

SUNDAY

8

 Libra
Air

 Scorpio
Water

 Sagittarius
Fire

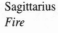 Capricorn
Earth

 Aquarius
Air

 Pisces
Water

OCTOBER

MONDAY 9 ♒ ☽ 16:20

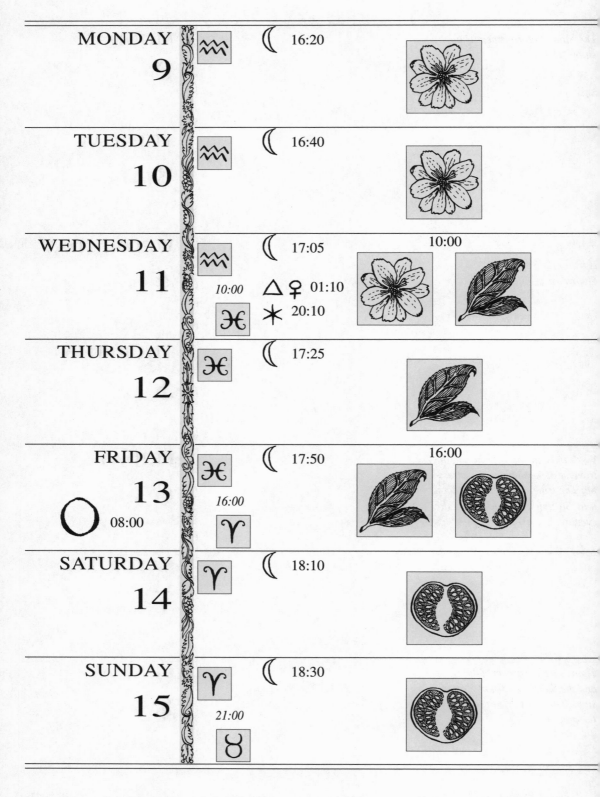

TUESDAY 10 ♒ ☽ 16:40

WEDNESDAY 11 ♒ ☽ 17:05
10:00 ♓
△ ♀ 01:10
✳ 20:10
10:00

THURSDAY 12 ♓ ☽ 17:25

FRIDAY 13 ♓ ☽ 17:50
○ 08:00
16:00 ♈
16:00

SATURDAY 14 ♈ ☽ 18:10

SUNDAY 15 ♈ ☽ 18:30
21:00 ♉

♈ Aries *Fire*   ♉ Taurus *Earth*   ♊ Gemini *Air*   ♋ Cancer *Water*   ♌ Leo *Fire*   ♍ Virgo *Earth*

OCTOBER

	MONDAY **9**
	TUESDAY **10**
The aspect of the Moon and Venus is trine (120°); then the Moon and Saturn are sextile (60°) later on.	**WEDNESDAY** **11**
	THURSDAY **12**
Full Moon.	**FRIDAY** **13**
	SATURDAY **14**
	SUNDAY **15**

 Libra
Air

 Scorpio
Water

 Sagittarius
Fire

 Capricorn
Earth

 Aquarius
Air

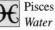 Pisces
Water

OCTOBER

MONDAY
16

♉   ☾ 19:10

     ♂ 06:20

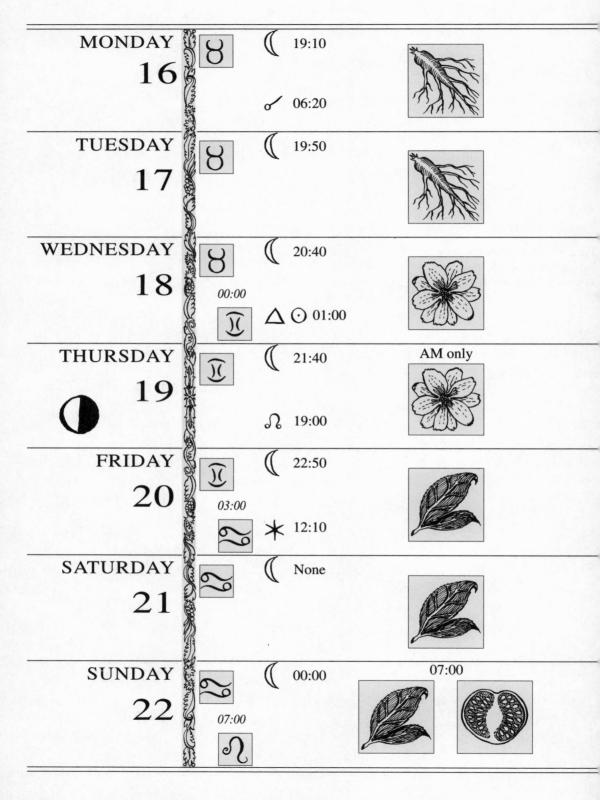

TUESDAY
17

♉   ☾ 19:50

WEDNESDAY
18

♉   ☾ 20:40

00:00

♊   △ ☉ 01:00

THURSDAY
19

♊   ☾ 21:40

AM only

♌ 19:00

FRIDAY
20

♊   ☾ 22:50

03:00

♋   ✳ 12:10

SATURDAY
21

♋   ☾ None

SUNDAY
22

♋   ☾ 00:00

07:00

07:00

♌

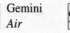

OCTOBER

The Moon and Saturn are in con-junction at the outset of the day.

MONDAY
16

TUESDAY
17

The change in elements happens in the middle of the night. The Moon and Sun form a trine aspect.

WEDNESDAY
18

The crossing of the north node is the reason for working in the morn-ing only.

THURSDAY
19

Moon-Saturn sextile aspect is har-monious.

FRIDAY
20

SATURDAY
21

SUNDAY
22

 Libra
Air

 Scorpio
Water

 Sagittarius
Fire

 Capricorn
Earth

 Aquarius
Air

 Pisces
Water

OCTOBER

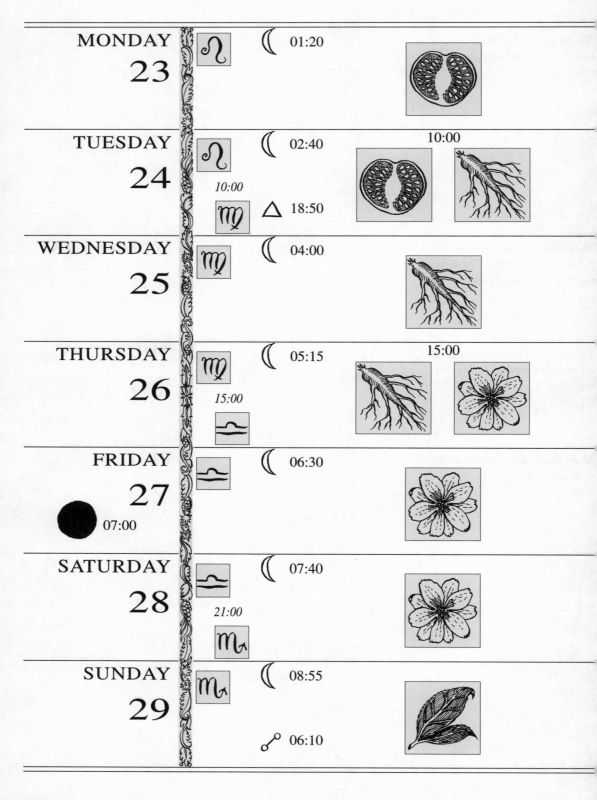

MONDAY 23   ♌   ☾ 01:20

TUESDAY 24   ♌   ☾ 02:40   10:00

10:00

♍   △ 18:50

WEDNESDAY 25   ♍   ☾ 04:00

THURSDAY 26   ♍   ☾ 05:15   15:00

15:00

♎

FRIDAY 27   ♎   ☾ 06:30

● 07:00

SATURDAY 28   ♎   ☾ 07:40

21:00

♏

SUNDAY 29   ♏   ☾ 08:55

☍ 06:10

 Aries *Fire*   **Taurus** *Earth*    **Gemini** *Air*   **Cancer** *Water*   **Leo** *Fire*   **Virgo** *Earth*

OCTOBER

	MONDAY **23**
There is a Moon-Saturn trine aspect at the end of the afternoon. The element-signs change in the morning.	**TUESDAY** **24**
	WEDNESDAY **25**
There is a progression through the elements from root plants to flowering plants.	**THURSDAY** **26**
New Moon. Good for harvesting crops that are to be stored over winter.	**FRIDAY** **27**
	SATURDAY **28**
The Moon has an oppositional aspect to Saturn.	**SUNDAY** **29**

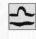 Libra
Air

  Scorpio
Water

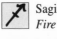 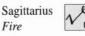 Sagittarius
Fire

 Capricorn
Earth

 Aquarius
Air

 Pisces
Water

OCTOBER/NOVEMBER

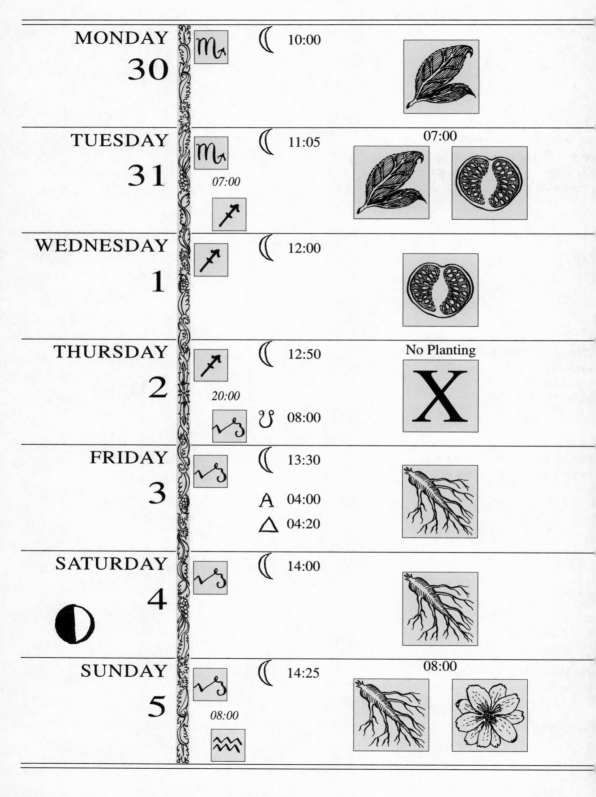

MONDAY 30 — ♏⚳ · ☾ 10:00

TUESDAY 31 — ♏⚳ · ☾ 11:05 · 07:00 ♐ · 07:00

WEDNESDAY 1 — ♐ · ☾ 12:00

THURSDAY 2 — ♐ 20:00 ♑ · ☾ 12:50 · ☊ 08:00 · No Planting X

FRIDAY 3 — ♑ · ☾ 13:30 · A 04:00 · △ 04:20

SATURDAY 4 — ♑ · ☾ 14:00

SUNDAY 5 — ♑ 08:00 ♒ · ☾ 14:25 · 08:00

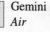

OCTOBER/NOVEMBER

	MONDAY **30**
The change in ruling elements happens at the beginning of the day.	**TUESDAY** **31**
	WEDNESDAY **1**
No planting: the Moon crosses its south node.	**THURSDAY** **2**
The Moon is at its apogee and there is a trine aspect of the Moon and Saturn in the early hours.	**FRIDAY** **3**
	SATURDAY **4**
	SUNDAY **5**

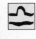 Libra *Air*   Scorpio *Water*   Sagittarius *Fire*   Capricorn *Earth*   Aquarius *Air*   Pisces *Water*

NOVEMBER

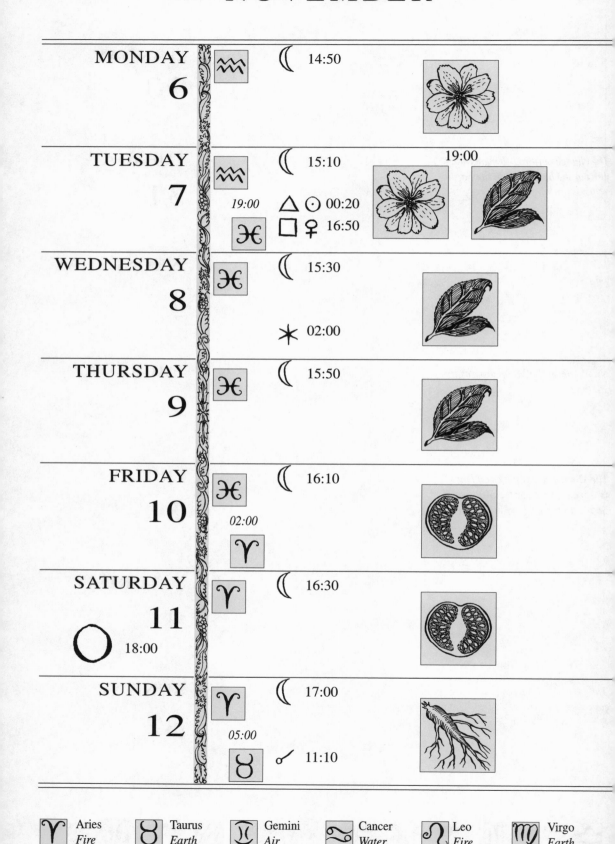

MONDAY 6
♒ ☾ 14:50

TUESDAY 7
♒ ☾ 15:10
19:00 △ ☉ 00:20
♓ □ ♀ 16:50
19:00

WEDNESDAY 8
♓ ☾ 15:30
✳ 02:00

THURSDAY 9
♓ ☾ 15:50

FRIDAY 10
♓ ☾ 16:10
02:00 ♈

SATURDAY 11
♈ ☾ 16:30
◯ 18:00

SUNDAY 12
♈ ☾ 17:00
05:00 ♉ ⚹ 11:10

♈ Aries *Fire*   ♉ Taurus *Earth*   ♊ Gemini *Air*   ♋ Cancer *Water*   ♌ Leo *Fire*   ♍ Virgo *Earth*

NOVEMBER

MONDAY

6

TUESDAY

7

The Moon forms a trine aspect with the Sun, then a square aspect with Venus later in the day.

WEDNESDAY

8

The Moon forms a sextile aspect with Saturn.

THURSDAY

9

FRIDAY

10

SATURDAY

11

Full Moon: the optimum period for sowing.

SUNDAY

12

The Moon and Saturn are in conjunction (0°).

 Libra
Air

 Scorpio
Water

 Sagittarius
Fire

 Capricorn
Earth

 Aquarius
Air

 Pisces
Water

NOVEMBER

MONDAY **13**	♉	☽ 17:40	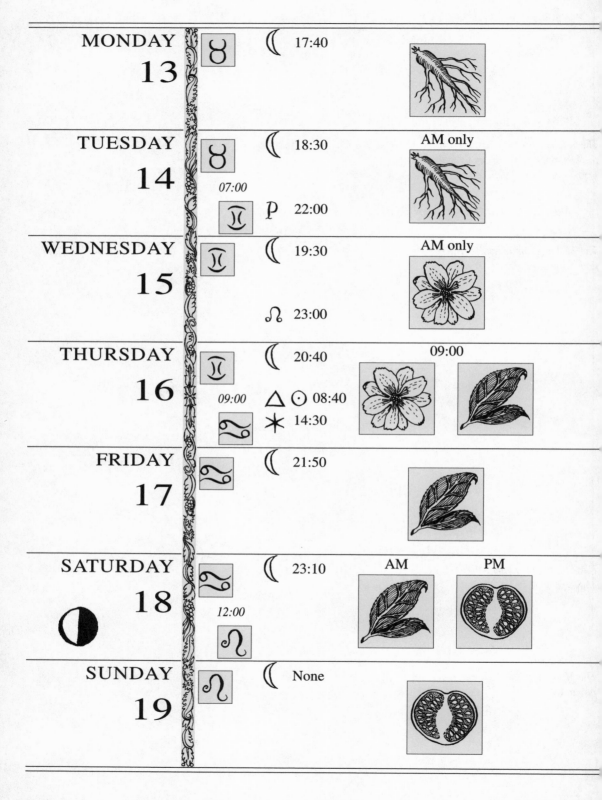
TUESDAY **14**	♉ *07:00* ♊	☽ 18:30 ℞ 22:00	AM only
WEDNESDAY **15**	♊	☽ 19:30 ♌ 23:00	AM only
THURSDAY **16**	♊ *09:00* ♋	☽ 20:40 △ ☉ 08:40 ✳ 14:30	09:00
FRIDAY **17**	♋	☽ 21:50	
SATURDAY **18**	♋ *12:00* ♌	☽ 23:10	AM PM
SUNDAY **19**	♌	☽ None	

NOVEMBER

	MONDAY **13**
The Moon is at its perigee, restrict work to the morning.	**TUESDAY** **14**
The Moon crosses its north node: again morning working only.	**WEDNESDAY** **15**
The Moon and Sun form a trine aspect. The ruling signs change early in the morning. There is a Moon-Saturn sextile aspect later in the day: good for perennials.	**THURSDAY** **16**
	FRIDAY **17**
There is progression from leaf plants (Water) to fruit- and seed-bearing plants (Fire) in the middle of the day.	**SATURDAY** **18**
	SUNDAY **19**

 Libra
Air

 Scorpio
Water

 Sagittarius
Fire

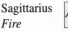 Capricorn
Earth

 Aquarius
Air

 Pisces
Water

NOVEMBER

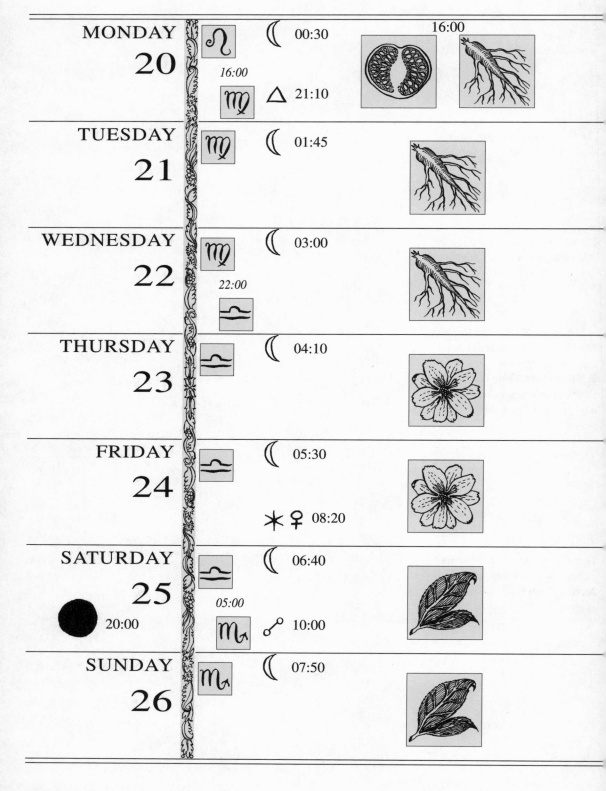

MONDAY 20
♌ | ☽ 00:30 | 16:00
16:00 ♍ | △ 21:10

TUESDAY 21
♍ | ☽ 01:45

WEDNESDAY 22
♍ | ☽ 03:00
22:00 ♎

THURSDAY 23
♎ | ☽ 04:10

FRIDAY 24
♎ | ☽ 05:30
✳ ♀ 08:20

SATURDAY 25
♎ | ☽ 06:40
05:00 ♏ | ☍ 10:00
● 20:00

SUNDAY 26
♏ | ☽ 07:50

 ♈ Aries *Fire*   ♉ Taurus *Earth*   ♊ Gemini *Air*   ♋ Cancer *Water*  ♌ Leo *Fire*   ♍ Virgo *Earth*

NOVEMBER

The Moon forms a trine with Saturn. Elements change in the afternoon.

MONDAY
20

TUESDAY
21

WEDNESDAY
22

THURSDAY
23

The Moon forms a sextile aspect with Venus. This is a good flower day.

FRIDAY
24

New Moon. It formed an oppositional aspect with Saturn earlier in the day.

SATURDAY
25

SUNDAY
26

 Libra
Air

 Scorpio
Water

 Sagittarius
Fire

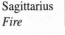 Capricorn
Earth

 Aquarius
Air

 Pisces
Water

NOVEMBER/DECEMBER

MONDAY 27 ♏ ☾ 08:50 15:00
15:00 ♐

TUESDAY 28 ♐ ☾ 09:50

WEDNESDAY 29 ♐ ☾ 10:40 No Planting
☊ 13:00 **X**

THURSDAY 30 ♐ ☾ 11:25
03:00 ♑ △ 07:40

FRIDAY 1 ♑ ☾ 12:00
A 00:00

SATURDAY 2 ♑ ☾ 12:30 16:00
16:00 ♒

SUNDAY 3 ♒ ☾ 12:50

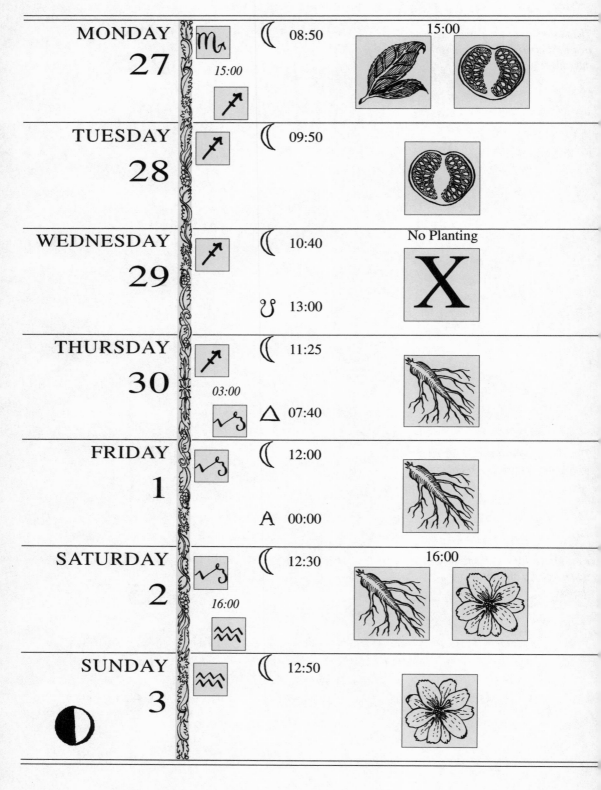

 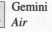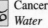

NOVEMBER/DECEMBER

The change in ruling elements happens towards the end of the day.

MONDAY
27

TUESDAY
28

The Moon crosses its south node in the middle of the day, so no planting through its entirety.

WEDNESDAY
29

Moon-Saturn trine. The element-signs have changed before sunrise.

THURSDAY
30

The Moon reaches its apogee.

FRIDAY
1

SATURDAY
2

SUNDAY
3

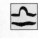 Libra
Air

 Scorpio
Water

 Sagittarius
Fire

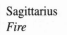 Capricorn
Earth

 Aquarius
Air

 Pisces
Water

DECEMBER

MONDAY 4 — ♒ ☾ 13:10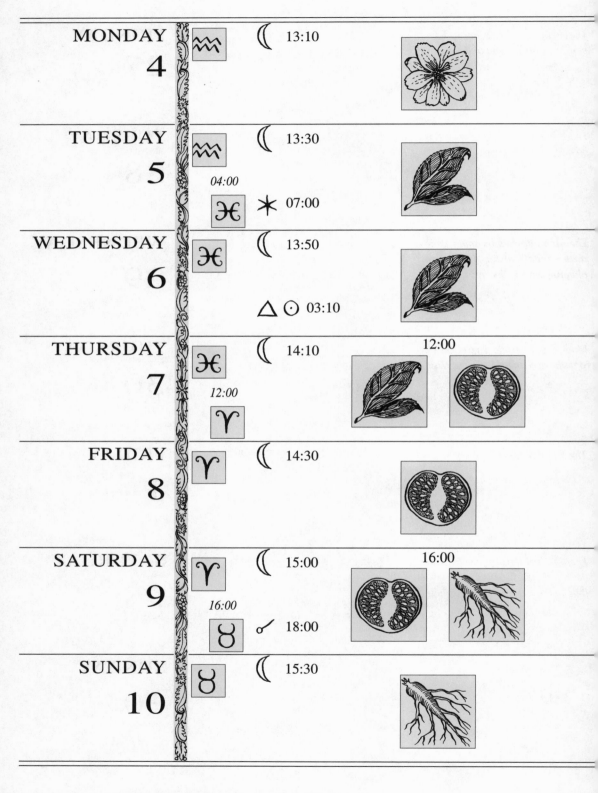

TUESDAY 5 — ♒ ☾ 13:30
04:00 ♓ ✳ 07:00

WEDNESDAY 6 — ♓ ☾ 13:50
△ ☉ 03:10

THURSDAY 7 — ♓ ☾ 14:10 · 12:00
12:00 ♈

FRIDAY 8 — ♈ ☾ 14:30

SATURDAY 9 — ♈ ☾ 15:00 · 16:00
16:00 ♉ ☌ 18:00

SUNDAY 10 — ♉ ☾ 15:30

 Aries
Fire

 Taurus
Earth

 Gemini
Air

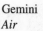 Cancer
Water

 Leo
Fire

 Virgo
Earth

DECEMBER

	MONDAY **4**
There is a sextile aspect between the Moon and Saturn.	**TUESDAY** **5**
The aspect of the Moon and the Sun is trine (120°).	**WEDNESDAY** **6**
	THURSDAY **7**
	FRIDAY **8**
There is a change in elements in the afternoon. Moon-Saturn conjunction (0°) a few hours later.	**SATURDAY** **9**
	SUNDAY **10**

 Libra
Air
 Scorpio
Water
 Sagittarius
Fire
 Capricorn
Earth
 Aquarius
Air
 Pisces
Water

DECEMBER

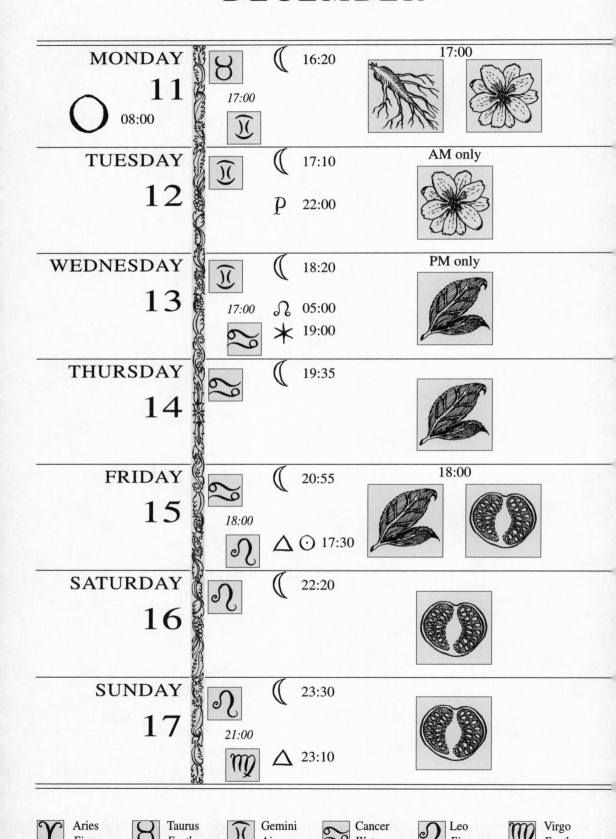

MONDAY 11

○ 08:00

♉

☾ 16:20

17:00

♊

17:00

TUESDAY 12

♊

☾ 17:10

℞ 22:00

AM only

WEDNESDAY 13

♊

17:00

♋

☾ 18:20

♌ 05:00

✳ 19:00

PM only

THURSDAY 14

♋

☾ 19:35

FRIDAY 15

♋

18:00

♌

☾ 20:55

△ ☉ 17:30

18:00

SATURDAY 16

♌

☾ 22:20

SUNDAY 17

♌

21:00

♍

☾ 23:30

△ 23:10

| ♈ Aries *Fire* | ♉ Taurus *Earth* | ♊ Gemini *Air* | ♋ Cancer *Water* | ♌ Leo *Fire* | ♍ Virgo *Earth* |

DECEMBER

Full Moon. The change in elements happens at the end of the afternoon.

MONDAY

11

The Moon is at its perigee: so no work in the afternoon.

TUESDAY

12

The Moon crosses its north node in the early hours: work in the afternoon. The Moon and Saturn are sextile.

WEDNESDAY

13

THURSDAY

14

The ruling signs change after work is done. There is a Moon and Sun trine.

FRIDAY

15

SATURDAY

16

The Moon is trine to Saturn.

SUNDAY

17

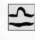 Libra
Air

 Scorpio
Water

 Sagittarius
Fire

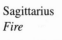 Capricorn
Earth

 Aquarius
Air

 Pisces
Water

DECEMBER

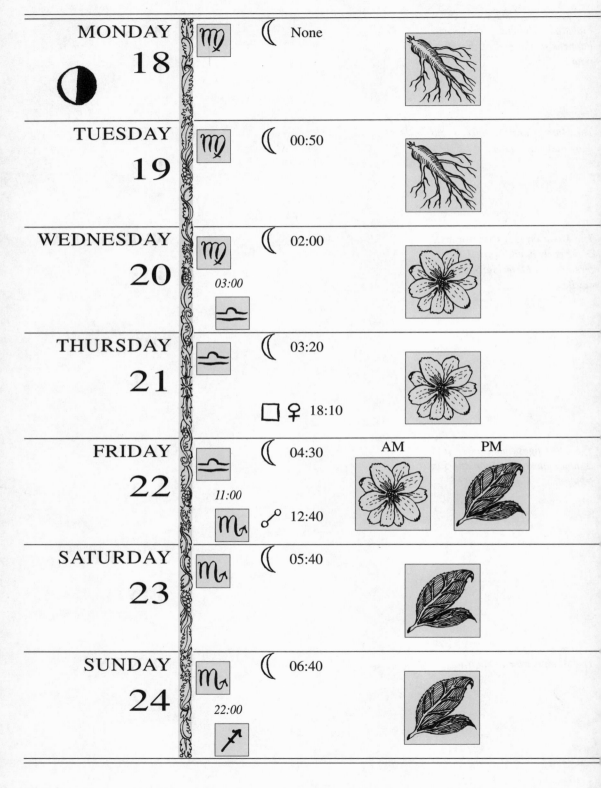

MONDAY 18 — ♍ ☽ None

TUESDAY 19 — ♍ ☽ 00:50

WEDNESDAY 20 — ♍ ☽ 02:00 — *03:00* ♎

THURSDAY 21 — ♎ ☽ 03:20 — □ ♀ 18:10

FRIDAY 22 — ♎ ☽ 04:30 — *11:00* ♏ ☌ 12:40 — AM / PM

SATURDAY 23 — ♏ ☽ 05:40

SUNDAY 24 — ♏ ☽ 06:40 — *22:00* ♐

 ♈ Aries *Fire*   ♉ Taurus *Earth*  ♊ Gemini *Air*   ♋ Cancer *Water*  ♌ Leo *Fire*   ♍ Virgo *Earth*

DECEMBER

MONDAY

18

TUESDAY

19

WEDNESDAY

20

The Moon forms a square aspect with Venus. Winter solstice.

THURSDAY

21

There is a progression from flower to leaf plants in the morning. The Moon is in opposition to Saturn.

FRIDAY

22

SATURDAY

23

SUNDAY

24

 Libra
Air

 Scorpio
Water

 Sagittarius
Fire

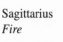 Capricorn
Earth

 Aquarius
Air

 Pisces
Water

DECEMBER

MONDAY
25

● 15:00

♐   ☽ 07:40

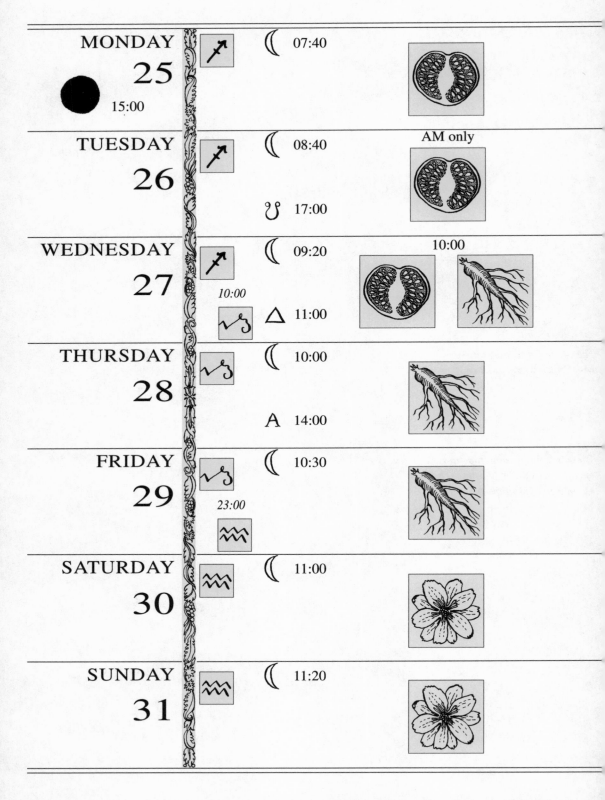

TUESDAY
26

♐   ☽ 08:40

      ☋ 17:00

AM only

WEDNESDAY
27

♐   ☽ 09:20

10:00
♑   △ 11:00

10:00

THURSDAY
28

♑   ☽ 10:00

      A 14:00

FRIDAY
29

♑   ☽ 10:30

23:00
♒

SATURDAY
30

♒   ☽ 11:00

SUNDAY
31

♒   ☽ 11:20

♈ Aries *Fire*	♉ Taurus *Earth*	♊ Gemini *Air*	♋ Cancer *Water*	♌ Leo *Fire*	♍ Virgo *Earth*

DECEMBER

New Moon.	**MONDAY** **25**
The Moon crosses its south node, so only work in the morning.	**TUESDAY** **26**
The change from fruit (Fire) to root (Earth) element occurs. There is a Moon-Saturn trine aspect.	**WEDNESDAY** **27**
The Moon reaches the apogee of its orbit.	**THURSDAY** **28**
	FRIDAY **29**
	SATURDAY **30**
The last day of the millennium (by proper counting).	**SUNDAY** **31**

 Libra
Air

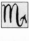 Scorpio
Water

 Sagittarius
Fire

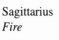 Capricorn
Earth

 Aquarius
Air

 Pisces
Water

NOTES

NOTES

NOTES

NOTES

NOTES

NOTES